METHODS IN MOLECULAR BIOLOGY

Series Editor
John M. Walker
School of Life and Medical Sciences
University of Hertfordshire
Hatfield, Hertfordshire, AL10 9AB, UK

For further volumes:
http://www.springer.com/series/7651

Vaccines for Invasive Fungal Infections

Methods and Protocols

Edited by

Markus Kalkum and Margarita Semis

Department of Molecular Immunology,
Beckman Research Institute of City of Hope, Duarte, CA, USA

Humana Press

Editors
Markus Kalkum
Department of Molecular Immunology
Beckman Research Institute of City of Hope
Duarte, CA, USA

Margarita Semis
Department of Molecular Immunology
Beckman Research Institute of City of Hope
Duarte, CA, USA

ISSN 1064-3745 ISSN 1940-6029 (electronic)
Methods in Molecular Biology
ISBN 978-1-4939-7103-9 ISBN 978-1-4939-7104-6 (eBook)
DOI 10.1007/978-1-4939-7104-6

Library of Congress Control Number: 2017943158

Cover illustration: Electron micrograph of an *Aspergillus fumigatus* conidiophore (spore head). Diameters of mature spores are approximately 1.4 μm. The leftmost image shows phagocytes (purple) attacking fungal hyphae (bluish-grey band) of *A. fumigatus*. Courtesy of Dr. Marcia Miller, Electron Microscopy Facility, Diana Diaz-Arevalo & Markus Kalkum, Department of Molecular Immunology, Beckman Research Institute of the City of Hope.

Printed on acid-free paper

This Humana Press imprint is published by Springer Nature
The registered company is Springer Science+Business Media LLC
The registered company address is: 233 Spring Street, New York, NY 10013, U.S.A.

Preface

Invasive mycoses are severe fungal infections that threaten the lives of thousands of patients with immunosuppressive conditions. As such, the disease targets the Achilles heel of hematopoietic stem cell transplantations for the treatment of leukemia, lymphoma, and other hematological malignancies. The most common etiological agents of mycoses are *Aspergillus* and *Candida* species, which therefore lie in the main focus of this book, followed by *Cryptococcus*, dimorphic fungi, and members of *Mucoraceae* family of fungi. Mycosis vaccines offer the promise to stop deadly fungal infections in their tracks. However, vaccination also has to accommodate the immunosuppressive state of the patient to be protected. Hence, delivery and routes to achieve protective immunization are of critical importance. Considerable research has been conducted for the development of mycosis vaccines in a variety of animal models, and attempts at translation of at least two antifungal vaccines into the clinic are currently being undertaken.

Methods in Molecular Biology's *Invasive Mycoses Vaccines* aims to provide interested researchers with detailed background information, laboratory protocols, and assessment strategies. The book is sectioned into five parts that describe experimental approaches for (1) vaccine candidate discovery, (2) improved vaccine design and delivery, (3) assessment of critical endpoints, (4) analysis of mechanisms of mycosis vaccine protection, and (5) key methods for clinical translation.

In conclusion, our volume, *Invasive Mycoses Vaccines: Methods and Protocols*, should provide the standard reference for vaccine researchers, including those who aspire to strengthen their knowledge and desire to acquire a particular technique.

Duarte, CA, USA

Markus Kalkum
Margarita Semis

Contents

Contributors

MASAHIRO ABE • *Department of Chemotherapy and Mycoses, National Institute of Infectious Diseases, Tokyo, Japan*

EJAJ AHMAD • *Interdisciplinary Biotechnology Unit, Aligarh Muslim University, Aligarh, India*

MOHD AJMAL • *Department of Anatomy, JNMC, Aligarh Muslim University, Aligarh, India*

ANDRÉ C. AMARAL • *Tropical Pathology and Public Health Institute, Federal University of Goiás, Goiânia, Goiás, Brazil*

ANTERO SILVA RIBEIRO DE ANDRADE • *Centro de Desenvolvimento da Tecnologia Nuclear (CDTN), Cidade Universitária-Campus da UFMG, Belo Horizonte, MG, Brazil*

SHANJANA AWASTHI • *Department of Pharmaceutical Sciences, College of Pharmacy, University of Oklahoma Health Sciences Center, Oklahoma City, OK, USA*

ASIM AZHAR • *Interdisciplinary Biotechnology Unit, Aligarh Muslim University, Aligarh, India*

ANAMELIA L. BOCCA • *Institute of Biological Sciences, University of Brasilia, Brasilia, FD, Brazil*

ASHOK K. CHATURVEDI • *Department of Biology and The South Texas Center for Emerging Infectious Diseases, University of Texas, San Antonio, TX, USA*

RUPANJALI CHAUDHURI • *IBM India Private Limited, Bangalore, India*

KARL V. CLEMONS • *California Institute for Medical Research, San Jose, CA, USA; Division of Infectious Diseases and Geographic Medicine, Department of Medicine, Stanford University, Stanford, CA, USA*

PAULO S.R. COELHO • *Departamento de Biologia Celular e Molecular e Bioagentes Patogênicos, Faculdade de Medicina de Ribeirão Preto, Universidade de São Paulo, Ribeirão Preto, SP, Brazil*

STEFANIA CONTI • *Unit of Microbiology and Virology, Department of Biomedical, Biotechnological and Translational Sciences (S.Bi.Bi.T.), University of Parma, Parma, Italy*

DIANA DIAZ-AREVALO • *Fundación Instituto de Inmunología de Colombia, FIDIC, Bogotá, Colombia; Universidad de Ciencias Aplicadas y Ambientales, UDCA, Bogotá, Colombia*

FUSUN DIKENGIL • *Program in Molecular Medicine, University of Massachusetts Medical School, Worcester, MA, USA*

MARIA SUELI S. FELIPE • *Institute of Biological Sciences, University of Brasilia, Brasilia, DF, Brazil; Genomic Science and Biotechnology, Catholic University of Brasilia, Brasilia, DF, Brazil*

FABRÍCIO FREITAS FERNANDES • *Departamento de Biologia Celular e Molecular e Bioagentes Patogênicos, Faculdade de Medicina de Ribeirão Preto, Universidade de São Paulo, São Paulo, SP, Brazil*

WILLIAM W. HOPE • *Antimicrobial Pharmacodynamics and Therapeutics, Department of Molecular and Clinical Pharmacology, Institute of Translational Medicine, University of Liverpool, Liverpool, UK*

YAN HU • *Department of Oral Biology, Guanghua School of Stomatology, Guangdong Provincial Key Laboratory of Stomatology, Sun Yat-sen University, Guangzhou, China*
CHIUNG-YU HUNG • *Department of Biology, South Texas Center for Emerging Infectious Diseases and Immune Defense Core, University of Texas, San Antonio, TX, USA*
BRADY J. HURTGEN • *Department of Biology, University of Texas, San Antonio, TX, USA; Department of Microbiology and Immunology, University of Texas Health Science Center, San Antonio, TX, USA*
MARKUS KALKUM • *Department of Molecular Immunology, Beckman Research Institute of City of Hope, Duarte, CA, USA*
NAZOORA KHAN • *Interdisciplinary Biotechnology Unit, Aligarh Muslim University, Aligarh, India*
NINA KHANNA • *Infection Biology Laboratory, Division of Infectious Diseases and Hospital Epidemiology, Departments of Biomedicine and Clinical Research, University Hospital of Basel, Basel, Switzerland*
YUKI KINJO • *Department of Chemotherapy and Mycoses, National Institute of Infectious Diseases, Tokyo, Japan*
TAISE NATALI LANDGRAF • *Faculdade de Filosofia, Ciências e Letras de Ribeirão Preto, Universidade de São Paulo, São Paulo, SP, Brazil*
SALOMÉ LEIBUNDGUT-LANDMANN • *Section of Immunology, Institute of Virology, University of Zürich, Zürich, Switzerland*
STUART M. LEVITZ • *Department of Medicine, University of Massachusetts Medical School, Worcester, MA, USA*
WENQING LI • *Department of Oral Biology, Guanghua School of Stomatology, Guangdong Provincial Key Laboratory of Stomatology, Sun Yat-sen University, Guangzhou, China*
LING LU • *Jiangsu Key Laboratory for Microbes and Functional Genomics, Jiangsu Engineering and Technology Research Center for Microbiology, College of Life Sciences, Nanjing Normal University, Nanjing, China*
WALTER MAGLIANI • *Unit of Microbiology and Virology, Department of Biomedical, Biotechnological; Translational Sciences (S.Bi.Bi.T.), University of Parma, Parma, Italy*
MARIFE MARTINEZ • *California Institute for Medical Research, San Jose, CA, USA*
ESTEFÂNIA MARA DO NASCIMENTO MARTINS • *Centro de Desenvolvimento da Tecnologia Nuclear (CDTN), Cidade Universitária-Campus da UFMG, Belo Horizonte, MG, Brazil*
ZEYNEP MIRZA • *Program in Molecular Medicine, University of Massachusetts Medical School, Worcester, MA, USA*
YOSHITSUGU MIYAZAKI • *Department of Chemotherapy and Mycoses, National Institute of Infectious Diseases, Tokyo, Japan*
ALINE FERREIRA OLIVEIRA • *Departamento de Biologia Celular e Molecular e Bioagentes Patogênicos, Faculdade de Medicina de Ribeirão Preto, Universidade de São Paulo, Ribeirão Preto, SP, Brazil; Universidade Paulista, Ribeirão Preto, SP, Brazil; Universidade Paulista, São José do Rio Pardo, SP, Brazil*
GARY R. OSTROFF • *Program in Molecular Medicine, University of Massachusetts Medical School, Worcester, MA, USA*
MOHAMMAD OWAIS • *Interdisciplinary Biotechnology Unit, Aligarh Muslim University, Aligarh, India*
ADEMÍLSON PANUNTO-CASTELO • *Faculdade de Filosofia, Ciências e Letras de Ribeirão Preto, Universidade de São Paulo, São Paulo, SP, Brazil*

RUTA PETRAITIENE • *Transplantation-Oncology Infectious Diseases Program, Division of Infectious Diseases, Department of Medicine, Weill Cornell Medicine, Cornell University, New York, NY, USA*
VIDMANTAS PETRAITIS • *Transplantation-Oncology Infectious Diseases Program, Division of Infectious Diseases, Department of Medicine, Weill Cornell Medicine, Cornell University, New York, NY, USA*
LUCIANO POLONELLI • *Unit of Microbiology and Virology, Department of Biomedical, Biotechnological and Translational Sciences (S.Bi.Bi.T.), University of Parma, Parma, Italy*
SRINIVASAN RAMACHANDRAN • *CSIR-Institute of Genomics and Integrative Biology, New Delhi, India*
ALICE M. RIBEIRO • *Institute of Biological Sciences, University of Brasilia, Brasilia, DF, Brazil*
MARIA CRISTINA ROQUE-BARREIRA • *Departamento de Biologia Celular e Molecular e Bioagentes Patogênicos, Faculdade de Medicina de Ribeirão Preto, Universidade de São Paulo, São Paulo, SP, Brazil*
BERND ROSCHITZKI • *Functional Genomics Center Zürich, University of Zürich & ETH Zurich, Zürich, Switzerland*
ESTHER SEGAL • *Department of Clinical Microbiology and Immunology, Sackler School of Medicine, Tel Aviv University, Tel Aviv, Israel*
SEIJI SHIBASAKI • *General Education Center and Graduate School of Pharmacy, Hyogo University of Health Sciences, Kobe, Japan*
THIAGO APARECIDO DA SILVA • *Departamento de Biologia Celular e Molecular e Bioagentes Patogênicos, Faculdade de Medicina de Ribeirão Preto, Universidade de São Paulo, São Paulo, SP, Brazil*
ERNESTO R. SOTO • *Program in Molecular Medicine, University of Massachusetts Medical School, Worcester, MA, USA*
DAVID A. STEVENS • *California Institute for Medical Research, San Jose, CA, USA; Division of Infectious Diseases and Geographic Medicine, Department of Medicine, Stanford University, Stanford, CA, USA*
CLAUDIA STUEHLER • *Infection Biology Laboratory, Department of Biomedicine, University and University Hospital of Basel, Basel, Switzerland*
CARLOS P. TABORDA • *Department of Microbiology, Institute of Biomedical Sciences, University of São Paulo, São Paulo, SP, Brazil; Laboratory of Medical Mycology IMTSP/LIM53/HCFMUSP, University of São Paulo, São Paulo, SP, Brazil*
SHOGO TAKATSUKA • *Department of Chemotherapy and Mycoses, National Institute of Infectious Diseases, Tokyo, Japan*
LUIZ R. TRAVASSOS • *Department of Microbiology, Immunology and Parasitology, Federal University of São Paulo, São Paulo, SP, Brazil*
MITSUYOSHI UEDA • *Division of Applied Life Sciences, Graduate School of Agriculture, Kyoto University, Kyoto, Japan*
KEIGO UENO • *Department of Chemotherapy and Mycoses, National Institute of Infectious Diseases, Tokyo, Japan*
MAKOTO URAI • *Department of Chemotherapy and Mycoses, National Institute of Infectious Diseases, Tokyo, Japan*

Thomas J. Walsh • *Transplantation-Oncology Infectious Diseases Program, Division of Infectious Diseases, Department of Medicine, Weill Cornell Medicine, Cornell University, New York, NY, USA; Department of Pediatrics, Weill Cornell Medicine, Cornell University, New York, NY, USA; Department of Microbiology and Immunology, Weill Cornell Medicine, Cornell University, New York, NY, USA; The Henry Schueler Foundation, Chicago, IL, USA; Weill Cornell Medical Center, New York, NY, USA*

Li Wang • *Institute of Genetics and Cytology, School of Life Sciences, Northeast Normal University, Changchun, China*

Yicun Wang • *Jilin Provincial Key Laboratory on Molecular and Chemical Genetic, The Second Hospital of Jilin University, Changchun, China*

Floyd L. Wormley Jr. • *Department of Biology and The South Texas Center for Emerging Infectious Diseases, University of Texas, San Antonio, TX, USA*

Chi Zhang • *Jiangsu Key Laboratory for Microbes and Functional Genomics, Jiangsu Engineering and Technology Research Center for Microbiology, College of Life Sciences, Nanjing Normal University, Nanjing, China*

Swaleha Zubair • *Women's College, Aligarh Muslim University, Aligarh, India*

Part I

Discovery and Testing of Vaccine Candidates

Chapter 1

Mouse Immunization with Radioattenuated Yeast Cells of *Paracoccidioides brasiliensis*

Estefânia Mara do Nascimento Martins and Antero Silva Ribeiro de Andrade

Abstract

Paracoccidioides brasiliensis is the agent of paracoccidioidomycosis, the most prevalent mycosis in Latin America, and currently there is no effective vaccine. The present chapter describes the methodology to obtain radioattenuated yeast cells of *P. brasiliensis* and a protocol to evaluate protective response elicited by this immunogen in experimental paracoccidioidomycosis. The radioattenuated yeast provides a valuable tool for immunological studies in experimental paracoccidioidomycosis and vaccine research.

Key words *Paracoccidioides brasiliensis*, Gamma irradiation, Attenuation, Live vaccine, Immunization, Paracoccidioidomycosis

1 Introduction

The use of vaccines in preventing infectious diseases has been applied against a broad range of infectious agents, but the complexity of eukaryotic systems, like fungi, presents additional challenges. Successful resolution of the diseases caused by pathogenic fungi is dependent on the coordinated interaction of many constituents of the host immune response [1]. Live attenuated vaccines can be an alternative tool to achieve this goal. The advantages of using live attenuated vaccines are that the pathogen induces strong and broad responses involving multiple arms of the immune response that recapitulates natural immunity to disease. Live vaccines can expose their antigens sequentially to the host as in a natural infection and can express antigens produced only during the infection; avoiding problems associated with single immunization with protein or killed agents [2].

The potential of irradiation as a tool for creating highly effective attenuated vaccines has been recognized since the 1950s. Gamma and X irradiation have consistently proved successful as attenuating agents for a remarkably wide range of helminthes,

Markus Kalkum and Margarita Semis (eds.), *Vaccines for Invasive Fungal Infections: Methods and Protocols*, Methods in Molecular Biology, vol. 1625, DOI 10.1007/978-1-4939-7104-6_1, © Springer Science+Business Media LLC 2017

nematodes, and protozoa's species. Irradiated pathogens frequently lose their virulence, but retain the metabolic activities and morphology, and consequently are able to induce a high level of immunity during its abbreviated lifespan in the host. However, they die before reaching the stages associated with pathogenicity. In some cases, the radioattenuated pathogens are more immunogenic than the normal counterparts [3].

A main concern with live attenuated vaccines is their risk of virulence reversion. However, the gamma radiation has proven to be a viable strategy to attenuate microorganisms. Appropriate gamma radiation doses cause an extensive DNA fragmentation beyond repair capacity of the cell repair mechanisms. The DNA damage led to an irreversible loss of *Paracoccidioides brasiliensis* yeast reproductive ability [4] and virulence [5].

P. brasiliensis is a thermally dimorphic fungus agent of paracoccidioidomycosis (PCM), a deep-seated systemic infection of humans, and currently there is no effective vaccine. The disease has a high incidence in Latin American countries, especially Brazil, Venezuela, Colombia, and Argentina [6, 7]. Herein, we describe the detailed protocols to obtain radioattenuated yeast cells of *P. brasiliensis* and for their use as an immunogen to elicit a protective response in experimental Paracoccidioidomycosis (PCM). By this process yeasts cells lose the reproductive ability and pathogenicity, while retaining the morphology, the synthesis, and secretion of proteins, the oxidative metabolism and the expression of the antigens present in the native yeast [4, 8]. The radioattenuated yeast cells are able to induce a long-lasting protection against highly infective yeast forms of *P. brasiliensis* [5, 9]. The immunization with radioattenuated yeast cells is a powerful tool for understanding the factors that contribute to protective immunity in experimental PCM and open new perspectives for research of fungal vaccines.

2 Materials

2.1 Culture

1. *P. brasiliensis* isolate (strain Pb18) (American Type Culture Collection (ATCC)–Rockville, MD, USA).
2. Yeast peptone dextrose agar medium (YPD).
3. Incubator at 35 °C.

2.2 Yeast Cell Counting

1. Phosphate buffer saline (PBS).
2. Vortex mixer.
3. Hemocytometer.

2.3 Yeast Viability Analysis

1. Janus green vital dye.
2. Vortex mixer.
3. Hemocytometer.

2.4 Recovery of *P. brasiliensis* Virulence

1. *P. brasiliensis* yeast cell (Pb 18) cultures.
2. Phosphate Buffer Saline (PBS).
3. Ultra-fine 8 mm needle Insulin Syringe.
4. Male Balb/c mice 6–8 week old mice.
5. Surgical instruments (tweezers and scissors).
6. Organ macerator.
7. Sterile 90 × 15 mm polystyrene petri dish.
8. Brain infusion agar medium (BHIA).
9. Gentamicin.
10. Fetal bovine serum (FBS).
11. *P. brasiliensis* spent culture medium (*see* **Note 9**).
12. Incubator at 35 °C.

2.5 Yeast Cell Attenuation by Gamma Irradiation

1. *P. brasiliensis* yeast cell (Pb 18) isolated in agar YPD medium.
2. Uniform source of ^{60}Co gamma rays (Centro de Desenvolvimento da Energia Nuclear/Comissão Nacional da Energia Nuclear (CDTN/CNEN)–Belo Horizonte, MG, BRAZIL).

2.6 Yeast Growth Analysis

1. *P. brasiliensis* yeast cell (Pb 18) cultures.
2. Phosphate Buffer Saline (PBS).
3. Brain infusion agar medium (BHIA).
4. Gentamicin.
5. Fetal bovine serum (FBS).
6. *P. brasiliensis* spent culture medium (*see* **Note 9**).
7. Centrifuge.
8. Incubator at 35 °C.

2.7 Virulence Assessment of Radioattenuated Yeast Cells

1. Male Balb/c and athimic male Nude/Nude mice.
2. Nonirradiated yeast cell (Pb 18) of *P. brasiliensis.*
3. Radioattenuated yeast cell (LevRad) of *P. brasiliensis.*
4. Phosphate Buffer Saline (PBS).
5. Ultra-fine 8 mm needle Insulin Syringe.
6. Xylazine.
7. Ketamine.
8. Surgical instruments (tweezers and scissors).
9. Organ macerator.
10. Brain infusion agar medium (BHIA).
11. Gentamicin.

12. Fetal bovine serum (FBS).
13. *P. brasiliensis* spent culture medium (*see* **Note 9**).
14. Incubator at 35 °C.

2.8 Mouse Immunization and Challenge

1. Male Balb/c mice.
2. Nonirradiated yeast cell (Pb 18) of *P. brasiliensis.*
3. Radioattenuated yeast cell (LevRad) of *P. brasiliensis.*
4. Phosphate Buffer Saline (PBS).
5. Ultra-fine 8 mm needle Insulin Syringe.
6. Surgical instruments (tweezers and scissors).
7. Xylazine.
8. Ketamine.

2.9 Colony-Forming Unit Recovery

1. Surgical instruments (tweezers and scissors).
2. Organ macerator.
3. Phosphate buffer saline (PBS).
4. Brain infusion agar medium (BHIA).
5. Gentamicin.
6. Fetal bovine serum (FBS).
7. *P. brasiliensis* spent culture medium (*see* **Note 9**).
8. Incubator at 35 °C.

2.10 Histopathology

1. 10% buffered formalin.
2. Paraffin.
3. Hematoxylin-eosin dye.
4. Optical microscopy.

2.11 Antibody Response to Radioattenuated Yeast Cells

1. Maxisorp™ 96 well surface plates.
2. MEXO antigens (*see* **Note 18**).
3. Carbonate/bicarbonate buffer.
4. Phosphate Buffer Saline (PBS).
5. 5% casein solution from bovine milk in water (Sigma-Aldrich).
6. Anti-mouse IgG-peroxidase conjugate (Sigma-Aldrich).
7. Anti-mouse IgG1 and IgG2a (heavy chain specific) antibody (Sigma-Aldrich).
8. Tetramethylbenzidine (TMB).
9. Automated ELISA reader.

2.12 Cytokine Transcript Level Detection by Real-Time PCR

1. Trizol LS Reagent.
2. Chloroform.
3. Isopropyl Alcohol.
4. Ethanol.
5. RQ1 RNase-free DNAse.
6. Spectrophotometer.
7. Superscript III RNase Reverse Transcriptase.
8. 96-well plate for Real-Time PCR.
9. Plate seals.
10. PowerUp Syber Green PCR Master Mix
11. Water, PCR grade.
12. Set of primers and constitutive gene (Integrated DNA Technologies (IDT)—Coralville, Lowa, USA).
13. Microcentrifuge for plate.
14. Quantitative PCR instrument.

2.13 Citokine Measurement by ELISA

1. Cytokine assay kit containing capture antibody, detection antibody, recombinant standard, streptavidin conjugated to horseradish-peroxidase (Streptavidin-HRP) (R&D System).
2. Maxisorp™ 96-well surface plates (NUNC™ Brand Products).
3. Phosphate Buffer Saline (PBS).
4. Tween 20.
5. Bovine serum albumin (BSA).
6. Substrate solution (R&D System).
7. Sulfuric acid solution.
8. Automated ELISA reader.

3 Methods

3.1 *P. brasiliensis* Yeast Cell (Pb 18) Culture

1. Seed *P. brasiliensis* yeast cell (Pb18 strain) in YPD agar medium at 35 °C (*see* **Note 1**).
2. Subculture the yeast cells every 7–8 days (*see* **Note 2**).

3.2 Yeast Cell Counting

1. Transfer the *P. brasiliensis* yeast cells to a PBS solution, pH 7.4.
2. Homogenize by vortexing the mixture to disperse cell clusters (*see* **Note 3**).
3. Perform the counting in a hemocytometer.

3.3 Yeast Cell Viability Analysis

1. Determine the yeast cell viability by using the modified vital dye Janus green method [10] (*see* **Note 4**).

2. Add 20 μL of 0.05% dye solution to an equal volume of the fungal cell suspension (1:1, v/v).
3. Allow the cell suspension to interact with the dye for 6–8 min. Viable cells remained unstained and dead cells stained blue (*see* **Note 5**).
4. Perform the counting in a hemocytometer.

3.4 Recovery of P. brasiliensis Virulence (See Note 6)

1. Inoculate the male BALB/c mice (*see* **Note 7**) by the orbital plexus with 1×10^7 yeast cells of *P. brasiliensis* in a 50 μL final volume of sterile PBS, pH 7.4.
2. Euthanize the mice 7 days after infection establishment.
3. Remove and homogenize their lungs in 1 mL of sterile PBS, pH 7.4.
4. Plate 300 μL of the macerate on a high plating efficiency medium (*see* **Notes 8** and **9**).
5. Incubate the plate at 35 °C for 20 days.
6. Recover the colonies that grow.

3.5 Gamma Irradiation

1. Perform the gamma irradiation of *P. brasiliensis* yeast cells in YPD agar medium, in the presence of oxygen at room temperature, using a uniform source of ^{60}Co gamma rays.
2. The irradiation dose and dose rate may be, respectively, 6.5 kGy and 950 Gy h^{-1} (*see* **Note 10**).
3. Use for irradiation 4–5 days growth cultures. Adequate control cultures must be maintained outside the source.
4. The reproductive capacity and viability of irradiated cells should be monitored after irradiation to confirm that attenuation was achieved.

3.6 Yeast Growth Analysis

1. Transfer nonirradiated (control) and irradiated yeast cells to PBS solution, pH 7.4.
2. Homogenize by vortexing and count the viable cells in a hemocytometer.
3. Spread the suspensions, containing 10^2 (control cells) to 10^7 (irradiated cells) colony-forming units (CFU) on a high plating efficiency medium.
4. Incubate the plates at 35 °C for 7 days and, next, count the colonies (Fig. 1).
5. The 6.5 kGy is the lowest gamma radiation dose necessary to eliminate the reproductive capacity of *P. brasiliensis* yeast cells. As shown in Fig. 2, the 6.5 kGy irradiated yeast cells were unable to form colonies, even if a large inoculum (10^7 cells) and incubation time (40 days) were used. However, cell viability is maintained according to the Janus green analysis.

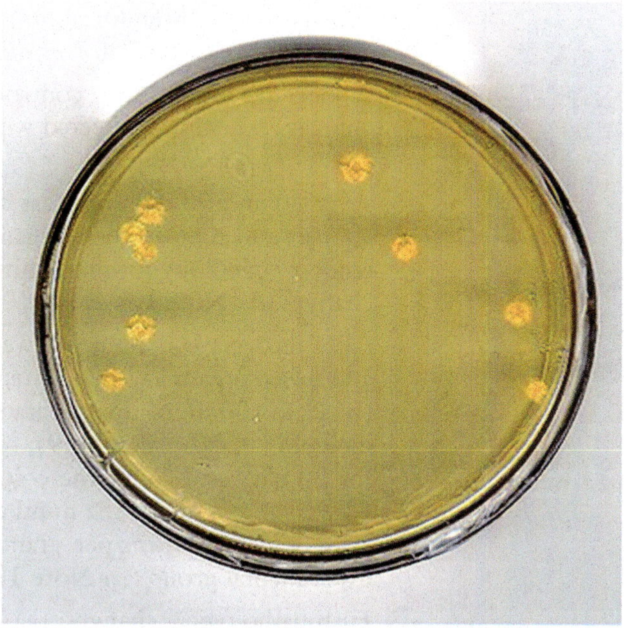

Fig. 1 Typical *Paraccocidioides brasiliensis* colonies growing on petri dishes with a high plating efficiency medium

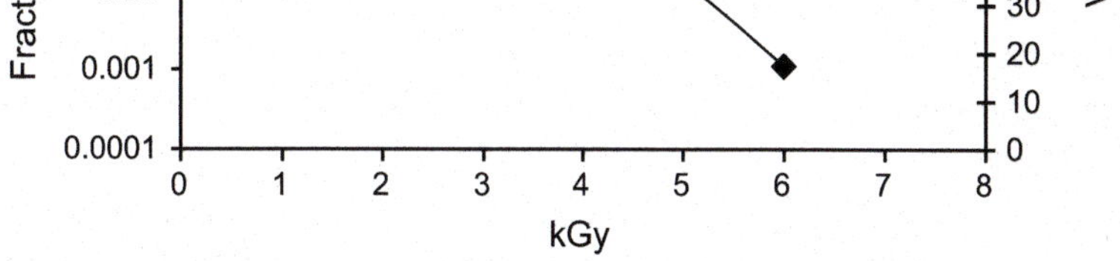

Fig. 2 Effect of gamma irradiation on reproductive capacity and viability of yeast cells of *P. brasiliensis*. Yeast cells were irradiated with increasing doses of external gamma radiation and the fraction of colony-forming units (CFU) determined (◆). The viability was measured by Janus green method (■). The *bars* represent the standard deviations of triplicate determinations

3.7 Virulence Assessment of Radioattenuated Yeast Cells

1. Evaluate the radioattenuated yeast cell infectivity in immunocompromised and immunocompetent mice (*see* **Note 11**).
2. Anesthetize mice by intramuscular (im) injection with 40 μL of a solution containing 57% of ketamine at 80 mg/Kg and 43% of xylazine at 15 mg/kg prior to the inoculation in the ocular plexus.

3. Inoculate mice by endovenous route with 3×10^5 viable radio-attenuated yeast cells of *P. brasiliensis* (*see* **Note 12**).
4. As negative and positive controls use, respectively, uninfected animals and animals infected with nonirradiated virulent yeast cells of *P. brasiliensis*.
5. After 30 and 90 days of yeast cell inoculation, euthanize the animals and remove their organs (lung, liver, and spleen) for recovery of colony-forming units (CFU) and histopathological changes (*see* **Note 13**).
6. CFU recovery: (a) Remove, weigh, and macerate lung, liver, and spleen organs in 1 mL of sterile PBS, pH 7.4 (*see* **Note 14**); (b) Plate 100 μL of the macerated on a high plating efficiency medium (*see* **Notes 8** and **9**); (c) Incubate the plate at 35 °C for 20 days and count the colony-forming units (CFU); (d) Express the results as the number of $\log_{10}$ CFU of viable yeast cells of *P. brasiliensis* per gram of tissue per mouse in each experimental group (*see* **Note 15**).
7. Histopathological changes: (a) Fix the organs excised in 10% formalin; (b) Embed the organs in paraffin for sectioning; (c) Stain the section with hematoxylin and eosin (H&E) and Grocott's methenamine nitrate (Grocott) (*see* **Note 16**); (d) Analyze organs alteration and fungal load by optical microscopy.
8. The radioattenuated yeast cell inability to cause infection, even in immunocompromised animals, is demonstrated in Fig. 3. No CFU were recovered nor histopathological changes were observed in any organs (lung, spleen, and liver) obtained from immunocompetent and immunocompromised mice.

3.8 Mouse Immunization and Intratracheal Challenge

1. Anesthetize mice by intramuscular (im) injection with 40 μL of a solution containing 57% of ketamine at 80 mg/Kg and 43% of xylazine at 15 mg/kg prior to the immunization and intratracheal challenge.
2. Immunize male BALB/c mice twice or three times, at 2 weeks intervals, by the ocular plexus with the injection of 10^5 radioattenuated yeast cells of *P. brasiliensis* in 50 μL of sterile PBS, pH 7.4, without any adjuvant.
3. Thirty days after immunization, perform the intratracheal challenge using 3×10^5 viable yeast forms of virulent *P. brasiliensis* in 50 μL of sterile PBS, pH 7.4 (*see* **Note 17**).

3.9 Protection Assay

1. Recover the colony-forming units (CFU) and analyze histopathological changes from lung, spleen, and liver at 30 and 90 days after intratracheal challenge as described in Subheading 3.7, **steps 4–6**.
2. Use organs collected from uninfected and infected mice with nonirradiated virulent yeast cells of *P. brasiliensis* as negative and positive controls, respectively.

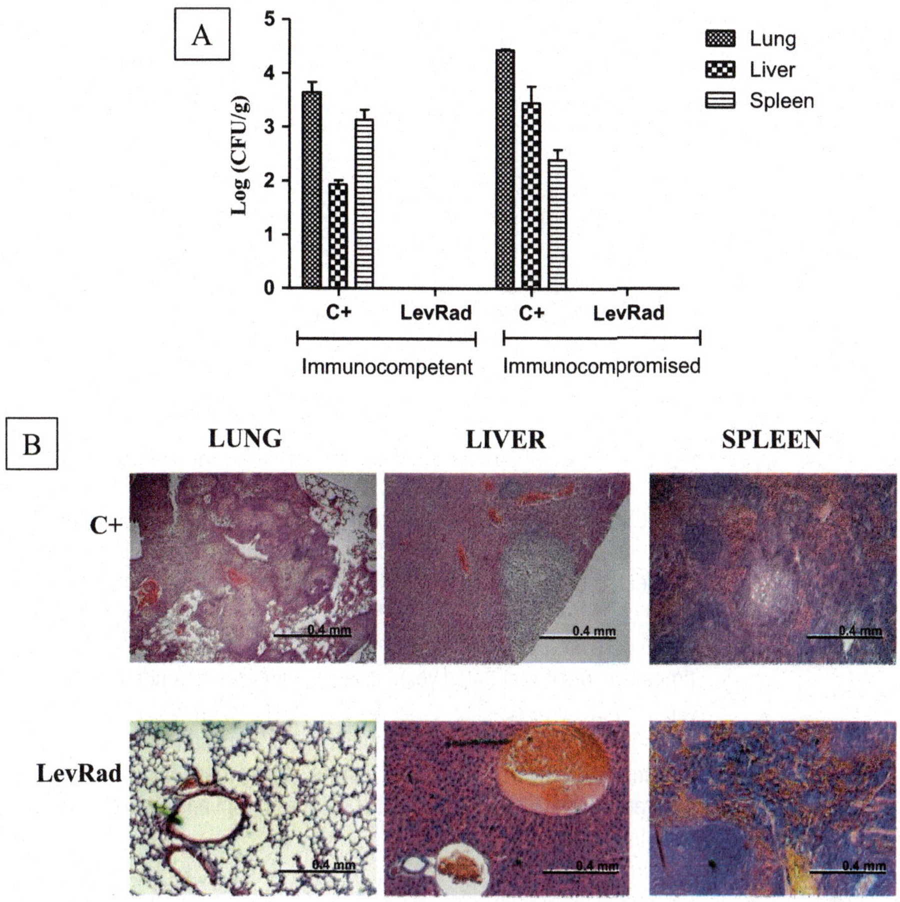

Fig. 3 CFU recovery in organs of immunocompetent and immunocompromised mice (**a**) and histopathological changes in organs of immunocompetent mice (**b**). Mice were inoculated by endovenous (i.v) with 3×10^5 viable radioattenuated yeast cell of *P. brasiliensis* (LevRad). Positive control was inoculated with virulent nonirradiated yeast cell of *P. brasiliensis* (C+). The organs CFU were estimated 30 days after inoculation. Data are reported as Log_{10} (CFU/g) mean ± SD in each experimental group ($n = 10$). Histopathology analyses showed the tissues of immunocompetent mice inoculated with LevRad free of yeast, granulomas, or inflammation. No CFU nor histopathology changes, or yeast cells were detected in the tissues of immunocompetent and immunocompromised mice inoculated with LevRad. Immunocompetent mice infected with nonirradiated yeast cell presented in their lungs intense coalescent multifocal interstitial granulomatous pneumonia. The liver showed a mild multifocal granuloma and the spleen a small unifocal granuloma

3. Report the data as the number of $\log_{10}$ CFU of viable yeast cells of *P. brasiliensis* per gram of tissue per mouse in each experimental group.
4. The best results concerning protection are achieved when mice are immunized three times, consecutively, at two-week intervals. Mice with local or disseminated disease were able to control effectively the PCM, as shown 90 days post-challenge (Fig. 4).

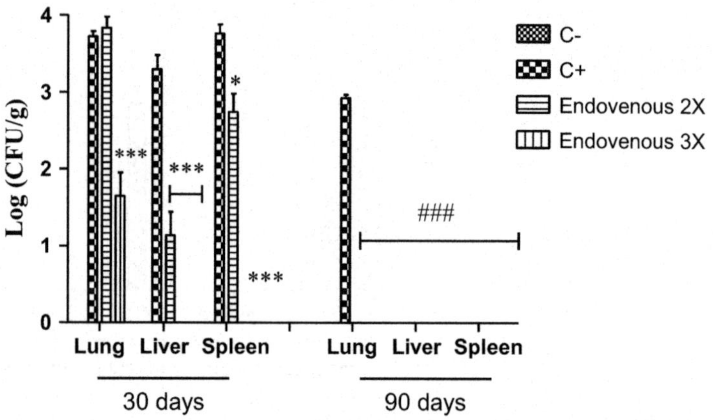

Fig. 4 CFU recovery from organs of infected mice immunized with viable radioattenuated yeast cells. Mice were challenged with virulent nonirradiated yeast cells of *P. brasiliensis* by intratracheal (i.t) 30 days after immunization. The organs CFU were estimated 30 and 90 days after challenge. Negative control (C−) uninfected mice; positive control (C+) infected mice with virulent nonirradiated yeast cells of *P. brasiliensis*; infected mice immunized twice with radioattenuated yeast cells by endovenous (Endovenous 2×); infected mice immunized three times with radioattenuated yeast cells by endovenous (Endovenous 3×). Data are reported as Log_{10} (CFU/g) mean ± SD in each experimental group ($n = 10$). The symbols (***) and (*) represent significant difference ($p < 0.001$ and $p < 0.05$, respectively) in relation to positive control. The symbol (###) represents significant difference ($p < 0.001$) in relation to positive control and mice challenged 30 days after immunization

3.10 Antibody Response Evaluation

1. Enzyme-linked immunosorbent assay (ELISA) using MEXO antigen (*see* **Note 18**) is usually performed to determine the antibody response in immunized mice and immunized mice after challenge.
2. Allow all reagents to reach room temperature before use. Gently mix all liquid reagents prior to use.
3. Perform ELISA using Maxisorp™ surface plates.
4. Coat the plate overnight at 4 °C with 0.5 μg per well of MEXO antigen in 0.05 M carbonate/bicarbonate buffer pH 9.6.
5. Wash the wells five times with 0.005 M PBS containing 0.5% Tween 20.
6. Add 150 μL of PBS, pH 7.4 containing 1.6% casein for 1 h at 37 °C.
7. Wash the wells five times with 0.005 M PBS containing 0.5% Tween 20.
8. Add 100 μL of diluted sera in PBS, pH 7.4 containing 25% casein, for 1 h at 37 °C.
9. Wash the wells five times with 0.005 M PBS containing 0.5% Tween 20.

10. Add 100 μL of diluted peroxidase-conjugated goat anti-mouse IgG, IgG2a, and IgG1 antibodies to wells. Cover plate and incubate at room temperature for 1 h at 37 °C (*see* **Note 19**).
11. Wash the wells five times with 0.005 M PBS containing 0.5% Tween 20.
12. Add 100 μL of tetramethylbenzidine (TMB) to each well for developing color at room temperature in the dark for 10–30 min.
13. Add 20 μL of stop solution (1 M sulfuric acid solution) to each well. The solution in the wells should change from blue to yellow.
14. Read the absorbance of each well at 490 nm.
15. Report data as mean ± standard deviations of optical density (490 nm) at 1:100 serum dilution in each experimental group ($n = 10$) (Fig. 5a–c).

3.11 Cytokine Detection by Real-Time PCR

1. Remove lungs from immunized and infected mice and frozen them in liquid nitrogen or–80 °C.
2. Use lungs collected from uninfected animal and infected with nonirradiated virulent yeast cells of *P. brasiliensis* as negative and positive controls, respectively.
3. Homogenize the lungs in 1 mL Trizol LS Reagent (*see* **Note 20**).
4. Incubate the homogenized samples for 5 min at 15–30 °C to permit the complete dissociation of nucleoprotein complex.
5. Add 200 μL of chloroform to each 1 mL of the lung homogenate and then incubate at room temperature for 2–3 min.
6. Centrifuge at 12,000 × *g* for 10 min at 2–8 °C.
7. Transfer the aqueous phase to a fresh tube and add 5 mL of isopropanol per 1 mL of Trizol, mix manually, and incubate the tube at room temperature for 10 min (*see* **Note 21**).
8. Centrifuge at 12,000 × *g* for 10 min at 2–8 °C to precipitate RNA.
9. Remove the supernatant and wash the RNA pellets once with at least 1 mL of 75% ethanol. Mix the sample by vortexing and centrifuge at no more than 7,500 × *g* for 5 min at 2–8 °C.
10. Briefly, dry the RNA pellets at room temperature for 5–10 min (*see* **Note 22**).
11. Dissolve RNA sample adding RNAse-free water and incubate for 10 min at 55–60 °C.
12. Incubate the isolated RNA with 10 U of DNAse (RNAse free) for 30 min at 37 °C.

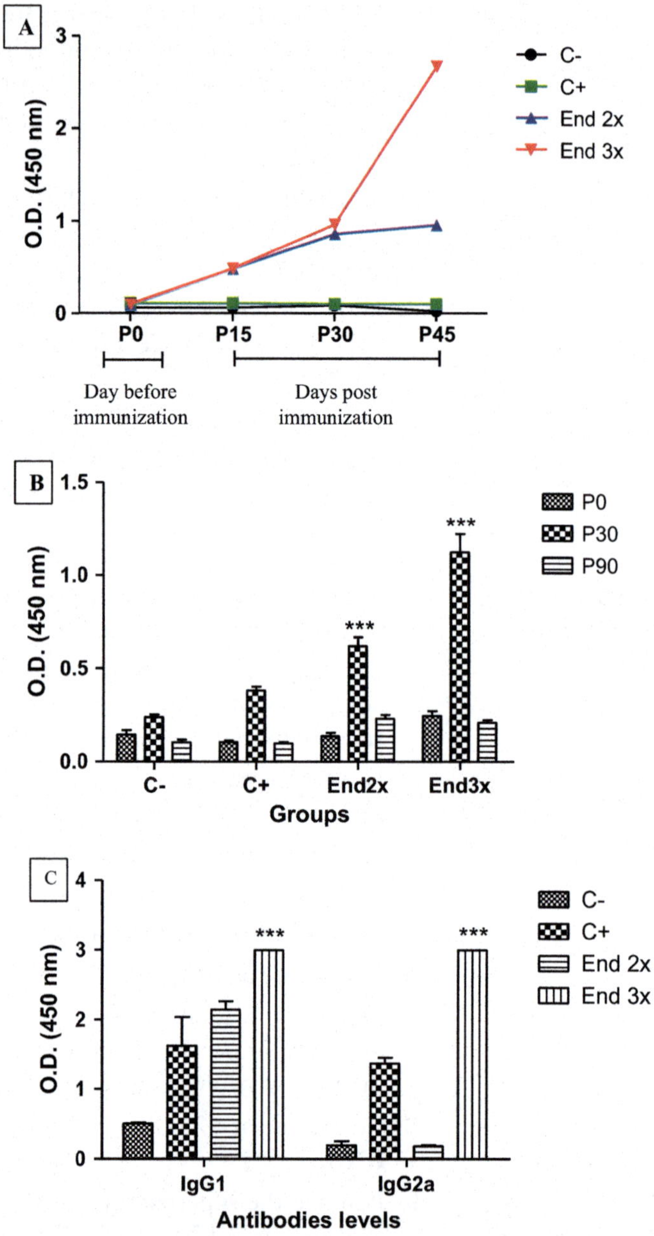

Fig. 5 (**a**) IgG production in serum from mice immunized twice (End 2×) or three times (End 3×) by endovenous with radioattenuated yeast cells of *P. brasiliensis*. Negative control (C−) uninfected mice; positive control (C+) infected mice with virulent nonirradiated yeast cells of *P. brasiliensis*. Antibody responses against MEXO were determined by ELISA just before (P0), as well as at 15 (P15), 30 (P30), and 45 (P45) days after mice immunization (**a**) and at 30 (P30) and 90 (P90) days after immunized mice challenged (**b**). IgG1 and IgG2a isotypes production against MEXO were determined by ELISA at 30 days after immunized mice challenged (**c**). The symbol (***) represents significant difference ($p < 0.001$) in relation to the other groups

13. Quantify the RNA sample by photometer and check the quality by agarose gel electrophoresis to ensure the absence of degradation.
14. For reverse transcription: (a) Mix and briefly centrifuge each component before use; (b) Add in a 0.2–0.5 mL tube about 2 μg of Total RNA per 20 μL cDNA reaction, 1 μL of 0.5 μg/μL Oligo (dT), 1 μL 10 mM dNTP Mix and DEPC-treated water to 10 μL; (c) Incubate the tube at 95 °C for 5 min, then place on ice for at least 1 min; (d) Add 10 μL of cDNA synthesis mix containing 2 μL of 10× RT buffer, 4 μL of 25 mM $MgCl_2$, 2 μL of 0.1 M DTT, 1 μL of RNaseOUT™ (40 U/μL) and 1 μL SuperScript® III RT (200 U/μL) to each tube prepared above; (e) Mix gently and incubate in the PCR machine programmed as follows: 50 °C for 50 min and then 85 °C for 5 min; (f) Store cDNA synthesis reaction at −30 °C to −10 °C or use for PCR immediately.
15. For real-time PCR: (a) Pipette 5 μL of diluted cDNA into all wells. Use 1-10 ng cDNA for each reaction; (b) Add 20 μL of real-time PCR mix containing 5 μL of each primer pair (See Note 23) and 10 μL of PowerUp Syber Green Master Mix into triplicate wells; (c) Seal plate with optical film; (d) Centrifuge briefly to spin down the contents and eliminate any air bubbles; (e) Set the Real Time PCR condition as follows: begin with 50 °C for 2 min and 95 °C for 2 min and then 40 cycles of amplification (95 °C for 15 s followed by 60 °C for 1 min) using an ABI PRISM 7900 apparatus (Applied Biosystems). Perform dissociation curves at 95 °C for 15 s and 60 °C for 15 s; (g) Cytokine transcript levels were assessed through the comparative Ct method, using uninfected mice as the calibrator and reporter. A twofold increase was determined as the baseline to differentiate the gene expressed from the calibrator. Data was reported as mean ± standard deviations of relative expression of cytokine in relation to β-actin from the lungs of ten animals per group (Fig. 6).

3.12 Cytokine Measurement by ELISA

1. Dilute the purified anti-cytokine capture antibody in Binding Solution, according to the instructions of the manufacturer (*see* **Note 24**).
2. Add 100 μL of diluted antibody to the wells of an enhanced protein-binding ELISA plate.
3. Seal the plate to prevent evaporation and incubate it overnight at 4 °C.
4. Wash the plate three times with PBS, pH 7.4 containing 0.5% Tween 20 (PBS/Tween 20).
5. Block nonspecific binding by adding 200 μL of PBS, pH 7.4 containing 1% BSA (PBS/BSA) per well.

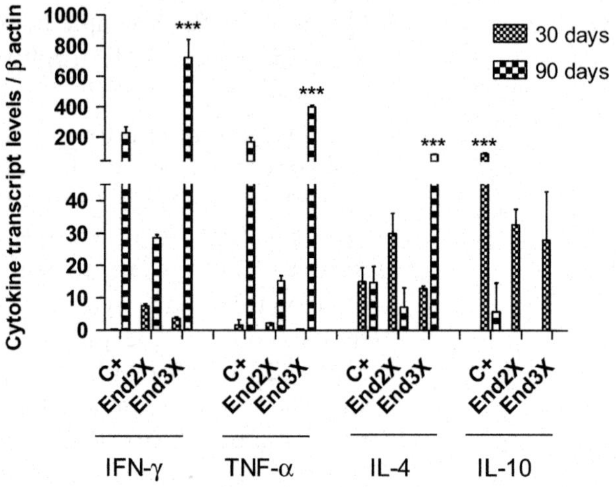

Fig. 6 Cytokine transcript levels from organs of infected mice immunized twice (End 2×) or three times (End 3×) by endovenous with viable radioattenuated yeast cells of *P. brasiliensis*. Positive control (C+) infected mice with virulent nonirradiated yeast cells of *P. brasiliensis.* The cytokine transcript levels were quantified through Real-Time PCR at 30 and 90 days after the challenge of immunized mice. Data were reported as mean ± SD of relative expression of cytokine in relation to β –actin from the lungs of ten animals per group. For IFN-γ, TNF-α, and IL-4 the symbol (***) represents significant difference (*p* < 0.001) in relation to C+. For IL-10, the symbol (***) represents significant difference ($p < 0.001$) in relation to End2× and End3×

6. Seal the plate and incubate it at room temperature for 1–2 h.
7. Wash three times with PBS/Tween 20.
8. Add 100 μL standards and splenocyte culture supernatants samples diluted in PBS/BSA per well (*see* **Note 25**).
9. Seal the plate and incubate it at room temperature for 1–2 h or overnight at 4 °C.
10. Wash four times with PBS/Tween 20.
11. Add 100 μL of diluted streptavidin-HRP (1:2000 (v/v) in PBS/BSA) per well.
12. Seal the plate and incubate it for 20 min at room temperature.
13. Wash four times with PBS/Tween 20.
14. Add 100 μL of color development solution to each well (*see* **Note 26**).
15. Seal the plate and incubate it in the dark for 20 min at room temperature.
16. Add 20 μL of stop solution to each well (1 M sulfuric acid solution). The solution color in the wells should change from blue to yellow.

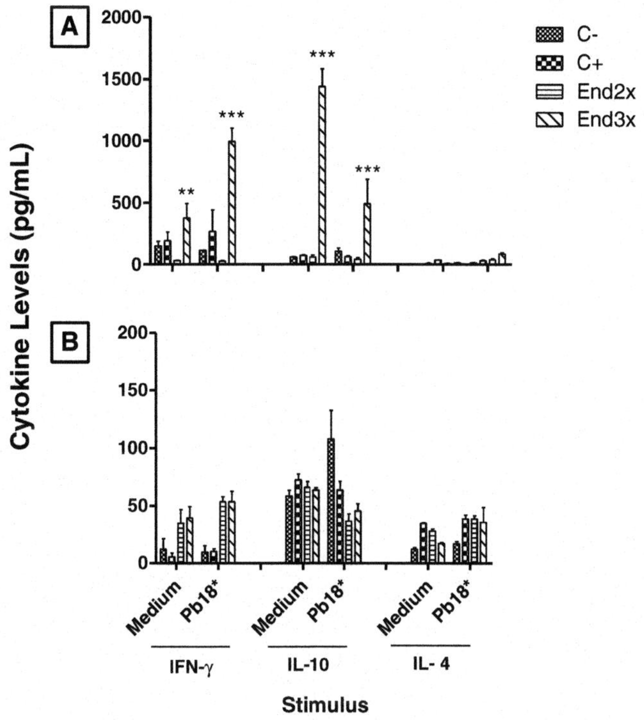

Fig. 7 Cytokine levels measured on splenocyte culture supernatants from infected mice immunized twice (End 2×) or three times (End 3×) by endovenous with viable radioattenuated yeast cells of *P. brasiliensis*. Balb/c mice were euthanized 30 (**a**) and 90 (**b**) days after challenge. The splenocytes were extracted and cultured (5×10^6 cells/well) in complete RPMI for 72 h, at 37 °C and 5% CO_2, in the absence or presence of attenuated yeast cell extract of *P. brasiliensis* culture as a stimulus (Pb18*). Negative control (C−) uninfected mice; positive control (C+) infected mice with virulent nonirradiated yeast cells of *P. brasiliensis*. Data were reported as mean ± SD of cytokine levels on splenocyte culture supernatants extracted from ten animals per group. For IFN- γ and IL-10 the symbols (**) and (***) represent significant difference ($p < 0.05$ and $p < 0.001$, respectively) in relation to the other groups

17. Read the absorbance of each well with a microplate reader set to 450 nm.
18. Report data as mean ± standard deviations of optical density (450 nm) at culture supernatant in each experimental group (Fig. 7a, b).

4 Notes

1. *P. brasiliensis* culture (strain Pb 18) may be maintained in liquid or solid YPD medium. The fungus must be weekly subcultures; otherwise, cells will lose their viability.

2. The temperature of the incubator should be checked frequently. Fungal growth is highly sensitive to temperature variations.
3. The *P. brasiliensis* yeast grows forming cell aggregates in culture medium. The cell cluster should be disrupted by vortexing to obtain single cells. Use cycles of 30 s of agitation alternating with 1.0 min of rest to avoid damaging the cells.
4. Viability analysis using vital dye must be carried out before every assay. We suggest the introduction of the dye during the cell counting.
5. Allow the cell suspension to interact with the dye not more than 8 min. We usually stained the concentrated cell suspension before its dilution to have an overview of the cell viability. Repeat the cell viability counting to certify that cells are dead and not overstained.
6. The recovery of the *P. brasiliensis* yeast cell virulence is crucial when the experiment demands highly infectious fungi. The *P. brasiliensis* yeast cell virulence recovery is usually performed in immunocompetent mice using a loaded fungal suspension. However, in some cases, it is necessary to use immunosuppressed mice to establish infection.
7. We suggest the use of male mice in experimental paracoccidioidomycosis (PCM). According to the literature, it is well known that the female presents resistance to disease, due to hormonal factors.
8. Prepare high plating efficiency medium as follows: add 37 g of Brain infusion agar medium (BHIA) to 910 mL of distilled water. Autoclave the BHIA medium for 15 min at 121 °C and cool it to 56 °C. Then, add 4% fetal calf serum, 5% *P. brasiliensis* spent culture medium (Pb18) as a growth factor, and 40 mg/mL of gentamycin.
9. *P. brasiliensis* spent culture medium is prepared by culturing the fungus (strain Pb 18), at 35 °C for 5 days on Brain infusion agar medium (BHIA) supplemented with 1% glucose. Suspend 5 mL of the pelleted yeast cells in 45 mL of distilled water and autoclave. Leave the suspension rest for 24 h at room temperature and centrifuge at 1000 × *g* for 15 min. Use the supernatant as the extract.
10. Gamma radiation doses ranging from 6.5 to 7.5 kG and dose rates between 750 and 1500 Gy/h may also be used to obtain the *P. brasiliensis* attenuation in the described culture conditions.
11. The cells must be counted and the viability estimated before the fungal inoculation. Do not use inoculum with viability less than 80%.

12. Use an ultra-fine 8 mm needle insulin syringe to inoculate the yeast cells by the ocular plexus. The inoculation should be performed carefully to avoid artery clog and inoculum lost.
13. The organs removed must be carefully divided into two parts: one for the CFU recovery and the other for histopathology.
14. Use a syringe plunger to macerate part of the organ in order to avoid damage and fungi death. Fix the other part immediately in 10% formalin for histopathological analyses.
15. The organs were collected, weighed, and macerated in 1 mL of sterile PBS, pH 7.4. The suspensions (100 μL) were plated on the high plating efficiency medium. The data was reported as $\log_{10}$ CFU per gram of tissue per mouse in each experimental group as follows:

$$\Upsilon = CFU / \left(W_{(g)} / 10\right) \times 1_{(g)} \text{or} \Upsilon = A / B$$

where Υ = CFU recovered per gram of tissue per mouse in each experimental group, A = CFU recovered in each animal organ, and B = organ weight that was macerated in 1 mL of sterile PBS (g) divided per 10.
16. The slides were stained with hematoxylin and eosin (H&E) and Grocott's methenamine nitrate (Grocott) at cellular morphology facility (Instituto de Ciências Biológicas/Universidade Federal de Minas Geais (ICB/UFMG)—Belo Horizonte/MG/Brazil).
17. We suggest an experiment standardization when working with other fungi. In our study, we immunized the Balb/c male mice two or three times, at two-week intervals, and challenged them 30 days later.
18. Prepare MEXO antigen as follows: homogenize by vortexing the nonirradiated *P. brasiliensis* colonies in PBS, pH 7.4. Centrifuge the suspension at 12,000 rpm for 30 min at 4 °C. Filter the supernatant using a 0.45 mm sterile filter. Quantify the protein by the Braford method and store at −20 °C.
19. Anti-mouse IgG-whole molecule-peroxidase conjugate and peroxidase-conjugated goat anti-mouse IgG, IgG2a and IgG1 antibodies were used at a dilution of 1:5000 (v/v) in PBS, pH 7.4 containing 25% casein.
20. Homogenize sample using a power homogenizer. Process or freeze tissue samples immediately upon extraction (Ambion RNA by life technologies' instructions [11]).
21. RNA remains exclusively in the aqueous phase. Save the interphase and organic phenol-chloroform phase if isolation of DNA or protein is desired (Ambion RNA by life technologies' instructions [11]).

22. The RNA is often invisible prior to centrifugation, and forms a gel-like pellet on the side and bottom of the tube. Do not allow the RNA to dry completely, because the pellet can lose solubility. Partially dissolve RNA samples to an A260/280 ratio <1.6 (Ambion RNA by life technologies' instructions [11]).
23. Cytokines and beta-actin-specific primers were designed as in Giulietti et al. [12]. It is important to set the concentration of each primer before its use. For optimal performance in Fast and Standard modes, use 300–800nM for each primer. All quantifications were normalized to the housekeeping gene beta-actin. A non-template control with no genetic material was included to eliminate contamination or nonspecific reactions.
24. Binding Solution: 0.1 M Na_2HPO_4, adjust to pH 9.0 when working with IFN—γ or to pH 6.0 to mouse IL10 and mouse TNF-α.
25. To perform the isolation of murine splenocytes: (a) Place the spleen in a small Petri dish (35 × 10mm) containing a cell strainer and 1 mL of sterile media (i.e., RPMI 1640); (b) Use a syringe plunger to macerate the spleen; (c) Transfer the homogenized cell suspension into a universal tube, complete the full volume with PBS, pH 7.4, and centrifuge twice at 400 × *g* for 10 min at room temperature; (d) Perform cell lysis by adding 1 mL of PBS 10×, pH 6.8, followed immediately by the addition of 9 mL of sterile deionized water; (e) Centrifuge at 400 × *g* for 5 min and aspirate the supernatant; (f) Resuspend the cells completely in PBS, pH 7.4. Centrifuge at 400 × *g* for 5 min and aspirate the supernatant. Then, resuspend cells in RPMI-1640 medium to a final known volume; (g) Count live cells using a hemocytometer and light microscope.
26. Prepare a working concentration of TMB substrate solution within 15 min prior to use. Mix equal volumes of Substrate Reagent A (H_2O_2) and Substrate Reagent B (Tetramethylbenzidine).

Acknowledgments

The authors acknowledge the Laboratory of Mycology from Microbiology Department and Laboratory of Molecular and Cellular Immunology from Biochemistry and Immunology Department, Institute of Biological Sciences/Federal University of Minas Gerais (ICB/UFMG) and Radiobiology Laboratory form Center of Nuclear Technology Development (CDTN), Brazil. This work was supported by the Brazilian agencies CNPq, CAPES, FAPEMIG, and CNEN.

References

1. Cutler JE, Deepe GS, Klein BS (2007) Advances in combating fungal diseases: vaccines on the threshold. Nat Rev Microbiol 5:13–18
2. Reina-San-Martin B, Cosson A, Minoprio P (2000) Lymphocyte polyclonal activation: a pitfall for vaccine design against infectious agents. Parasitol Today 16:62–67
3. Wales A, Kusel JR (1992) Biochemistry of irradiated parasites vaccines: suggested models for their mode of action. Parasitol Today 8:358–363
4. Demicheli MC, Goes AM, Andrade ASR (2007) Ultrastructural changes in *Paracoccidioides brasiliensis* yeast cells attenuated by gamma irradiation. Mycoses 50:397–402
5. Martins EMN, Sgarbi SR, Fernandes VC, Costa MMS, Goes AM, Andrade ASR (2007) Immunization with radioattenuated yeast cells of *Paracoccidioides brasiliensis* induces a long lasting protection in BALB/c mice. Vaccine 25:7893–7899
6. Brummer E, Castañeda E, Restrepo A (1993) Paracoccidioidomycosis: an update. Clin Microbiol 6:89–117
7. Shikanaii-Yasuda MA, Filho FQ, Mendes RP, Colombo AL, Moretti AL (2006) Guidelines in paracoccidioidomycosis. Rev Soc Bras Med Trop 39:297–310
8. Demicheli MC, Reis BS, Goes AM, Andrade ASR (2006) *Paraccocidioides brasiliensis*: attenuation of yeast cells by gamma irradiation. Mycoses 49:184–189
9. Martins EMN, Reis BS, Resende MA, Andrade ASR, Goes AM (2009) Mice immunization with radioattenuated yeast cells of *Paracoccidiodes brasiliensis*: influence of the number of immunizations. Mycopathologia 168:51–58
10. Sano A, Kurita N, Labuki K, Coelho R, Takeo K, Nishimura K, Miyaji M (1993) Comparative study of four different staining methods for estimation of live yeast form cells of *Paracoccidioides brasiliensis*. Mycopathologia 124:157–161
11. Life Technologies. Trizol® Reagent. 2012. Disponível em: www.lifetechnologies.com. Acesso em: 13 junho 2016
12. Giulietti A, Overbergh L, Valckx D, Decallonne RB, Mathieu C (2001) As overview of real-time quantitative PCR: applications to quantify cytokine gene expression. Methods 25:386–401

Chapter 2

Heat-Killed Yeast as a Pan-Fungal Vaccine

Marife Martinez, Karl V. Clemons, and David A. Stevens

Abstract

Fungal infections continue to rise worldwide. Antifungal therapy has long been a mainstay for the treatment of these infections, but often can fail for a number of reasons. These include acquired or innate drug resistance of the causative agent, poor drug penetration into the affected tissues, lack of cidal activity of the drug and drug toxicities that limit therapy. In some instances, such as coccidioidal meningitis, therapy is life-long. In addition, few new antifungal drugs are under development. In light of this information a preventative vaccine is highly desirable. Although numerous investigators have worked toward the development of fungal vaccines, none have become commercially available for use in humans. In the course of our studies, we have discovered that heat-killed yeast (HKY) of *Saccharomyces cerevisiae* can be used as a vaccine and have shown that it has efficacy in the prevention and reduction of five different fungal infections when used experimentally in mice, which raises the possibility of a pan-fungal vaccine preparation. In our studies we grow *S. cerevisiae* in broth and heat-kill the organism at 70 ° C for 3 h. The number of dead yeast cells is adjusted and mice are vaccinated subcutaneously beginning 3–7 weeks prior to infection. After infection, efficacy is assessed on the basis of survival and residual burden of the fungus in the target organs. Alternatively, efficacy can be assessed solely on fungal burden at a predetermined time postinfection. Although itself it is unlikely to be moved toward commercialization, HKY can be used a positive control vaccine for studies on specific molecular entities as vaccines, and as a guidepost for the key elements of potential, more purified, pan-fungal vaccine preparations.

Key words Heat-killed yeast, *Saccharomyces*, Vaccine, Murine model, Aspergillosis, Pan-fungal vaccine

1 Introduction

Antifungal vaccines are a desirable product for the prevention of invasive fungal infections. Their use could be relevant in the prevention of endemic mycoses such as coccidioidomycosis, where infection occurs naturally in both immunocompetent and immunodeficient persons in the geographic area of endemicity. In addition, an antifungal vaccine could be useful against opportunistic infections that occur in immunocompromised persons. As an example the vaccination of patients prior to chemotherapy-induced neutropenia for bone marrow transplants, or prior to high-dose steroid treatments, may result

Markus Kalkum and Margarita Semis (eds.), *Vaccines for Invasive Fungal Infections: Methods and Protocols*, Methods in Molecular Biology, vol. 1625, DOI 10.1007/978-1-4939-7104-6_2,

in sufficient carryover of protective immunity to prevent or at least reduce the severity of opportunistic infection of *Aspergillus* until the patient has recovered his own immune response. It is also possible that antifungal vaccines could be used therapeutically, but little work has been performed on this aspect.

Over the years there have been a variety of preparations tested as possible vaccines. These include killed organisms, attenuated strains of an organism, specific proteins from an organism, and other cellular components. Primarily, each of these has been directed at a single specific fungal infection, with cross-reactivities not assessed. However, cross-protection against some fungal infections by immunization with heterologous fungi has long been known [1]. Likewise, cross-protection by glycan vaccine preparations from different species has been shown [1–3]. A vaccine composed of conjugated laminarin (β-glucan) induced antibody-mediated protection against candidiasis, cryptococcosis, and aspergillosis, suggesting that it is possible to immunize with a cross-reacting antigen against evolutionarily distant infectious agents [2]. In studies using a protein chip comprised of 4800 full-length fusion proteins from *S. cerevisiae*, we found many of these proteins were cross-reactive with the sera of mice infected with *Candida albicans*, *Coccidioides posadasii*, and *Paracoccidioides brasiliensis*, as well as the sera from HKY vaccinated mice [4]. Furthermore, using proteomic technologies highly homologous proteins were found in comparisons of cell wall proteins from 13 different fungi [5]. Taken together, these data are highly suggestive that the goal of a pan-fungal vaccine is possible.

During the course of studies on potential vaccines against aspergillosis using *S. cerevisiae* expressing a specific protein from *Aspergillus fumigatus*, we noted that the yeast vector alone provided protection [6]. This observation led to various studies where we showed that the heat-killed yeast (HKY) of *S. cerevisiae* as a vaccine protects mice against *Aspergillus*, *Coccidioides*, *Candida*, *Cryptococcus*, and *Rhizopus* [7–11], making it a prototype crude panfungal vaccine. Furthermore, we showed that the HKY induced a significant and specific Th1 immune response, as well as antibodies against β-glucan and mannan [12].

Here, we describe the preparation and testing of the HKY vaccine. As noted above, we have used this preparation against five different experimental fungal infections and shown protection. In addition, we have used HKY as the positive control for examining possible vaccine candidates of glycans and glucan-BSA conjugates for protection in murine models of coccidioidomycosis and aspergillosis [6, 13–17]. Adult mice are vaccinated subcutaneously with HKY at various times prior to infection using a split dose scheme of giving one-half of the total dose in two different sites on the dorsal surface. The number of doses used and dosage depends on the infection model, but we have routinely used three doses given

1 week apart beginning 4 weeks prior to infection, with our standard dose being 6 × 10^7 HKY per dose, which equates to 2.5 mg of HKY [7]. For testing of the potency of the HKY preparation we present the use of a systemic model of aspergillosis performed in CD-1 mice. Testing against other models of fungal infection and the specifics of the model may require empiric determination of the HKY regimen that is most effective, as was done in our other studies [6–11].

2 Materials

1. *Saccharomyces cerevisiae* culture (*see* **Note 1**).
2. *Aspergillus fumigatus* (*see* **Note 2**).
3. Incubator shaker.
4. Water bath capable of heating to more than 70 ° C.
5. Sabouraud dextrose agar with 50 mg of chloramphenicol per liter as agar plates (SDAc).
6. Potato dextrose agar plates.
7. YPD agar, 1% yeast extract, 1% peptone, 2% dextrose, and 2% agar; YPD broth same with no agar.
8. Hemacytometer.
9. Sterile plastic centrifuge tubes 15 and 50 ml capacities.
10. Five-week-old female CD-1 mice from the virus antibody-free colony (VAF) purchased from Charles River Laboratories (*see* **Note 3**).
11. Tuberculin syringes and 26-gauge needles.
12. Sterile saline with 100 U penicillin and 100 μg streptomycin per ml added.
13. Sterile phosphate buffered saline (pH 7) and sterile water.
14. Sterile saline with 0.05% Tween 80.
15. Sterile saline.
16. Glycerol.
17. Dissecting instruments—dissecting scissors and forceps.
18. Copeland jar with 70% ethanol (for dipping scissors and forceps) and a squeeze bottle of 70% isopropanol used to wet the fur.
19. Sterile tubes used to make dilutions of tissue homogenates.
20. Sterile 100 × 15 mm petri plates and 60 × 15 mm petri plates.
21. Mechanical tissue homogenizer with a probe for 5 ml volumes.

3 Methods

3.1 HKY Preparation

1. Recover *S. cerevisiae* strain 96–108 from the −80 °C freezer and culture on yeast-extract peptone dextrose (YPD) agar for 72 h at 37 °C.
2. Culture one loop-full in YPD broth for an additional 24 h at 37 °C and 170 rpm.
3. Harvest the cells by centrifugation at 1000 × *g* for 15 min and wash by centrifugation three times with PBS.
4. Count the cells using a hemacytometer and adjust the suspension to obtain a count of 4×10^8 yeast cells/ml in suspension in a 50 ml centrifuge tube.
5. Kill the yeast cell by heating the suspension at 70 °C for 3 h.
6. Determine the viability of the heat-killed cells by plating cells on Sabouraud Dextrose Agar (SDAc) with chloramphenicol.
7. Store the HKY in a refrigerator for further use (*see* **Note 4**).

3.2 Vaccination

1. Use groups of 10 CD-1 female mice (6 weeks old at the time of the first vaccination dose). Give the first vaccine dose 28 days prior to infection.
2. Use the 4×10^8 HKY/ml suspension and with a tuberculin syringe with a 26-gauge needle give each mouse 0.15 ml HKY split into two sites (0.075 ml per site) as a subcutaneous injection on the dorsal surface. This results in the standard dose of HKY used as 6×10^7 HKY per dose per mouse or 2.5 mg per dose.
3. Perform booster doses 1 week apart for a total of three doses given on days 28, 21, and 14 prior to infection (*see* **Note 5**).

3.3 Preparation of Aspergillus Fumigatus 10AF for Systemic Murine Model

1. Revive the organism from frozen storage (−80 °C). Thaw a frozen vial. Put two drops, each of 50 μl, onto Potato Dextrose Agar (PDA) plates ($n = 2$). Mark vial as thawed once and return vial to the freezer (vials are used only twice). Incubate plates at 35 °C for 4–5 days or until sporulation is sufficient (entire colony shows a green coloration) (*see* **Note 6**).
2. Harvesting conidia (in a Class 2 Biosafety cabinet): Use a 50 ml centrifuge tube. Add ~15 ml of sterile saline with 0.05% Tween 80.
3. With a sterile transfer pipette, aspirate (1–2 ml at a time) saline/Tween solution (from the 50 ml tube) and pour in the plate (over the green "lawn" of conidia).
4. Using the same transfer pipette, carefully scrape off conidia, then suction and collect in the tube.

5. Repeat this until a heavy suspension of conidia has been obtained.
6. Enumerating conidia/ml: Make about 7–8 serial tenfold dilutions of the harvested conidia stock. Plate 0.5 ml duplicates of dilutions 10^{-4}, 10^{-5}, 10^{-6}, 10^{-7}, and 10^{-8} onto Sabouraud Dextrose Agar (SDAc) plates with chloramphenicol. Incubate plates at 35 °C for 48 h and count the colonies.
7. Also enumerate the number of conidia in the suspension by hemacytometer count.
8. Store conidial suspensions at 4 ° C and it can be used for several weeks. Conidial counts should be confirmed for each use of the suspension.

3.4 Infection Model

1. Dilute the stock suspension of conidia with saline to 3.2×10^7 conidia/ml. Each mouse will be given 0.25 ml of this suspension, which equates to 8×10^6 conidia/mouse.
2. All mice are infected intravenously. Use a tuberculin syringe with a 26-gauge needle and give 0.25 ml of the conidial suspension.
3. Tally survival on a daily basis (*see* **Note** 7).
4. At day 10–12 postinfection euthanize all surviving mice using an approved method (CO_2 anoxia is approved in our institution).
5. Aseptically remove the kidneys and brains of mice for determination of fungal burdens.
6. Weigh each organ in a 60 mm petri plate.
7. Place each weighed organ in 5 ml of saline with penicillin and streptomycin.
8. Homogenize the organ using mechanical method.
9. Dilute the homogenate using tenfold serial dilutions (approximately three are sufficient).
10. Plate sample dilutions on SDA with chloramphenicol.
11. Incubate at 37 ° C for 18–24 h and count colonies.
12. Determine the fungal burden as the number of CFU per entire organ or CFU per gram of organ weight.
13. Assess vaccine efficacy based on survival using a log rank test and on comparative CFU using a Mann-Whitney U test.

4 Notes

1. We recommend that archival aliquots of the strain of *S. cerevisiae* to be used be kept frozen at −80 °C in 40% glycerol. Multiple vials should be frozen and each vial used a minimum of times to avoid repeated freezing and thawing. Cultures are

grown in YPD agar slants at 37 ° C for 24 h. Cells are harvested by adding the 40% glycerol solution to the slants to suspend the yeast. One milliliter aliquots of the yeast suspension are pipetted into cryovials (use caps with an O-ring) and placed in the freezer. We also recommend the use of a wild-type clinical strain of *S. cerevisiae* rather than a commercial strain such as Red Star. The clinical strains are more robust in growth and induce better protection.

2. We recommend that archival stocks of the strain of *A. fumigatus* to be used be kept frozen at −80 °C. Multiple vials should be frozen and each vial used a minimum of times to avoid repeated freezing and thawing. The method described [18] is used. In brief, organisms are grown at 35 °C on potato dextrose agar until they are well sporulated, usually 4–7 days. Conidia are harvested from the plate by gently washing with 0.2% Tween 80 in PBS (PBST) (5–10 ml per plate) and gently scraping the surface of the colony to dislodge the conidia. The conidial suspension is collected in a separate sterile tube.

   For long-term storage at −80 °C, 1 ml of 10% glycerol in PBST is added to 2 ml of conidial suspension. The resulting suspension is mixed using a vortex mixer and 1 ml volumes pipetted into cryovials with O-rings in the caps. These tubes are frozen at −80 °C. The strain of *A. fumigatus* we use is 10AF (ATCC 90240), which has been used by our laboratory for various models of aspergillosis in studies of antifungal drugs and vaccines [6, 8, 14, 15, 19]. Other standard strains, such as Af293, could also be used.

3. Mice are housed five mice per cage and we use ten mice to comprise each group (i.e., control or treatment) in an experiment, because this allows robust nonparametric statistics. All caging equipment, bedding (hardwood chip), and food should be sterilized prior to use. The drinking water used in our facility is acidified, although sterile water can also be used. Caging should be changed at least twice weekly and animals handled using clean latex gloves or surgical gloves.

   We have chosen to use outbred female CD-1 mice in our studies. However, there is no reason that male CD-1 mice could not be used. Should a different strain of mice (e.g., BALB/c, C57BL/6, etc.) be needed for specific studies, the investigator will need to perform pilot studies to ascertain relative resistance.

4. We recommend the HKY suspension not be stored for more than 3 months, at which time a new suspension should be prepared. We also recommend that at least 50–100 ml of suspension be prepared to ensure that the same suspension can be used throughout a single experiment, or multiple experiments if done within the 3 months.

5. We have found that this regimen of vaccine dosing repeatedly provides significant protection against systemic murine aspergillosis. Other regimens have been tested successfully as well as have higher dosages of HKY [8]. Also, it should be noted that granulomatous bumps in the skin at the site of injection can occur. We have noted no erosion or ulceration of the skin during our studies.
6. It has been our experience that growth of *A. fumigatus* to be used in animal models is best done on PDA. Although growth from SDA is good, we have found that the virulence of the organism is highly variable and inconsistent. We have not observed this inconsistency when conidial suspension is recovered from PDA plate growth.
7. The model used in this example will result in mortality of control mice beginning usually on day 3 or 4 postinfection. In accord with the institutional requirements and under the advice of the attending veterinarian, criteria for euthanasia should be determined and followed closely. Weight loss of greater than 30% (percentage may differ at individual institutions) is usually considered a basis for euthanasia.

References

1. Kong YC, Levine HB (1967) Experimentally induced immunity in the mycoses. Bacteriol Rev 31(1):35–53
2. Torosantucci A, Chiani P, Bromuro C, De Bernardis F, Palma AS, Liu Y, Mignogna G, Maras B, Colone M, Stringaro A, Zamboni S, Feizi T, Cassone A (2009) Protection by anti-beta-glucan antibodies is associated with restricted beta-1,3 glucan binding specificity and inhibition of fungal growth and adherence. PLoS One 4(4):e5392
3. Torosantucci A, Bromuro C, Chiani P, De Bernardis F, Berti F, Galli C, Norelli F, Bellucci C, Polonelli L, Costantino P, Rappuoli R, Cassone A (2005) A novel glyco-conjugate vaccine against fungal pathogens. J Exp Med 202(5):597–606
4. Coelho PSR, Im H, Clemons KV, Snyder MP, Stevens DA (2015) Evaluating common humoral responses against fungal infections with yeast protein microarrays. J Proteome Res 14:3924–3931. doi:10.1021/acs.jproteome.5b00365
5. Champer J, Ito JI, Clemons KV, Stevens DA, Kalkum M (2016) Proteomic analysis of pathogenic fungi reveals highly expressed conserved cell wall proteins. J Fungi 2(1). doi:10.3390/jof2010006
6. Stevens DA, Clemons KV, Liu M (2011) Developing a vaccine against aspergillosis. Med Mycol 49(Suppl 1):S170–S176. doi:10.3109/13693786.2010.497775
7. Capilla J, Clemons KV, Liu M, Levine HB, Stevens DA (2009) *Saccharomyces cerevisiae* as a vaccine against coccidioidomycosis. Vaccine 27(27):3662–3668. doi:10.1016/j.vaccine.2009.03.030. S0264-410X(09)00436-8 [pii]
8. Liu M, Capilla J, Johansen ME, Alvarado D, Martinez M, Chen V, Clemons KV, Stevens DA (2011) *Saccharomyces* as a vaccine against systemic aspergillosis: 'the friend of man' a friend again? J Med Microbiol 60(Pt 10):1423–1432. doi:10.1099/jmm.0.033290-0. jmm.0.033290-0 [pii]
9. Liu M, Clemons KV, Johansen ME, Martinez M, Chen V, Stevens DA (2012) *Saccharomyces* as a vaccine against systemic candidiasis. Immunol Investig 41(8):847–855. doi:10.3109/08820139.2012.692418
10. Luo G, Gebremariam T, Clemons KV, Stevens DA, Ibrahim AS (2014) Heat-killed yeast protects diabetic ketoacidotic-steroid treated mice from pulmonary mucormycosis. Vaccine 32(29):3573–3576. doi:10.1016/j.vaccine.2014.04.086

11. Majumder T, Liu M, Chen V, Martinez M, Alvarado D, Clemons KV, Stevens DA (2014) Killed *Saccharomyces cerevisiae* protects against lethal challenge of *Cryptococcus grubii*. Mycopathologia 178(3-4):189–195. doi:10.1007/s11046-014-9798-5
12. Liu M, Clemons KV, Bigos M, Medovarska I, Brummer E, Stevens DA (2011) Immune responses induced by heat killed *Saccharomyces cerevisiae*: a vaccine against fungal infection. Vaccine 29(9):1745–1753. doi:10.1016/j.vaccine.2010.12.119. S0264-410X(10)01906-7 [pii]
13. Liu M, Clemons K, Bystricky S, Stevens D (2010) Glycans and conjugates as vaccines against coccidioidomycosis. Paper presented at the 50th interscience conference on antimicrobial agents and chemotherapy, Boston, MA, Sept. 2010. Abstract no. G1-1657
14. Liu M, Machova E, Nescakova Z, Medovarska I, Clemons KV, Martinez M, Chen V, Bystricky S, Stevens DA (2012) Vaccination with mannan protects mice against systemic aspergillosis. Med Mycol 50(8):818–828. doi:10.3109/13693786.2012.683539
15. Clemons KV, Danielson ME, Michel KS, Liu M, Ottoson NC, Leonardo SM, Martinez M, Chen V, Antonysamy MA, Stevens DA (2014) Whole glucan particles as a vaccine against murine aspergillosis. J Med Microbiol 63(Pt 12):1750–1759. doi:10.1099/jmm.0.079681-0
16. Clemons KV, Antonysamy MA, Danielson ME, Michel KS, Martinez M, Chen V, Stevens DA (2015) Whole glucan particles as a vaccine against systemic coccidioidomycosis. J Med Microbiol 64(10):1237–1243. doi:10.1099/jmm.0.000138
17. Clemons KV, Hanson LH, Perlman AM, Stevens DA (1990) Efficacy of SCH39304 and fluconazole in a murine model of disseminated coccidioidomycosis. Antimicrob Agents Chemother 34(5):928–930
18. Denning DW, Clemons KV, Stevens DA (1992) Quantitative preservation of viability of *Aspergillus fumigatus*. J Med Vet Mycol 30(6):485–488
19. Clemons KV, Grunig G, Sobel RA, Mirels LF, Rennick DM, Stevens DA (2000) Role of IL-10 in invasive aspergillosis: increased resistance of IL-10 gene knockout mice to lethal systemic aspergillosis. Clin Exp Immunol 122(2):186–191

Chapter 3

Immunoinformatics as a Tool for New Antifungal Vaccines

Rupanjali Chaudhuri and Srinivasan Ramachandran

Abstract

Immunoinformatics aids in screening for vaccine candidates, which can be experimentally tested for their efficacy. This chapter describes methods to use immunoinformatics to screen fungal vaccines candidates. Surface-localized molecules called adhesins could elicit immune response and serve as efficient vaccine candidates. The screening process is patterned on two steps, namely, a First Layer screen mostly used for value addition and prioritization based on characteristics of known antigens and a Second Layer highly focussed on core immunoinformatics analysis involving the binding and interactions of the molecules of the immune system. Together they offer a comprehensive objective evaluation of vaccine candidates selection in silico for fungal pathogens.

Key words Immunoinformatics, Adhesins, Immune response, Vaccine candidates

1 Introduction

Among the opportunistic fungal infections in immunocompromised patients, *Candida albicans* and *Candida glabrata* are very common [1]. Other major fungal pathogens include *Aspergillus fumigatus, Blastomyces dermatitidis, Coccidiodes immitis, Coccidiodes posadasii, Histoplasma capsulatum*, and *Paracoccidioides brasiliensis* [2–6]. It is being realized that either a therapeutic or preventive vaccine could be useful for at-risk patients [7, 8]. Because the complete genome sequences and the encoded proteins of pathogens are available, it is prudent to computationally screen for potential antigenic proteins, a process called "reverse vaccinology" [9–11]. The advantages of time and offer of entire range of potential antigens of reverse vaccinology are immensely rewarding [12]. Surface-localized adhesins act as major virulence factors aiding in the establishment of infections by pathogens. Therefore, immunization with adhesins can combat fungal infections at early stage of infection by blocking their function, namely, in the pathogen's adherence to the host cell.

Markus Kalkum and Margarita Semis (eds.), *Vaccines for Invasive Fungal Infections: Methods and Protocols*, Methods in Molecular Biology, vol. 1625, DOI 10.1007/978-1-4939-7104-6_3, © Springer Science+Business Media LLC 2017

A few fungal vaccine formulations include adhesins for example, agglutinin-like sequence proteins in *Candida albicans*, 43 kDa glycoprotein in *Paracoccidioides brasiliensis*, BAD-1 (WI adhesin) protein in *Blastomyces dermatitidis*, and spherule outer wall glycoprotein in *Coccidioides immitis*. The spherule outer wall glycoprotein in *Coccidioides immitis* has undergone trials in humans, whereas the rest have shown efficacy in mouse experimental models [13–21].

The adhesin vaccine candidates (both predicted and experimentally tested) can be further evaluated for their potential antigenicity using immunoinformatics. Immunoinformatics refers to collection of databases and prediction algorithms using immunological information of the molecules of interest (*see* **Note 1**). This chapter outlines the principles and methods to screen most probable fungal adhesin vaccine candidates using immunoinformatics (*see* **Note 6**).

2 Materials and Methods

2.1 Rationale

The experience gained during initial applications of reverse vaccinology can be used by implementing an integrative approach for prediction of multiple features of proteins. We collected the known adhesins from the literature and also predicted novel adhesins using the FungalRV adhesin predictor (*see* **Notes 2** and **7**). Together, this list of proteins offers a wide window for the evaluation of potential antigens. Subsequently, the following analyses were carried out: prediction of homologs (orthologs and paralogs), of transmembrane topologies, of motifs (beta helix supersecondary structural motifs), of subcellular localization, of similarity against Human proteins, of antigenic regions, and of conserved domains. These data are organized as "First Layer" Immunoinformatics data (*see* **Note 3**). The "Second Layer Immunoinformatics data" constitute the epitopes and allergens predictions data (*see* **Notes 3–6**). This type of structuring of the data simplifies the user protocol by excluding those candidates, which do not pass the criteria from First Layer data. However, because the processes of development of immunoinformatics algorithms are ongoing, we have included the complete data for all the adhesins (known and predicted) for future evaluations. This analysis for fungal vaccine candidates using immunoinformatics techniques has been incorporated into FungalRV, a portal for Adhesin prediction and immunoinformatics of human fungal pathogens [9] (*see* **Notes 2** and **7**).

2.2 First Layer

2.2.1 List of Adhesins

An example of getting the list of Adhesins is shown in Fig. 1. The pathogen *Aspergillus fumigatus* was selected from the pull down list of pathogens and then the push button Get Adhesin List is pressed. A new window in the browser displays the list of known and predicted adhesins containing the fields ORF_id, Organism,

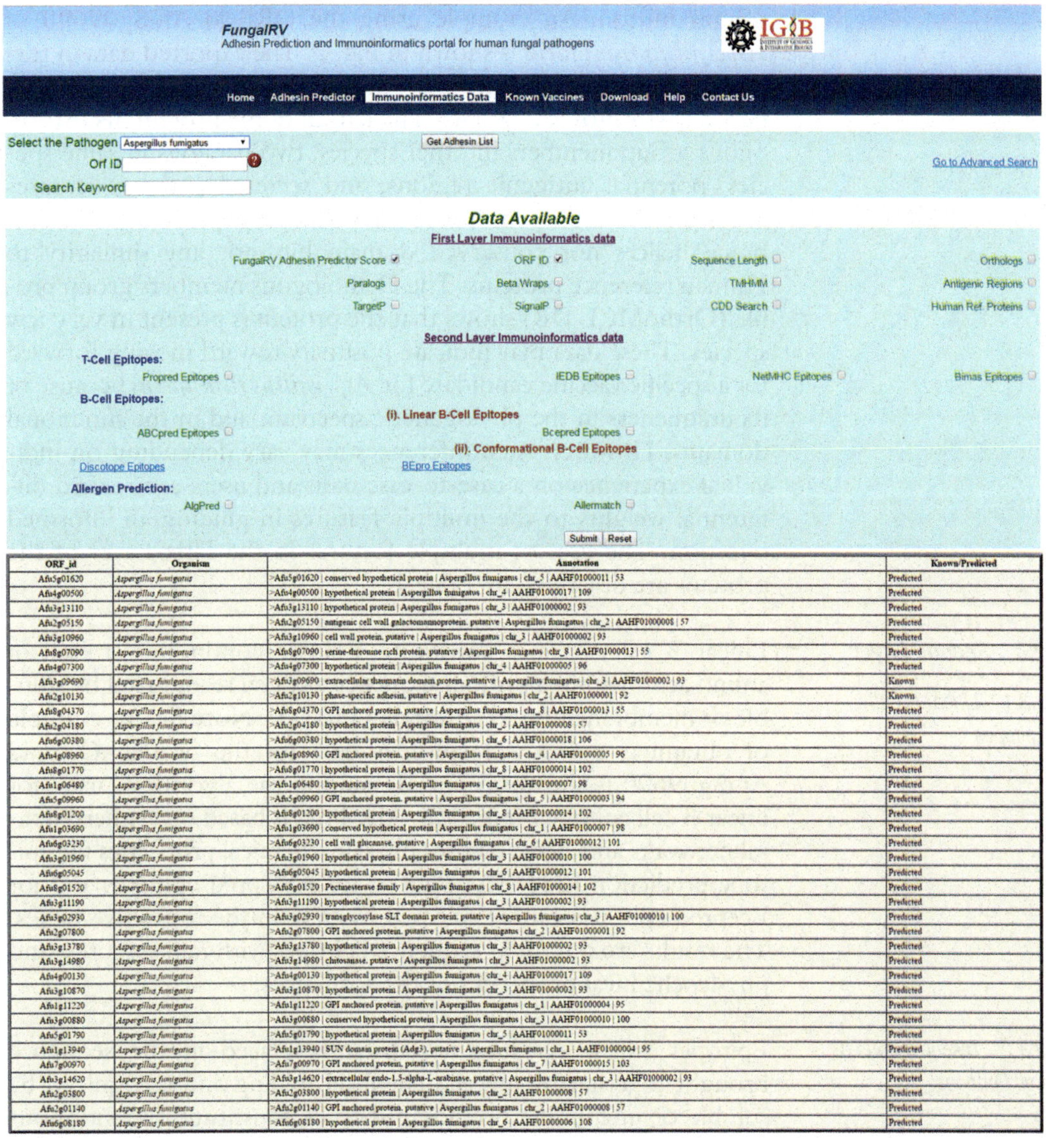

Fig. 1 Screen shots of FungalRV portal for getting the list of adhesins (known and predicted) of Aspergillus fumigatus. *Top*: selection in pull down menu. *Bottom*: output of the list of adhesins

Annotation, and whether the corresponding adhesins are known (from the literature) or predicted using the Fungal adhesin predictor algorithm (*see* **Notes 2** and 7).

2.2.2 Multiple Features Analyses

A given ORF_id can be selected and submitted in the Orf ID space bar along with the corresponding pathogen selection from pull down list in the Select the Pathogen menu bar. Subsequently, the fields of interest can be selected by tick in the respective boxes against the feature of the protein to be queried and press the submit button. An example using the ORF_id Afu3g09690 of *Aspergillus fumigatus* is shown in Fig. 2. The exported data in text format offers the full features of the given protein in the First Layer [22–27] (*see* **Notes 3** and **4**). The length of the protein, its orthologous group members in other species, two paralogs in same species, potential antigenic regions, and secreted pathway features predicted are displayed. There are no BetaWraps, nor transmembrane helices nor conserved domain hits nor any similarity to Human reference proteins. The Orthologous members group profile (OrthoMCL DB) shows that the protein is present in very few species. These data may indicate positivity toward moving forward for a specific vaccine candidate for *Aspergillus fumigatus* because of its uniqueness in the phylogenetic spectrum and in the functional domains. However, such inferences may vary depending on individual experience on a case-to-case basis and users can reward differential weights to the multiple features in guiding an informed selection. The uses of multiple features in the First Layer of the proteins are described in Table 1.

2.3 Second Layer

2.3.1 Linear B Cell Epitopes

Linear B cell epitopes constitute a single continuous stretch of amino acids within a protein sequence antigen recognized by soluble or membrane bound antibodies [12] (*see* **Note 5**). An example of obtaining the B cell epitopes data for the protein ORF_id Afu3g09690 is shown in Fig. 3. Among the algorithms used for linear B cell epitope prediction, ABCPred is based on artificial neural networks and BcePred uses physico-chemical properties for epitope prediction [28]. The options for ABCpred epitopes and for Bcepred epitopes can be selected by ticks in the respective boxes. The results are output as sequence epitopes with ranks, scores, and physicochemical properties of the sequences.

2.3.2 Discontinuous B Cell Epitopes

Epitopes whose residues are distantly placed in the sequence brought together by physico-chemical folding and recognized by soluble or membrane bound antibodies constitute discontinuous epitopes [12]. Discontinuous epitopes were predicted using Discotope 1.2, CEP, and BEPro servers based on the available crystal structures of antigens [29, 30]. An example in case of BEPro is shown in Fig. 4.

2.3.3 MHC Class I and Class II T Cell Epitopes

These are short regions presented on the surface of an antigen-presenting cell, where they are bound to MHC Class I molecules. An example of obtaining the MHC Class I T Cell epitopes data for the protein ORF_id Afu3g09690 is shown in Fig. 5. The output data consist of sequences of peptides predicted as HLA Classi, MHC Class-I, and MHC Class-II binding using the following algorithms [31–37]: Propred (promiscuous peptide binding using quantitative matrices from published literature), Bimas (half-time of dissociation to HLA class I molecules), NetMHC 3.0 (artificial

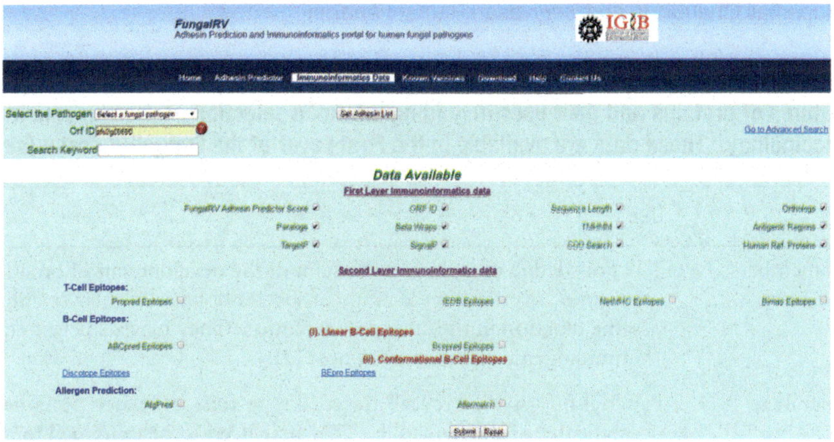


```
>Afu3g09690 | extracellular thaumatin domain protein, putative | Aspergillus fumigatus | chr_3 |
AAHF01000002 | 93
FungalRV_adhesin_predictor_score     1.001
ORF_id    Afu3g09690
Length    177
Orthomcl_Group    OG4_88813
Seq_id_of_best_hit afum|XP_754650
Percent_identity    100
Percent_match       100
No_of_Paralogs      2 (cluster no-171)
Best_Wrap           None
No_of_TM_Helices 0
Topology -

Antigenic_regions

#=======================================
#
# Sequence: Afu3g09690    from: 1   to: 177
# HitCount: 8
#=======================================

Max_score_pos at "*"

(1) Score 1.148 length 21 at residues 5->25
                *
 Sequence: KAFFAAAFATLSTALPHVIQR
           |              |
           5              25
 Max_score_pos: 21

(2) Score 1.141 length 10 at residues 134->143
            *
 Sequence: GGDCPSVNCK
           |     |
          134   143
 Max_score_pos: 140

(3) Score 1.137 length 26 at residues 33->58
                *
 Sequence: GGGVQIVNNLSQTVYAWSVADSVSDM
           |              |
           33             58
 Max_score_pos: 49

(4) Score 1.124 length 13 at residues 145->157
          *
 Sequence: GDTACAEAYLQPK
           |      |
          145    157
 Max_score_pos: 151

(5) Score 1.101 length 13 at residues 162->174
          *
 Sequence: THGCPINTSFVVN
           |      |
          162    174
 Max_score_pos: 170

(6) Score 1.094 length 9 at residues 91->99
          *
 Sequence: QSDVLQFEY
           |  |
           91 99
 Max_score_pos: 97

(7) Score 1.093 length 6 at residues 81->86
          *
 Sequence: VSIKLS
           | |
           81 86
 Max_score_pos: 84

(8) Score 1.046 length 7 at residues 125->131
          *
 Sequence: GFTVEPS
           | |
          125 131
 Max_score_pos: 129

Mitochondrial_Targeting_Peptide_Probability_from_TargetP     0.34
Signal_Peptide_Probability_from_TargetP     0.76
Other_from_TargetP  0.02
Localization_from_TargetP       Secretory Pathway
Reliability_Class_from_TargetP  3
Is_Signal_peptide_from_SignalP  YES
cdd_hits    No Conserved Domain found
Href_hits   No Hits found
```

Fig. 2 Screen shots of FungalRV portal for obtaining First Layer data of multiple features of proteins. *Top*: selection of pathogen in pull down menu and inputting the OrfID of the corresponding adhesin protein (Afu3g09690 in this example) and selection of multiple algorithms by ticks in the boxes. *Bottom*: output data, which can be exported in plain text format. Long output in browser rearranged for presentation in the given space

Table 1
Multiple features of proteins and their uses in guiding informed selection of vaccine candidates for "reverse vaccinology." These data are available in the First Layer of the FungalRV portal (*see* Note 6)

Feature	Use
Orthologs members	The knowledge of orthologs is useful in the development of broad-spectrum vaccines covering a wide range of species because of their retention of same function in the course of evolution. They may also elicit equivalent immunogenic response from host [20]
Paralogs members	Paralogs information reveals the total repertoire of related potential vaccine candidates of a given family. They may need to be examined for possibility of antigenic variations and of evasion of immunity by the pathogen [20]
Conserved domains	Conserved Domains information elaborates on the functionality of a protein and along with its family members lends support during informed selection. These sequences can be used for comparative analysis with other members with known information on antigen-antibody interactions [21]
Similarity to human reference proteins	Ideally, antigens selected must not have any observable similarity to human proteins in order to avoid generating an autoimmune response. At this time the most readily available data is the sequence similarity data at very low stringency (maximum E-value of 0.01 in BLASTP) [22]
BetaWrap	BetaWrap motifs are right-handed parallel beta-helix supersecondary structural motifs present in some proteins (toxins, virulence factors, adhesins) of pathogens. This value-added information is useful when prioritizing vaccine candidates [23]
Transmembrane helices	Although the presence of transmembrane domains is strongly indicative of the surface localization of a given protein, it is generally difficult to express and purify proteins with multiple transmembrane domains [24]
Subcellular localization	Potential antigens are generally surface localized. The subcellular localization predictions and SignalP predictions offer information on the potential extracellular localization of the given protein. This information can value add to the process of informed selection of potential antigens [25]
Antigenic regions	Knowledge of potential antigenic regions offers confidence in terms of the physico-chemical characteristics of a given protein and therefore its similarity to other antigens at this level. In addition, the potential antigenic sequences predicted could be used for developing constructs for testing [26]

neural networks (ANNs) and weight matrices), IEDB resource (Average Relative Binding Method (ARB)). The results are output in terms of ranks and scores, type of binding (Strong Binding (SB) or Weak Binding (WB)), IC_{50} in nM units.

2.3.4 Allergens

We also fetched potential allergen information, as it is desirable for a vaccine candidate to be non-allergic in a general sense. For this purpose Algpred, an allergen prediction algorithm, was used with a combined approach. This combined approach included finding

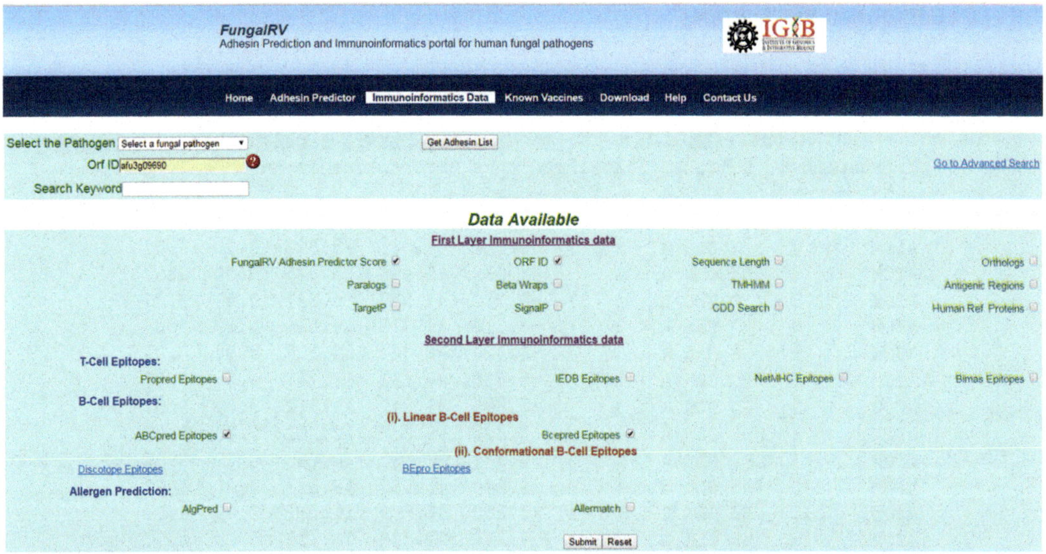

ABCpred Epitopes:
Export ABCPred Epitope Data

Orfid	Species	Rank	Sequence	Position	Score
Afu3g09690	Aspergillus fumigatus	1	GVSIKLSTKPDQSDVL	80	0.890
Afu3g09690	Aspergillus fumigatus	1	MSCIDMGTDSEFSKFG	110	0.890
Afu3g09690	Aspergillus fumigatus	2	LQPKDDHATHGCPINT	154	0.880
Afu3g09690	Aspergillus fumigatus	3	SQSGGDCPSVNCKAGD	131	0.870
Afu3g09690	Aspergillus fumigatus	4	GDTIYWDMSCIDMGTD	103	0.860
Afu3g09690	Aspergillus fumigatus	5	SGNSSASGGGVQIVNN	26	0.850
Afu3g09690	Aspergillus fumigatus	6	DVLQFEYTQSGDTIYW	93	0.820
Afu3g09690	Aspergillus fumigatus	6	SVSDMHTLSADGGSYS	54	0.820
Afu3g09690	Aspergillus fumigatus	7	YSEDWRTNSNGGGVSI	68	0.810
Afu3g09690	Aspergillus fumigatus	7	SQTVYAWSVADSVSDM	43	0.810
Afu3g09690	Aspergillus fumigatus	8	NCKAGDTACAEAYLQP	141	0.750
Afu3g09690	Aspergillus fumigatus	9	GVQIVNNLSQTVYAWS	35	0.740
Afu3g09690	Aspergillus fumigatus	10	ATLSTALPHVIQRSGN	13	0.720
Afu3g09690	Aspergillus fumigatus	11	HATHGCPINTSFVVNI	160	0.640
Afu3g09690	Aspergillus fumigatus	12	TKPDQSDVLQFEYTQS	87	0.560
Afu3g09690	Aspergillus fumigatus	13	TDSEFSKFGFTVEPSQ	117	0.500

Bcepred Epitopes:
Export Bcepred Epitope Data

Orfid	Species	Property	Sequence	Length
Afu3g09690	Aspergillus fumigatus	Hydrophilicity	QRSGNSSASGGG	12
Afu3g09690	Aspergillus fumigatus	Hydrophilicity	SADGGSYSED	10
Afu3g09690	Aspergillus fumigatus	Hydrophilicity	RTNSNGGGVS	10
Afu3g09690	Aspergillus fumigatus	Hydrophilicity	STKPDQSDV	9
Afu3g09690	Aspergillus fumigatus	Hydrophilicity	EYTQSGDT	8
Afu3g09690	Aspergillus fumigatus	Hydrophilicity	DMGTDSEFSK	10
Afu3g09690	Aspergillus fumigatus	Hydrophilicity	EPSQSGGDCPS	11
Afu3g09690	Aspergillus fumigatus	Hydrophilicity	NCKAGDTACAE	11
Afu3g09690	Aspergillus fumigatus	Hydrophilicity	QPKDDHATHG	10
Afu3g09690	Aspergillus fumigatus	Flexibility	HVIQRSGNSSASG	13
Afu3g09690	Aspergillus fumigatus	Flexibility	HTLSADG	7
Afu3g09690	Aspergillus fumigatus	Flexibility	EDWRTNSNG	9
Afu3g09690	Aspergillus fumigatus	Flexibility	IKLSTKPDQ	9
Afu3g09690	Aspergillus fumigatus	Flexibility	FEYTQSG	7
Afu3g09690	Aspergillus fumigatus	Flexibility	MGTDSEF	7
Afu3g09690	Aspergillus fumigatus	Flexibility	FTVEPSQSG	9
Afu3g09690	Aspergillus fumigatus	Accessibility	QRSGNSS	7
Afu3g09690	Aspergillus fumigatus	Accessibility	SYSEDWRTNSNGG	13
Afu3g09690	Aspergillus fumigatus	Accessibility	IKLSTKPDQSDVLQFEYTQSGDT	23
Afu3g09690	Aspergillus fumigatus	Accessibility	TDSEFSK	7
Afu3g09690	Aspergillus fumigatus	Accessibility	TVEPSQS	7
Afu3g09690	Aspergillus fumigatus	Accessibility	EAYLQPKDDHATH	13
Afu3g09690	Aspergillus fumigatus	Turns	RTNSNGG	7
Afu3g09690	Aspergillus fumigatus	Exposed Surface	KLSTKPDQSD	10
Afu3g09690	Aspergillus fumigatus	Exposed Surface	YLQPKDDH	8
Afu3g09690	Aspergillus fumigatus	Polarity	LQPKDDHATHG	11
Afu3g09690	Aspergillus fumigatus	Antigenic Propensity	LPHVIQRS	8
Afu3g09690	Aspergillus fumigatus	Antigenic Propensity	VQIVNNL	7
Afu3g09690	Aspergillus fumigatus	Antigenic Propensity	GVSIKLST	8
Afu3g09690	Aspergillus fumigatus	Antigenic Propensity	QSDVLQFEYT	10
Afu3g09690	Aspergillus fumigatus	Antigenic Propensity	DCPSVNCK	8
Afu3g09690	Aspergillus fumigatus	Antigenic Propensity	INTSFVVNIG	10

Fig. 3 Screen shots of FungalRV portal for obtaining data on B cell epitopes. *Top*: selection of pathogen in pull down menu and inputting the OrfID of the corresponding adhesin protein (Afu3g09690 in this example) and selection of multiple algorithms by ticks in the boxes. *Bottom*: output data, which can be exported in plain text format. Long output in browser truncated

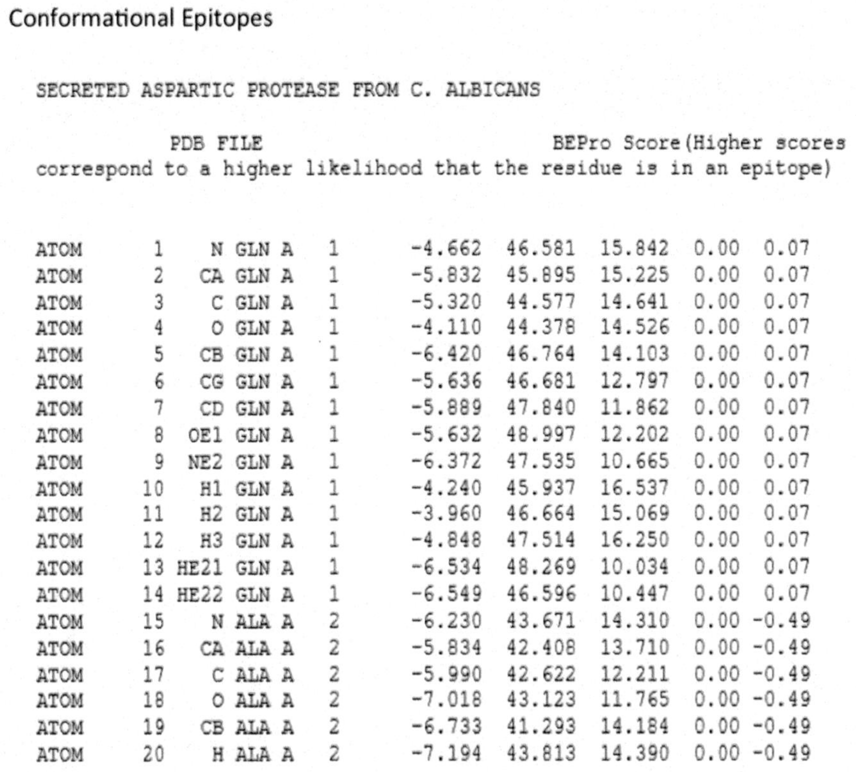

Conformational Epitopes

SECRETED ASPARTIC PROTEASE FROM C. ALBICANS

PDB FILE BEPro Score(Higher scores correspond to a higher likelihood that the residue is in an epitope)

```
ATOM     1    N GLN A   1     -4.662  46.581  15.842  0.00  0.07
ATOM     2   CA GLN A   1     -5.832  45.895  15.225  0.00  0.07
ATOM     3    C GLN A   1     -5.320  44.577  14.641  0.00  0.07
ATOM     4    O GLN A   1     -4.110  44.378  14.526  0.00  0.07
ATOM     5   CB GLN A   1     -6.420  46.764  14.103  0.00  0.07
ATOM     6   CG GLN A   1     -5.636  46.681  12.797  0.00  0.07
ATOM     7   CD GLN A   1     -5.889  47.840  11.862  0.00  0.07
ATOM     8  OE1 GLN A   1     -5.632  48.997  12.202  0.00  0.07
ATOM     9  NE2 GLN A   1     -6.372  47.535  10.665  0.00  0.07
ATOM    10   H1 GLN A   1     -4.240  45.937  16.537  0.00  0.07
ATOM    11   H2 GLN A   1     -3.960  46.664  15.069  0.00  0.07
ATOM    12   H3 GLN A   1     -4.848  47.514  16.250  0.00  0.07
ATOM    13 HE21 GLN A   1     -6.534  48.269  10.034  0.00  0.07
ATOM    14 HE22 GLN A   1     -6.549  46.596  10.447  0.00  0.07
ATOM    15    N ALA A   2     -6.230  43.671  14.310  0.00 -0.49
ATOM    16   CA ALA A   2     -5.834  42.408  13.710  0.00 -0.49
ATOM    17    C ALA A   2     -5.990  42.622  12.211  0.00 -0.49
ATOM    18    O ALA A   2     -7.018  43.123  11.765  0.00 -0.49
ATOM    19   CB ALA A   2     -6.733  41.293  14.184  0.00 -0.49
ATOM    20    H ALA A   2     -7.194  43.813  14.390  0.00 -0.49
```

Fig. 4 Screen shot of FungalRV portal for obtaining data on BEPro conformational epitopes. The example results are for a secreted aspartic protease from the pathogenic fungus *Candida albicans*

similarity to known allergic epitopes, searching Multiple EM for Motif Elicitation (MEME)/Motif Alignment and Search Tool (MAST) allergen motifs using MAST, search based on SVM modules and BLAST search against 2890 allergen-representative peptides [38, 39]. Additionally, Allermatch, an allergen prediction algorithm based on "Codex alimentarius and FAO/WHO Expert consultation on allergenicity of foods derived through modern biotechnology," was used [40]. An example output of allergen prediction for the protein ORF_id Afu3g09690 is shown in Fig. 6. It is apparent that this protein is not likely to be an allergen and hence could be pursued further as a potential vaccine candidate.

3 Notes

1. Immunoinformatics tools are the tools that can be used to obtain information on cells of immune system. Here, we have used immunoinformatics tools to collect B cell and T cell epitopes and allergen information.

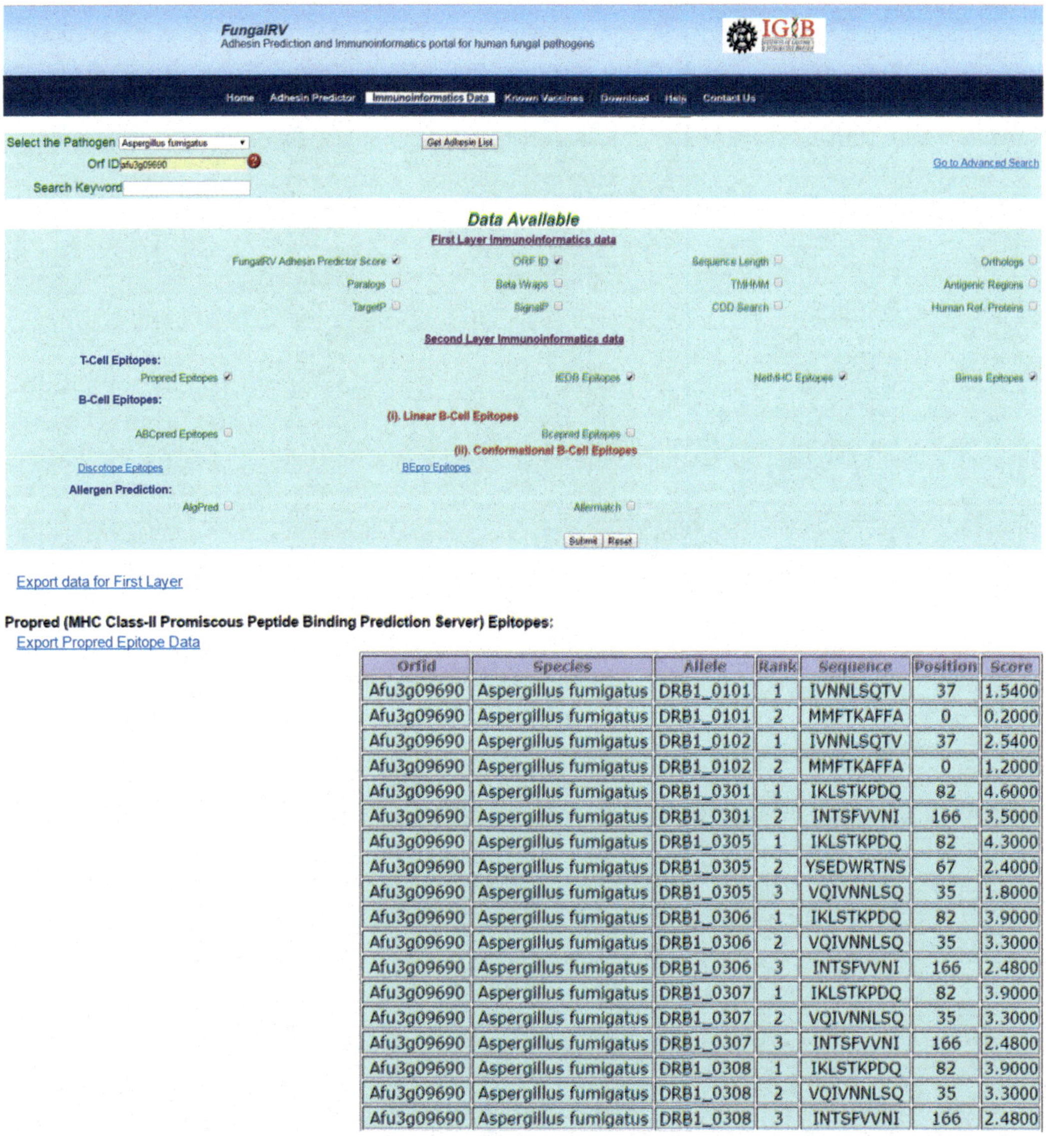

Orfid	Species	Allele	Rank	Sequence	Position	Score
Afu3g09690	Aspergillus fumigatus	DRB1_0101	1	IVNNLSQTV	37	1.5400
Afu3g09690	Aspergillus fumigatus	DRB1_0101	2	MMFTKAFFA	0	0.2000
Afu3g09690	Aspergillus fumigatus	DRB1_0102	1	IVNNLSQTV	37	2.5400
Afu3g09690	Aspergillus fumigatus	DRB1_0102	2	MMFTKAFFA	0	1.2000
Afu3g09690	Aspergillus fumigatus	DRB1_0301	1	IKLSTKPDQ	82	4.6000
Afu3g09690	Aspergillus fumigatus	DRB1_0301	2	INTSFVVNI	166	3.5000
Afu3g09690	Aspergillus fumigatus	DRB1_0305	1	IKLSTKPDQ	82	4.3000
Afu3g09690	Aspergillus fumigatus	DRB1_0305	2	YSEDWRTNS	67	2.4000
Afu3g09690	Aspergillus fumigatus	DRB1_0305	3	VQIVNNLSQ	35	1.8000
Afu3g09690	Aspergillus fumigatus	DRB1_0306	1	IKLSTKPDQ	82	3.9000
Afu3g09690	Aspergillus fumigatus	DRB1_0306	2	VQIVNNLSQ	35	3.3000
Afu3g09690	Aspergillus fumigatus	DRB1_0306	3	INTSFVVNI	166	2.4800
Afu3g09690	Aspergillus fumigatus	DRB1_0307	1	IKLSTKPDQ	82	3.9000
Afu3g09690	Aspergillus fumigatus	DRB1_0307	2	VQIVNNLSQ	35	3.3000
Afu3g09690	Aspergillus fumigatus	DRB1_0307	3	INTSFVVNI	166	2.4800
Afu3g09690	Aspergillus fumigatus	DRB1_0308	1	IKLSTKPDQ	82	3.9000
Afu3g09690	Aspergillus fumigatus	DRB1_0308	2	VQIVNNLSQ	35	3.3000
Afu3g09690	Aspergillus fumigatus	DRB1_0308	3	INTSFVVNI	166	2.4800

Fig. 5 Screen shots of FungalRV portal for obtaining data on MHC Class I and Class II epitopes. *Top*: selection of pathogen in pull down menu and inputting the OrfID of the corresponding adhesin protein (Afu3g09690 in this example) and selection of multiple algorithms by ticks in the boxes. *Bottom*: output data, which can be exported in plain text format. Long output in browser truncated

2. FungalRV is the webserver used to predict fungal adhesins and also to fetch immunoinformatics data on fungal adhesin vaccine candidates.

3. Both "First Layer" and "Second Layer" information should be analyzed to get list of most probable adhesion vaccine candidates.

NetMHC (HLA Class-I Peptide Binding Prediction Server) Epitopes by Weight Matrix Method:

Export NetMHC Weight Matrix Epitope Data

Orfid	Species	Allele	Pred_method	Position	Sequence	score	Bind_level
Afu3g09690	Aspergillus fumigatus	A01	Weight Matrix	90	QSDVLQFEY	16.90	SB
Afu3g09690	Aspergillus fumigatus	A01	Weight Matrix	98	YTQSGDTIY	14.80	SB
Afu3g09690	Aspergillus fumigatus	A01	Weight Matrix	115	GTDSEFSKF	13.10	WB
Afu3g09690	Aspergillus fumigatus	A0207	Weight Matrix	13	TLSTALPHV	12.90	SB
Afu3g09690	Aspergillus fumigatus	A0207	Weight Matrix	17	ALPHVIQRS	9.50	WB
Afu3g09690	Aspergillus fumigatus	A0209	Weight Matrix	30	ASGGGVQIV	16.00	SB
Afu3g09690	Aspergillus fumigatus	A0209	Weight Matrix	8	AAAFATLST	12.50	WB
Afu3g09690	Aspergillus fumigatus	A0217	Weight Matrix	17	ALPHVIQRS	27.30	SB
Afu3g09690	Aspergillus fumigatus	A03	Weight Matrix	79	GVSIKLSTK	9.20	WB
Afu3g09690	Aspergillus fumigatus	A23	Weight Matrix	3	TKAFFAAAF	8.80	WB
Afu3g09690	Aspergillus fumigatus	A24	Weight Matrix	97	EYTQSGDTI	9.20	WB
Afu3g09690	Aspergillus fumigatus	A26	Weight Matrix	58	HTLSADGGS	10.90	WB
Afu3g09690	Aspergillus fumigatus	A26	Weight Matrix	103	DTIYWDMSC	9.70	WB
Afu3g09690	Aspergillus fumigatus	A26	Weight Matrix	4	KAFFAAAFA	9.60	WB
Afu3g09690	Aspergillus fumigatus	A3004	Weight Matrix	154	QPKDDHATH	10.80	WB
Afu3g09690	Aspergillus fumigatus	A3004	Weight Matrix	115	GTDSEFSKF	10.20	WB
Afu3g09690	Aspergillus fumigatus	A32	Weight Matrix	40	NLSQTVYAW	15.50	SB
Afu3g09690	Aspergillus fumigatus	A3303	Weight Matrix	16	TALPHVIQR	17.10	SB
Afu3g09690	Aspergillus fumigatus	A3303	Weight Matrix	44	TVYAWSVAD	9.30	WB
Afu3g09690	Aspergillus fumigatus	B14	Weight Matrix	52	DSVSDMHTL	10.00	WB
Afu3g09690	Aspergillus fumigatus	B1503	Weight Matrix	22	IQRSGNSSA	13.90	SB
Afu3g09690	Aspergillus fumigatus	B1503	Weight Matrix	28	SSASGGGVQ	11.30	WB
Afu3g09690	Aspergillus fumigatus	B1503	Weight Matrix	29	SASGGGVQI	10.90	WB
Afu3g09690	Aspergillus fumigatus	B1503	Weight Matrix	60	LSADGGSYS	10.50	WB
Afu3g09690	Aspergillus fumigatus	B1503	Weight Matrix	75	SNGGGVSIK	9.50	WB
Afu3g09690	Aspergillus fumigatus	B1503	Weight Matrix	73	TNSNGGGVS	8.70	WB
Afu3g09690	Aspergillus fumigatus	B1508	Weight Matrix	98	YTQSGDTIY	11.30	WB
Afu3g09690	Aspergillus fumigatus	B1508	Weight Matrix	59	TLSADGGSY	11.10	WB
Afu3g09690	Aspergillus fumigatus	B1508	Weight Matrix	162	HGCPINTSF	8.70	WB
Afu3g09690	Aspergillus fumigatus	B1509	Weight Matrix	29	SASGGGVQI	10.00	WB

Export data for First Layer

IEDB resource (MHC Class-I Peptide Binding Prediction Server)

Export IEDB MHC Class I Epitope Data

Orfid	Species	Pred Method	Allele	Sequence	IC50[nM]
Afu3g09690	Aspergillus fumigatus	ARB	HLA A*0212	YLQPKDDHA	0.30864
Afu3g09690	Aspergillus fumigatus	ARB	HLA A*0250	YLQPKDDHA	0.500905
Afu3g09690	Aspergillus fumigatus	ARB	HLA A*0250	VLQFEYTQS	0.546352
Afu3g09690	Aspergillus fumigatus	ARB	HLA A*0206	TLSTALPHV	0.563862
Afu3g09690	Aspergillus fumigatus	ARB	HLA A*0211	YLQPKDDHA	0.610644
Afu3g09690	Aspergillus fumigatus	ARB	HLA A*0203	TLSTALPHV	0.671843
Afu3g09690	Aspergillus fumigatus	ARB	Mamu A*02	YTQSGDTIY	0.696768
Afu3g09690	Aspergillus fumigatus	ARB	Mamu A*01	FAAAFATLS	0.708639
Afu3g09690	Aspergillus fumigatus	ARB	Mamu A*01	SVSDMHTLS	0.736603
Afu3g09690	Aspergillus fumigatus	ARB	HLA B*5401	CPINTSFVV	0.766233
Afu3g09690	Aspergillus fumigatus	ARB	HLA B*1503	TQSGDTIYW	0.798699
Afu3g09690	Aspergillus fumigatus	ARB	HLA A*0211	ALPHVIQRS	1.06553
Afu3g09690	Aspergillus fumigatus	ARB	HLA A*6801	MGTDSEFSK	1.09025
Afu3g09690	Aspergillus fumigatus	ARB	Mamu A*02	LSTALPHVI	1.10939
Afu3g09690	Aspergillus fumigatus	ARB	HLA A*0250	ALPHVIQRS	1.1374
Afu3g09690	Aspergillus fumigatus	ARB	HLA A*3001	KAFFAAAFA	1.16221
Afu3g09690	Aspergillus fumigatus	ARB	HLA A*0206	SQTVYAWSV	1.17435
Afu3g09690	Aspergillus fumigatus	ARB	HLA A*0202	FFAAAFATL	1.31828
Afu3g09690	Aspergillus fumigatus	ARB	Mamu A*02	GTDSEFSKF	1.4551
Afu3g09690	Aspergillus fumigatus	ARB	HLA B*1503	IDMGTDSEF	1.46766
Afu3g09690	Aspergillus fumigatus	ARB	HLA A*0250	TLSTALPHV	1.51971
Afu3g09690	Aspergillus fumigatus	ARB	HLA B*1501	LQFEYTQSG	1.66613
Afu3g09690	Aspergillus fumigatus	ARB	HLA A*0216	YLQPKDDHA	1.80044
Afu3g09690	Aspergillus fumigatus	ARB	HLA A*6901	YAWSVADSV	1.83948
Afu3g09690	Aspergillus fumigatus	ARB	HLA B*1502	NSSASGGGV	1.92496
Afu3g09690	Aspergillus fumigatus	ARB	HLA A*0250	SQSGGDCPS	1.96113
Afu3g09690	Aspergillus fumigatus	ARB	HLA A*0250	MMFTKAFFA	2.04779
Afu3g09690	Aspergillus fumigatus	ARB	HLA A*3002	QSDVLQFEY	2.10516
Afu3g09690	Aspergillus fumigatus	ARB	HLA A*2602	DSVSDMHTL	2.20934

Fig. 5 (continued)

4. Prioritization on selection of antigens can be based on First Layer data, which offers value addition using multiple feature predictions analysis. For example, if a given protein is a *known or predicted adhesin* and the subcellular location algorithm also predicts it as *extracellular* then the two predictions value add and more priority could be assigned to the given protein.
5. The data in Second Layer is profuse by the nature of the immunoinformatics epitopes prediction algorithms. Therefore, it is advisable to use as much knowledge and experience as affordable before moving to use the Second Layer data.

Bimas (HLA Class-I Peptide Binding Prediction Server) Epitopes:

Export Bimas Epitope Data

Orfid	Organism	Allele	Rank	Position	Sequence	Score
Afu3g09690	Aspergillus fumigatus	A1	1	91	QSDVLQFEY	187.5000
Afu3g09690	Aspergillus fumigatus	A1	2	118	DSEFSKFGF	67.5000
Afu3g09690	Aspergillus fumigatus	A_0201	1	1	MMFTKAFFA	719.9360
Afu3g09690	Aspergillus fumigatus	A_0201	2	14	TLSTALPHV	159.9700
Afu3g09690	Aspergillus fumigatus	A_0201	3	43	SQTVYAWSV	52.8890
Afu3g09690	Aspergillus fumigatus	A24	1	98	EYTQSGDTI	50.0000
Afu3g09690	Aspergillus fumigatus	A68.1	1	80	GVSIKLSTK	120.0000
Afu3g09690	Aspergillus fumigatus	B_2705	1	24	QRSGNSSAS	200.0000
Afu3g09690	Aspergillus fumigatus	B_2705	2	43	SQTVYAWSV	60.0000
Afu3g09690	Aspergillus fumigatus	B_5101	1	47	YAWSVADSV	286.0000
Afu3g09690	Aspergillus fumigatus	B_5101	2	30	SASGGGVQI	242.0000
Afu3g09690	Aspergillus fumigatus	B_5101	3	165	CPINTSFVV	220.0000
Afu3g09690	Aspergillus fumigatus	B_5102	1	47	YAWSVADSV	1100.0000
Afu3g09690	Aspergillus fumigatus	B_5102	2	165	CPINTSFVV	726.0000
Afu3g09690	Aspergillus fumigatus	B_5102	3	30	SASGGGVQI	242.0000
Afu3g09690	Aspergillus fumigatus	B_5102	4	34	GGVQIVNNL	66.0000
Afu3g09690	Aspergillus fumigatus	B_5103	1	30	SASGGGVQI	133.1000
Afu3g09690	Aspergillus fumigatus	B_5103	2	47	YAWSVADSV	110.0000
Afu3g09690	Aspergillus fumigatus	B_5201	1	165	CPINTSFVV	165.0000
Afu3g09690	Aspergillus fumigatus	B_5801	1	116	GTDSEFSKF	58.0800
Afu3g09690	Aspergillus fumigatus	Cw_0401	1	7	FFAAAFATL	264.0000
Afu3g09690	Aspergillus fumigatus	Cw_0401	2	11	AFATLSTAL	200.0000
Afu3g09690	Aspergillus fumigatus	Kd	1	98	EYTQSGDTI	2400.0000
Afu3g09690	Aspergillus fumigatus	Kd	2	11	AFATLSTAL	1382.4000
Afu3g09690	Aspergillus fumigatus	Kd	3	7	FFAAAFATL	1152.0000
Afu3g09690	Aspergillus fumigatus	Kd	4	120	EFSKFGFTV	200.0000
Afu3g09690	Aspergillus fumigatus	Kd	5	34	GGVQIVNNL	115.2000
Afu3g09690	Aspergillus fumigatus	Kd	6	53	DSVSDMHTL	115.2000
Afu3g09690	Aspergillus fumigatus	Kd	7	67	SYSEDWRTN	72.0000
Afu3g09690	Aspergillus fumigatus	Kd	8	46	VYAWSVADS	60.0000
Afu3g09690	Aspergillus fumigatus	Kd	9	15	LSTALPHVI	57.6000
Afu3g09690	Aspergillus fumigatus	Ld	1	165	CPINTSFVV	60.0000

NetMHC (HLA Class-I Peptide Binding Prediction Server) Epitopes by Neural Network Method:

Export NetMHC Neural Network Epitope Data

Orfid	Species	Allele	Pred_method	Position	Sequence	Log_aff	Affinity	Bind_level
Afu3g09690	Aspergillus fumigatus	A1101	Neural Networks	79	GVSIKLSTK	0.68600	29.00	SB
Afu3g09690	Aspergillus fumigatus	A1101	Neural Networks	148	CAEAYLQPK	0.56300	113.00	WB
Afu3g09690	Aspergillus fumigatus	A1101	Neural Networks	16	TALPHVIQR	0.55500	123.00	WB
Afu3g09690	Aspergillus fumigatus	A1101	Neural Networks	12	ATLSTALPH	0.55200	127.00	WB
Afu3g09690	Aspergillus fumigatus	A0201	Neural Networks	0	MMFTKAFFA	0.80900	7.00	SB
Afu3g09690	Aspergillus fumigatus	A0201	Neural Networks	13	TLSTALPHV	0.75000	14.00	SB
Afu3g09690	Aspergillus fumigatus	A0201	Neural Networks	46	YAWSVADSV	0.67100	35.00	SB
Afu3g09690	Aspergillus fumigatus	A0201	Neural Networks	42	SQTVYAWSV	0.63700	50.00	WB
Afu3g09690	Aspergillus fumigatus	A0201	Neural Networks	104	TIYWDMSCI	0.48100	274.00	WB
Afu3g09690	Aspergillus fumigatus	A0101	Neural Networks	90	QSDVLQFEY	0.79200	9.00	SB
Afu3g09690	Aspergillus fumigatus	A0101	Neural Networks	98	YTQSGDTIY	0.67800	32.00	SB
Afu3g09690	Aspergillus fumigatus	A0301	Neural Networks	79	GVSIKLSTK	0.54700	134.00	WB
Afu3g09690	Aspergillus fumigatus	A0301	Neural Networks	0	MMFTKAFFA	0.51300	195.00	WB
Afu3g09690	Aspergillus fumigatus	B0702	Neural Networks	8	AAAFATLST	0.42600	495.00	WB
Afu3g09690	Aspergillus fumigatus	A6901	Neural Networks	46	YAWSVADSV	0.73100	18.00	SB
Afu3g09690	Aspergillus fumigatus	A6901	Neural Networks	145	DTACAEAYL	0.63700	51.00	WB
Afu3g09690	Aspergillus fumigatus	A6901	Neural Networks	104	TIYWDMSCI	0.51900	181.00	WB
Afu3g09690	Aspergillus fumigatus	A6901	Neural Networks	37	IVNNLSQTV	0.45500	363.00	WB
Afu3g09690	Aspergillus fumigatus	A6901	Neural Networks	13	TLSTALPHV	0.44100	423.00	WB
Afu3g09690	Aspergillus fumigatus	A6901	Neural Networks	0	MMFTKAFFA	0.43800	437.00	WB
Afu3g09690	Aspergillus fumigatus	A3101	Neural Networks	16	TALPHVIQR	0.66000	39.00	SB
Afu3g09690	Aspergillus fumigatus	A3101	Neural Networks	0	MMFTKAFFA	0.44800	393.00	WB
Afu3g09690	Aspergillus fumigatus	B1501	Neural Networks	59	TLSADGGSY	0.58000	94.00	WB
Afu3g09690	Aspergillus fumigatus	B1501	Neural Networks	98	YTQSGDTIY	0.50600	210.00	WB
Afu3g09690	Aspergillus fumigatus	B1501	Neural Networks	22	IQRSGNSSA	0.44000	429.00	WB
Afu3g09690	Aspergillus fumigatus	B5801	Neural Networks	90	QSDVLQFEY	0.59300	81.00	WB
Afu3g09690	Aspergillus fumigatus	A2403	Neural Networks	6	FFAAAFATL	0.47800	282.00	WB
Afu3g09690	Aspergillus fumigatus	A2601	Neural Networks	49	SVADSVSDM	0.55000	129.00	WB
Afu3g09690	Aspergillus fumigatus	A2601	Neural Networks	98	YTQSGDTIY	0.47400	295.00	WB
Afu3g09690	Aspergillus fumigatus	A3001	Neural Networks	4	KAFFAAAFA	0.45300	373.00	WB

Fig. 5 (continued)

6. A principal aim in going through these comprehensive analyses is to reduce potential failures and to maximize efficacy or success.
7. The online help can also be used for using Fungal portal: http://fungalrv.igib.res.in/help.html.

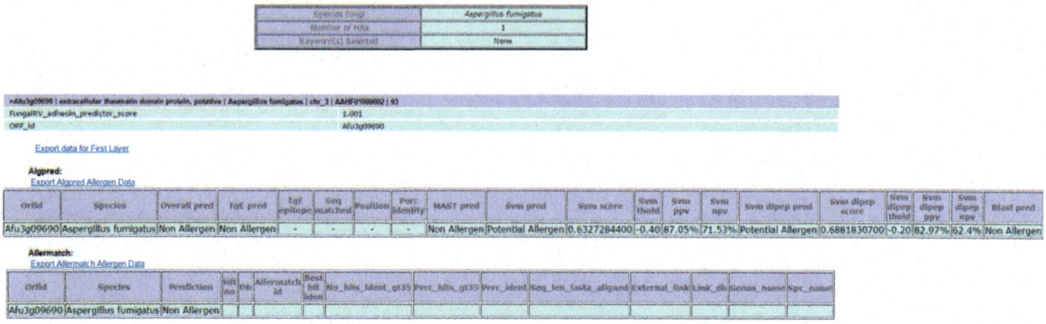

Fig. 6 Screen shots of FungalRV portal for obtaining data on Allergens prediction. *Top*: selection of pathogen in pull down menu and inputting the OrfID of the corresponding adhesin protein (Afu3g09690 in this example) and selection of multiple algorithms AlgPred and Allermatch by ticks in the boxes. *Bottom*: output data, which can be exported in plain text format

References

1. Pfaller MA, Diekema DJ (2007) Epidemiology of invasive candidiasis: a persistent public health problem. Clin Microbiol Rev 20:133–163
2. Dagenais TR, Keller NP (2009) Pathogenesis of aspergillus fumigatus in invasive aspergillosis. Clin Microbiol Rev 22:447–465
3. Latgé JP (1999) Aspergillus fumigatus and aspergillosis. Clin Microbiol Rev 12:310–350
4. Saubolle MA, McKellar PP, Sussland D (2007) Epidemiologic, clinical, and diagnostic aspects of coccidioidomycosis. J Clin Microbiol 45:26–30
5. Kauffman CA (2009) Histoplasmosis. Clin Chest Med 30:217–225
6. JA MK, Pappas PG (2009) Blastomycosis: new insights into diagnosis, prevention, and treatment. Clin Chest Med 30:227–239
7. Cutler JE, Deepe GS, Klein BS (2007) Advances in combating fungal diseases: vaccines on the threshold. Nat Rev Microbiol 5:13–28
8. Cassone A (2008) Fungal vaccines: real progress from real challenges. Lancet Infect Dis 8:114–124
9. Chaudhuri R, Ansari FA, Raghunandanan MV, Ramachandran S (2011) FungalRV: adhesin prediction and immunoinformatics portal for human fungal pathogens. BMC Genomics 12:192
10. Mora M, Veggi D, Santini L, Pizza M, Rappuoli R (2003) Reverse vaccinology. Drug Discov Today 8(10):459–464
11. Sette A, Rappuoli R (2010) Reverse vaccinology: developing vaccines in the era of genomics. Immunity 33(4):530–541
12. Vivona S, Gardy JL, Ramachandran S, Brinkman FS, Raghava GP, Flower DR, Filippini F (2008) Computer-aided biotechnology: from immuno-informatics to reverse vaccinology. Trends Biotechnol 26(4):190–200
13. Spellberg BJ, Ibrahim AS, Avenissian V, Filler SG, Myers CL, Fu Y, Edwards JE (2005) The anti-*Candida albicans* vaccine composed of the recombinant N terminus of Als1p reduces fungal burden and improves survival in both immunocompetent and immunocompromised mice. Infect Immun 73:6191–6193
14. Ibrahim AS, Spellberg BJ, Avanesian V, Fu Y, Edwards JE (2006) The anti-Candida vaccine based on the recombinant N-terminal domain of Als1p is broadly active against disseminated candidiasis. Infect Immun 74:3039–3041
15. Wüthrich M, Chang WL, Klein BS (1998) Immunogenicity and protective efficacy of the WI-1 adhesin of Blastomyces dermatitidis. Infect Immun 66:5443–5449
16. Wüthrich M, Filutowicz HI, Warner T, Klein BS (2002) Requisite elements in vaccine immunity to Blastomyces dermatitidis: plasticity uncovers vaccine potential in immune-deficient hosts. J Immunol 169:6969–6976
17. Braga CJ, Rittner GM, Muñoz Henao JE, Teixeira AF, Massis LM, Sbrogio-Almeida ME, Taborda CP, Travassos LR, Ferreira LC (2009) Paracoccidioides brasiliensis vaccine formulations based on the gp43-derived P10 sequence and the salmonella enterica FliC flagellin. Infect Immun 77:1700–1707
18. Pinto AR, Puccia R, Diniz SN, Franco MF, Travassos LR (2000) DNA-based vaccination against murine paracoccidioidomycosis using

the gp43 gene from Paracoccidioides brasiliensis. Vaccine 18:3050–3058
19. Hung CY, Ampel NM, Christian L, Seshan KR, Cole GT (2000) A major cell surface antigen of Coccidioides immitis which elicits both humoral and cellular immune responses. Infect Immun 68:584–593
20. Koonin EV (2005) Orthologs, paralogs, and evolutionary genomics. Annu Rev Genet 39:309–338
21. Hung CY, JJ Y, Seshan KR, Reichard U, Cole GT (2002) A parasitic phase-specific adhesin of Coccidioides immitis contributes to the virulence of this respiratory fungal pathogen. Infect Immun 70:3443–3456
22. Marchler-Bauer A, Anderson JB, Cherukuri PF, DeWeese-Scott C, Geer LY, Gwadz M, He S, Hurwitz DI, Jackson JD, Ke Z, Lanczycki CJ, Liebert CA, Liu C, Lu F, Marchler GH, Mullokandov M, Shoemaker BA, Simonyan V, Song JS, Thiessen PA, Yamashita RA, Yin JJ, Zhang D, Bryant SH (2005) CDD: a conserved domain database for protein classification. Nucleic Acids Res 33(Database issue):D192–D196
23. Altschul SF, Gish W, Miller W, Myers EW, Lipman DJ (1990) Basic local alignment search tool. J Mol Biol 215(3):403–410
24. Bradley P, Cowen L, Menke M, King J, Berger B (2001) BETAWRAP: successful prediction of parallel beta -helices from primary sequence reveals an association with many microbial pathogens. Proc Natl Acad Sci U S A 98(26):14819–14824
25. Krogh A, Larsson B, von Heijne G, Sonnhammer EL (2001) Predicting transmembrane protein topology with a hidden Markov model: application to complete genomes. J Mol Biol 305(3):567–580
26. Yu NY, Wagner JR, Laird MR, Melli G, Rey S, Lo R, Dao P, Sahinalp SC, Ester M, Foster LJ, Brinkman FS (2010) PSORTb 3.0: improved protein subcellular localization prediction with refined localization subcategories and predictive capabilities for all prokaryotes. Bioinformatics 26(13):1608–1615
27. Kolaskar AS, Tongaonkar PC (1990) A semi-empirical method for prediction of antigenic determinants on protein antigens. FEBS Lett 276(1–2):172–174
28. Saha S, Raghava GP (2007) Prediction methods for B-cell epitopes. Methods Mol Biol 409:387–394
29. Haste Andersen P, Nielsen M, Lund O (2006) Prediction of residues in discontinuous B-cell epitopes using protein 3D structures. Protein Sci 15(11):2558–2567
30. Sweredoski MJ, Baldi P (2008) PEPITO: improved discontinuous B-cell epitope prediction using multiple distance thresholds and half sphere exposure. Bioinformatics 24(12):1459–1460
31. Parker KC, Bednarek MA, Coligan JE (1994) Scheme for ranking potential HLA-A2 binding peptides based on independent binding of individual peptide side-chains. J Immunol 152(1):163–175
32. Singh H, Raghava GP (2003) ProPred1: prediction of promiscuous MHC class-I binding sites. Bioinformatics 19(8):1009–1014
33. Bui HH, Sidney J, Peters B, Sathiamurthy M, Sinichi A, Purton KA, Mothé BR, Chisari FV, Watkins DI, Sette A (2005) Automated generation and evaluation of specific MHC binding predictive tools: ARB matrix applications. Immunogenetics 57(5):304–314
34. Moutaftsi M, Peters B, Pasquetto V, Tscharke DC, Sidney J, Bui HH, Grey H, Sette A (2006) A consensus epitope prediction approach identifies the breadth of murine T(CD8+)-cell responses to vaccinia virus. Nat Biotechnol 24(7):817–819
35. Lundegaard C, Lamberth K, Harndahl M, Buus S, Lund O, Nielsen M (2008) NetMHC-3.0: accurate web accessible predictions of human, mouse and monkey MHC class I affinities for peptides of length 8-11. Nucleic Acids Res 36(Web Server):W509–W512
36. Zhang Q, Wang P, Kim Y, Haste-Andersen P, Beaver J, Bourne PE, Bui HH, Buus S, Frankild S, Greenbaum J, Lund O, Lundegaard C, Nielsen M, Ponomarenko J, Sette A, Zhu Z, Peters B (2008) Immune epitope database analysis resource (IEDB-AR). Nucleic Acids Res 36(Web Server issue):W513–W518
37. Wang P, Sidney J, Kim Y, Sette A, Lund O, Nielsen M, Peters B (2010) Peptide binding predictions for HLA DR, DP and DQ molecules. BMC Bioinformatics 11:568
38. Saha S, Raghava GP (2006) AlgPred: prediction of allergenic proteins and mapping of IgE epitopes. Nucleic Acids Res 34(Web Server issue):W202–W209
39. Björklund AK, Soeria-Atmadja D, Zorzet A, Hammerling U, Gustafsson MG (2005) Supervised identification of allergen-representative peptides for in silico detection of potentially allergenic proteins. Bioinformatics 21(1):39–50
40. Fiers MW, Kleter GA, Nijland H, Peijnenburg AA, Nap JP, van Ham RC (2004) Allermatch, a webtool for the prediction of potential allergenicity according to current FAO/WHO codex alimentarius guidelines. BMC Bioinformatics 5:133

Chapter 4

Rational Design of T Lymphocyte Epitope-Based Vaccines Against *Coccidioides* Infection

Brady J. Hurtgen and Chiung-Yu Hung

Abstract

Coccidioidomycosis is a potentially life-threatening mycosis endemic to the Southwestern USA and some arid regions of Central and South America. A vaccine against *Coccidioides* infection would benefit over 30-million people who reside in or visit the endemic regions. Vaccine candidates against systemic fungal infections come in many forms. Live attenuated vaccines are derived from disease-causing pathogens and generally stimulate excellent protective immunity. Since attenuated vaccines contain living microbes, there is a degree of unpredictability raising concerns regarding safety and stability. Generation of a subunit vaccine has initiated efforts to design a safe reagent suitable for administration to humans at risk of coccidioidomycosis. Epitope-based vaccines allow for eliciting specific protective immune responses and removal of potentially detrimental sequences to improve safety. This chapter describes methods for the identification of T cell epitopes derived from *Coccidioides* antigens, design, and production of a recombinant vaccine containing multiple T cell epitopes, and evaluation of its protective efficacy and vaccine immunity against pulmonary *Coccidioides* infection using a strain of transgenic mice that express a human MHC II molecule.

Key words *Coccidioides*, Coccidioidomycosis, HLA-DR4 transgenic mice, T Lymphocyte, Epitope-based vaccine, Fungal vaccine, Vaccine immunity

1 Introduction

1.1 Coccidioidomycosis and a Formalin-Killed Whole Cell Vaccine (FKS)

Coccidioides immitis and *Coccidioides posadasii* are the causative agents of coccidioidomycosis that is also known as San Joaquin Valley fever. Coccidioidomycosis is a fungal disease endemic to the Southwestern United States [1]. To date, no FDA-approved vaccine against *Coccidioides* infection exists. A handful of *Coccidioides* vaccine candidates have been evaluated in murine models of pulmonary coccidioidomycosis [2–10], while only a formalin-killed spherule vaccine (FKS) was further evaluated in a phase III double-blind human trial during the 1980s [11]. FKS-vaccinated mice were shown to be fully protected against a potentially lethal respiratory challenge with the pathogen. Despite its success as a protective reagent in mice and nonhuman primates, FKS failed to

Markus Kalkum and Margarita Semis (eds.), *Vaccines for Invasive Fungal Infections: Methods and Protocols*, Methods in Molecular Biology, vol. 1625, DOI 10.1007/978-1-4939-7104-6_4, © Springer Science+Business Media LLC 2017

demonstrate significant reduction in the incidence of coccidioidomycosis nor disease severity of the vaccinated population compared to the placebo group. This may have been due, at least in part, to an intense inflammatory reaction at the site of vaccination which necessitated adoption of a suboptimal dose of FKS, insufficient group size to accommodate the low infectious rate during the clinical trial, and lack of understanding the protective immunological mechanisms to optimize the vaccine formulation [11].

1.2 Protective Vaccine Immunity Against Pulmonary Coccidioidomycosis

We have applied a live, attenuated vaccine (ΔT) to explore the nature of vaccine immunity in mice during the initial 2 week period after intranasal challenge with a potentially lethal dose of *Coccidioides* spores. The live, attenuated strain of *C. posadasii* (ΔT) has lost the ability to endosporulate in vivo but is able to elicit protective immunity to coccidioidomycosis in disease susceptible C57BL/6 and BALB/c mice and a strain of human leukocyte antigen transgenic mice (HLA-DR4) [12, 13]. Host defenses mounted in response to invasion by dimorphic fungi are largely Th1 driven and disease exacerbation is a consequence of an imbalance between type 2 immunity and/or IL-10 and Th1 responses [14–19]. Many studies of coccidioidomycosis conducted before Th17 was discovered have reported IFN-γ production as a correlate of vaccine-induced protection in mice [18–22]. While mice lacking IFN-γ or IL-4 receptors developed comparable vaccine immunity without loss of ΔT vaccine-induced resistance, deficiency of the IL-17 receptor resulted in increased susceptibility of infection in immunized mice. These data support the concept that activation of CD4+ effector T cells including Th17 and Th1 cells can enhance recruitment of phagocytes to alveoli and promote early reduction of fungal burden while dampening inflammatory pathology at infection sites [23–25].

1.3 Design a Safe Subunit Vaccine

Attenuated vaccines contain living microbes. There is a degree of unpredictability raising safety and stability concerns for individuals with underlying conditions that compromise their cell-mediated immune system. As a result, these individuals could potentially display severe reactogenicity to immunization with a live, attenuated vaccine. Generation of a T cell epitope-based recombinant protein vaccine was initiated as a strategy for the design of a clinically acceptable reagent. Since the human population expresses a vast repertoire of major histocompatibility complex (MHC) molecules, a multivalent subunit vaccine that contains several antigenic epitopes can generate an enhanced immune response in a broader population compared to a single subunit vaccine that has limited human MHC restriction. Multi-epitope-based vaccines offer several advantages that include: (1) increased safety by minimizing deleterious portions of epitopes that are homologous to human proteins and unnecessary for vaccine-induced immune responses,

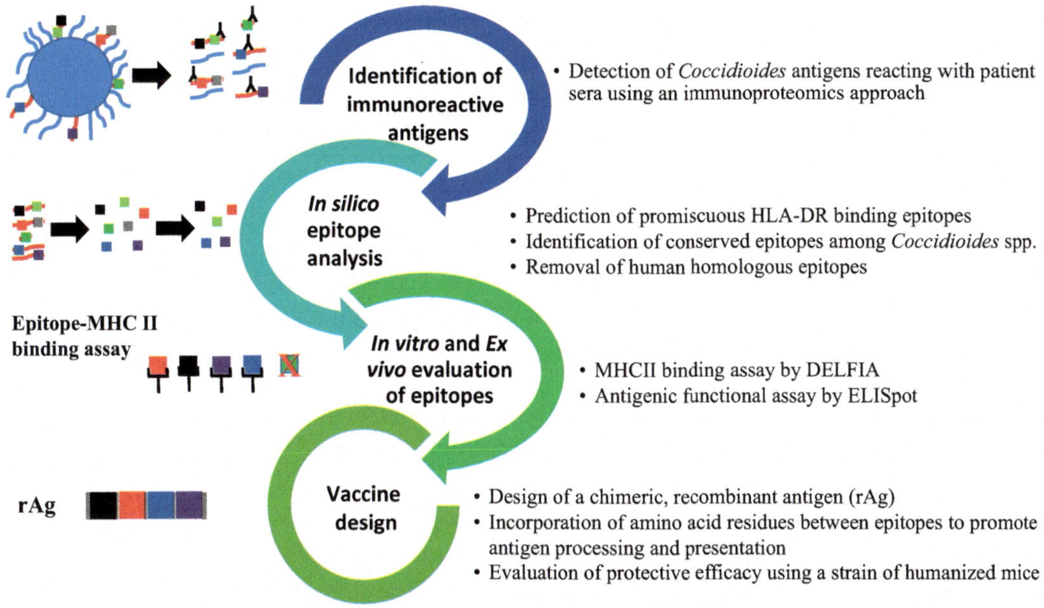

Fig. 1 Schematic illustration of the stepwise process in developing a T cell epitope based vaccine. Identification of candidate antigens derived from *Coccidioides* cell wall is conducted using an immunoproteomics approached as previously described [9]. Downstream in silico analysis of epitopes is carried out by first evaluating HLA-DR binding to identify predicted promiscuous HLA-DR binding epitopes (colored cubes). Epitopes are evaluated for *Coccidioides* spp. conservation, predicted SNPs, and human homology. Candidate epitopes are further discriminated by in vitro and ex vivo HLA binding assays (DELFIA and ELISpot to eliminate epitopes that lack high affinity binding (*green cube* with a *red cross*) to HLA molecules (*black* receptor). Final candidate epitopes are incorporated into a single recombinant antigen (rAg) for further evaluation

(2) the flexibility to incorporate a diverse set of epitopes from an array of microbial antigens into a single recombinant protein, and (3) the option to incorporate amino acids, motifs, or glycosylation patterns for enhanced antigen processing and immunogenicity. To design a vaccine that contains multiple T cell epitopes, individual epitopes must be initially identified. Methods to identify T cell epitopes of coccidioidal proteins have been previously described [8, 9, 26, 27]. Here, we present a methodological process that allows for rational epitope selection and vaccine design against *Coccidioides* spp. (*see* Fig. 1). This process begins with in silico analysis of identified, immunoreactive antigens for predicted promiscuous HLA-DR binding regions. Conserved and promiscuous epitopes are selected by ranking their binding affinity and functional ability to stimulate Th1 and Th17 cytokine production by T cells as determined by dissociation-enhanced lanthanide fluorescent immunoassay (DELFIA; [28]) and enzyme-linked immunospot (ELISpot) assays, respectively. Validated epitopes are incorporated into a unique amino acid sequence and expressed as a single recombinant

protein antigen (rAg). Purified rAg is then evaluated for its immunogenicity and protective efficacy in a strain of HLA transgenic mice [6].

2 Materials

Prepare all media and buffers using ultrapure, deionized (DI) water with resistivity of 18 MΩ·cm at 25 °C. Use only tissue-culture grade reagents. Store all reagents at 4 °C unless otherwise indicated.

2.1 Bioinformatic Analysis of Amino Acid Sequence of Select Proteins and Peptides

1. ProPred: MHC Class II binding peptide prediction server (http://www.imtech.res.in/raghava/propred/).
2. *Coccidioides* genome information is available in the following website: http://www.broadinstitute.org/annotation/genome/coccidioides_group/MultiHome.html.

   Genome databases for 8 and 6 isolates of *C. immitis* and *C. posadasii* are available in Genbank, respectively [29, 30].
3. RefSeq: NCBI Reference Sequence Database (http://blast.ncbi.nlm.nih.gov/Blast.cgi).

2.2 Cytokine ELISPOT Assay

1. Purified full-length recombinant antigens derived from aspartyl peptidase 1 (Pep1), alpha-mannosidase (Amn1), and phospholipase (Plb) of *Coccidioides posadasii* [9].
2. PBS pH 7.4.
3. PBST: PBS plus 0.05% Tween 20.
4. Synthetic unmethylated CpG oligodeoxynucleotide (ODN) dissolved in PBS at a concentration of 10 μg/μL (*see* **Note 1**).
5. Incomplete Freund's adjuvant (IFA).
6. 1 mL syringes (27 G) for vaccination.
7. HLA-DR4 (DRB1*0401) transgenic mice (Taconic Farm, *see* **Note 2**).
8. MultiScreen 96-well filtration plates.
9. 35% Ethanol: Dilute 35 mL of ethanol (200 proof, molecular biology grade) into 65 mL of DI H_2O.
10. Interferon-γ (INF-γ) capture antibody (Clone No. AN-18) diluted in PBS at a concentration of 1.0 μg/mL.
11. Complete HL-1 media (cHL_1)containing 3% (v/v) L-glutamine, 3% (v/v) gentamicin.
12. Peptide stimulants: 18-25mer peptides representing MHC II-binding epitopes (90% purity) or scrambled peptide (nonspecific control) were commercially synthesized and dissolved in cHL-1 medium at a concentration of 30 μg/mL. Store the peptide stock solutions in −20 °C freezer in 1 mL aliquots.

Thaw the required aliquots for each experiment one night before.

13. Positive stimulant: 1.0 μg/mL Concanavalin A (ConA) dissolved in cHL-1.
14. Sterile dissecting equipment.
15. Petri dish (100 × 15 mm diameter).
16. 70 μm cell strainers.
17. 40 μm cell strainers.
18. RPMI 1640.
19. Sterile 3 mL syringes.
20. Sterile plastic transfer pipets.
21. 50 mL conical tubes.
22. ACK red blood cell lysing buffer.
23. Hanks buffered salt solution (HBSS) without calcium, magnesium, and phenol red.
24. Sterile blocking solution: PBS containing 1% bovine serum albumin (BSA) Fraction V filtered through a sterile 0.2 micron-filter.
25. 0.4% trypan blue.
26. Hemocytometer, cover glasses, and light microscope.
27. CD90.2 microbeads (Miltenyi Biotec; Cat. #130-049-101) for purification of antigen-presenting cells (APCs).
28. $CD4^+$ T cell microbeads (Miltenyi Biotec; Cat. #130-104-454) for purification of $CD4^+$ T cells.
29. CO_2 Incubator.
30. IFN-γ detection antibody solution: 0.5 μg/mL anti-IFN-γ antibody (Clone No. R4–6A2) in sterile PBS containing 0.05% Tween 20, and 1% BSA.
31. Streptavidin/alkaline phosphatase (S/AP) solution: 0.1% (v/v) S/AP in sterile PBS containing 0.05% Tween 20, 1% BSA.
32. 5-bromo-4-chloro-3-indolyl-phosphate/nitro blue tetrazolium (BCIP/NBT) substrate.
33. ELISPOT plate imager/reader.

2.3 Recombinant Antigen (rAg) Design, Production, and Purification

1. ProPred: MHC Class II Binding Peptide Prediction Server.
2. Synthetic DNA fragment encoding rAg.
3. Bacterial p*ET28b* cloning vector for generating p*ET28b-rAg* construct.
4. *E. coli* host strain BL21(DE3).
5. Luria-Bertani (LB) broth containing 10 g/L tryptone, 5 g/L yeast extract, and 10 g/L sodium chloride, adjust the pH to

7.0 with 5 N NaOH; Aliquot 250 mL in 1 L flask covered with foil paper and autoclaved for 15 min at 121 °C and 18 psi.

6. Kanamycin stock solution at a concentration of 10 mg/mL in H_2O.
7. Sterile isopropyl β-d-1-thiogalactopyranoside (IPTG) stock solution at a concentration of 800 mM.
8. Soluble protein extraction buffer: 0.5 M NaH_2PO_4, 50 mM Tris, 1–10 mM imidazole, 250 mM NaCl pH 6.8 containing Halt™ Protease inhibitor cocktail.
9. Autoclaved 50 mL centrifuge tubes with silicon gasket and screw-cap.
10. Insoluble protein extraction buffer: 0.5 M NaH_2PO_4, 50 mM Tris, 1–10 mM imidazole, 250 mM NaCl, pH 6.8 containing Halt™ Protease inhibitor cocktail.
11. Nickel-NTA resin packed affinity chromatography columns.
12. Slide-A-Lyzer™ dialysis cassettes.
13. Endotoxin removal columns.
14. Pyrochrome® *Limulus* amebocyte lyase (LAL) kit.
15. Pierce™ BCA protein assay kit.
16. Microplate reader with temperature incubation and kinetic reading capabilities.
17. His-Tag ELISA detection kit (GenScript).
18. SDS-PAGE reagents and equipment.
19. Sonicator.
20. Spectrophotometer.
21. Shaking incubator with a temperature control unit.

2.4 Evaluation of rAg-Induced Protective Efficacy in HLA-DR Transgenic Mice

1. HLA-DR4 (DRB1*0401) transgenic mice (*see* **Note 2**).
2. Purified rAg at a concentration of at least 0.25 μg/μL in PBS buffer.
3. GYE agar plates containing 1% glucose, 0.5% yeast extract, 2% Bacto-agar. Add 5 g glucose plus 2.5 g yeast extract to 400 mL water in a 1 L flask and stir the solution until both ingredients are dissolved. Add water to a final volume of 500 mL and then add 10 g of Bacto-agar to the flask. Cover the flask with a piece of aluminum foil and autoclave for 15 min at 121 °C and 18 psi. Cool autoclaved medium to 55–60 °C and pour 25 mL into each Petri dish (100 × 15 mm) (*see* **Note 3**).
4. Autoclaved 5 mm diameter glass beads.
5. Cell lifters.
6. T-shaped spreaders.

7. Autoclaved 50 mL polycarbonate Oak Ridge centrifuge tubes with silicon gasket and screw-cap.
8. 1 mL syringes (27 G) for vaccination.
9. Centrifuges with covered rotors for 50 mL conical tubes, 96-well tissue culture plates, and 2.0 mL cryotubes.

3 Methods

3.1 Prediction of Promiscuous Epitopes Using Bioinformatic Analysis Tools

1. Identify cell-wall proteins of *Coccidioides posadasii* isolate C735 that react with IgG antibodies of patients with confirmed coccidioidomycosis and contain putative MHC II binding epitopes (Table 1 in [9]).
2. Screen full-length amino acid sequences of the putative antigens of *C. posadasii* to identify promiscuous HLA-DR binding epitopes using the ProPred algorithm [9, 31]. Set parameters at a 5% threshold and displayed in HTML II format.
3. Compile a list of *C. posadasii* peptides by flanking 5 amino acids (5 mers) at both ends of predicted, promiscuous epitopes identified by the ProPred analysis above.
4. TBLASTN search all available alleles of the identified peptides using the peptides of *C. posadasii* isolate C735 against 13 sequenced genomes of *Coccidioides spp.* (http://blast.ncbi.nlm.nih.gov/Blast.cgi?PAGE=Proteins) (*see* **Note 4**).
5. Screen nucleic acid regions that encode predicted epitopes for the presence of nonsynonymous coding single nucleotide polymorphisms (SNPs) by aligning the available, multiple nucleotide sequences of various isolates obtained from the *Coccidioides* genome databases. Use neighborhood quality standard (NQS) criteria [32] to reduce base-calling errors and alignment artifacts [29].
6. Verify epitope amino acid sequence displays low homology to human proteins by BLASTP searching the nonredundant NCBI Human protein database (RefSeq database). Ensure algorithm parameters are set to adjust for short input sequences.
7. Select for candidate epitopes that meet all of the following criteria: predicted promiscuous HLA-DR binders that bind >80% of the 51 HLA-DR alleles, >90% amino acid conservation among 14 *Coccidioides* isolates, low human homology (*E*-value >0.001), and contain a low number of SNPs. Rank the qualified peptides by their predicted promiscuous binding capacity.
8. Evaluate predicted epitopes for their binding capacity to HLA-DR molecules using a DELFIA method or an ELISA-based binding assay provided by a commercial service company. Synthesize candidate peptides identified in **step 7** to 90% purity

using commercial services. In the DELFIA binding assay, add peptide epitopes at incremental concentrations (10–10,000 nM) to compete with the MHC II-associated invariant chain peptide (CLIP) for binding to HLA-DR molecules. The readout for this assay is the concentration of synthetic peptide that prevents 50% of CLIP from binding to HLA-DR molecules. Peptides displaying an inhibitory concentration (IC^{50}) less than 3000 nM are selected for further functional analysis by an ELISpot assay described below. A total of eight peptides that belong to three *Coccidioides* antigens (i.e., Pep1, Amn1, and Plb) were selected.

3.2 Assessment of Immunogenicity of the Selected Peptides Using ELISpot Assays

1. Express and purify the recombinant *Coccidioides* antigens (rPep1, rAmn1, and rPlb) that contain the selected eight peptide epitopes as previously described [5, 8, 9, 21].
2. Calculate the required number of mice to harvest sufficient amounts of APCs and $CD4^+$ T cells for the assays. We routinely obtain 5–10 × 10^6 $CD4^+$ T cells and APCs each from a mouse spleen.
3. Prepare an experimental vaccine on the vaccination day by mixing 10 μg of each purified antigens in total of 49 μL PBS buffer, 10 μg of CpG in 1 μL PBS, and 50 μL of IFA per dose (total of 100 μL). Scale up for the required doses. Vortex the mixture until an emulsion forms. The mixture should not be separated into oil and liquid phases.
4. Vaccinate the required number of HLA-DR4 transgenic mice each with one dose of the prepared experimental vaccine by the subcutaneous (SC) route on the abdominal region using a 1 mL syringe with 27 gauge needle on week 0 (*see* Fig. 2a).
5. Prepare CpG + IFA (adjuvant control) following the same procedure, but omit the recombinant antigens. Mice immunized with the adjuvant alone are used as a negative control.
6. Administer a booster vaccination to both vaccinated and control mice using the same dose of vaccine described above 2 weeks post the first immunization.
7. Conduct ELISpot assays at 4 weeks after the booster vaccination (a total of 6 weeks from priming immunization).
8. Calculate the required well numbers on ELISpot filter 96-well plates for the assay, as shown in Fig. 2b. Three final concentrations (0.5, 1.0, and 10 μg/mL) of each synthetic peptide diluted in cHL-1 medium plus a negative (medium) and a positive control (1.0 μg/mL ConA) are tested in triplicate.
9. Prepare the required ELISpot filter plates by pre-wetting wells with 15 μL each of 35% ethanol (*see* **Notes 5** and **6**) 1 day prior to harvesting murine splenocytes (Day 0).
10. Decant ethanol by tapping 96-well plates on KimWipes.

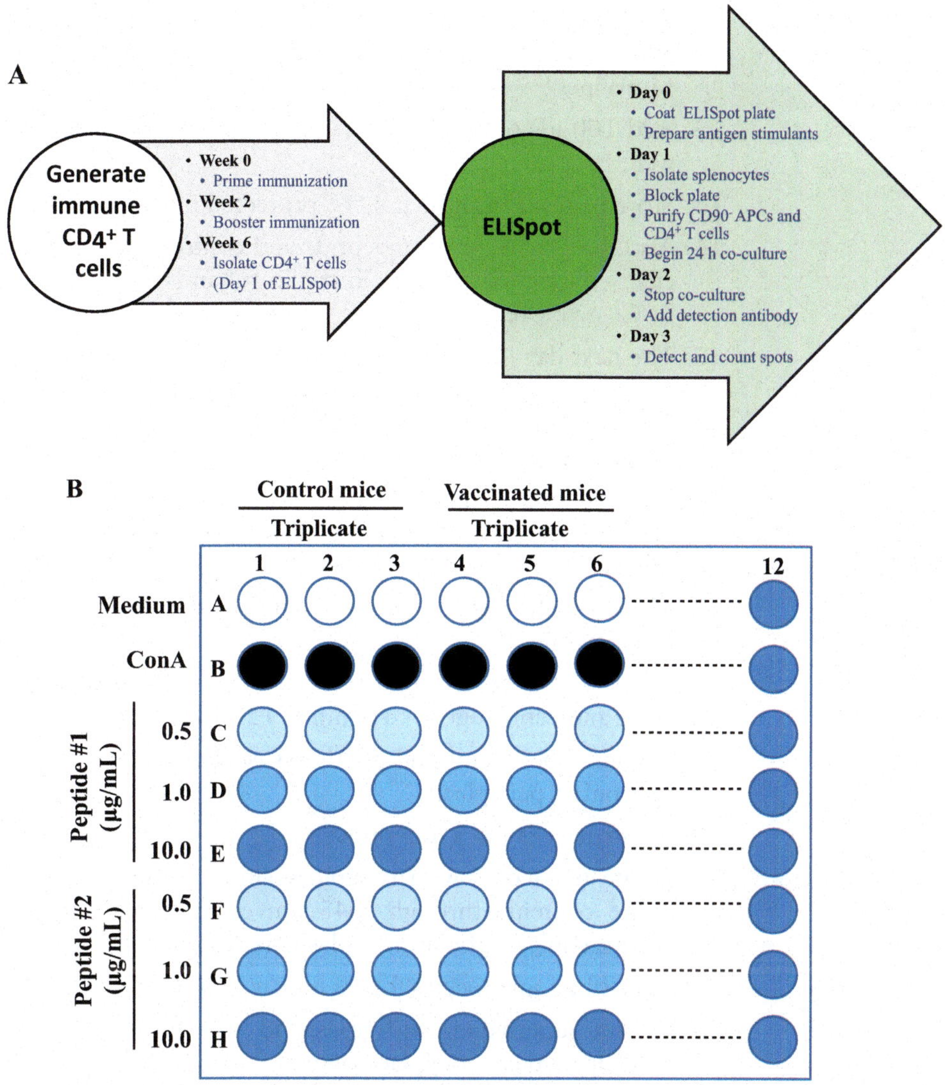

Fig. 2 ELISpot timeline and plate template. (**A**) Initial ELISpot assay is focused on generating immune $CD4^+$ T cells by immunizing HLA-DR transgenic mice at weeks 0 and 2 with an antigen or a mixture of antigens of interest that contains epitopes to be evaluated in downstream ELISpot assays (week 6). One day prior to the ELISpot assay (day 0), 96-well filter plates and antigen stimulants are prepared. At day 1, splenocytes are isolated from naive and immunized mice to isolate $CD90^-$ APCs and $CD4^+$ T cells, respectively. The plates are treated with a blocking solution containing 1% BSA. During the blocking step APCs and T cells are purified. APCs, $CD4^+$ T cells, and antigens of interest are cocultured for 24 h. On day two plates are washed and the cytokine detection antibody is added. Subsequently, plates are incubated for additional 24 h. On day 3, IFN-γ producing cells (*spots*) are detected and counted. (**B**) An ELISpot plate template is illustrated to include negative/positive controls and antigen peptides of interest. All stimulants are tested in triplicate

11. Wash wells twice with 350 μL PBS by decanting liquid into a waste container and gently tapping the 96-well plates onto KimWipes.
12. Add 100 μL of anti-IFN-γ capture antibody solution to each well.
13. Store plates overnight at 4 °C, protected from light.
14. Also, on Day 0, prepare peptide and control stimulants (sufficient volumes for analysis in triplicate) and store overnight at 4 °C (*see* **Note 7**).
15. The next day (Day 1) dissect spleens of euthanized mice from immunized and adjuvant control mice for purification of $CD4^+$ T cells and naive mice for isolating $CD90^-$ APCs using sterile dissecting equipment.
16. Place the spleens into a 70 μm cell strainer that has been placed in a culture plate containing 10–15 mL ice-cold RPMI per spleen.
17. Mechanically disrupt the spleen using the back of a sterile 3 mL syringe.
18. Transfer isolated cells to a 50 mL conical tube using a transfer pipet and centrifuge for 10 min at 1200 × *g*, 4 °C.
19. Decant supernatant and gently resuspend cells in 3 mL ACK lysis buffer per spleen.
20. Incubate cells for 5 min on ice.
21. Dilute lysed cells with twofold volume RPMI and filter the entire contents through a 45 μm cell strainer placed on a 50 mL conical tube using a plastic transfer pipet.
22. Centrifuge splenocytes for 10 min at 1200 × *g*, 4 °C.
23. Decant supernatant and resuspend cells in 10 mL ice-cold HBSS per spleen and place on ice.
24. Remove antibody-coated plates from 4 °C storage, decant liquid into a waste container, and tap plate against KimWipes to remove residual liquid.
25. Wash plates four times with PBS (300 μL/well), decanting and removing liquid as described above.
26. Add 200 μL blocking buffer to each well, protect plates from light, and incubate without shaking for 1 h at room temperature.
27. Return to cell purification process and dilute an aliquot of splenocytes in trypan blue to determine viable cell numbers using a hemocytometer.
28. Centrifuge cells for 10 min at 1200 × *g*, 4 °C, and decant supernatant.

29. Follow manufacturer's protocols to purify untouched $CD90^-$ APCs and $CD4^+$ T cells.
30. Determine absolute cell numbers of purified $CD90^-$ APCs and $CD4^+$ T cells by diluting cells in trypan blue and counting with a hemocytometer.
31. Centrifuge cells for 10 min at 1200 × *g* at 4 °C.
32. Decant supernatant and resuspend cells in cHL-1 media so that APCs and $CD4^+$ T cell concentrations are 5×10^6 and 4×10^6 cells/mL, respectively.
33. Temporarily store cells on ice.
34. Continue to prepare 96-well ELISpot plates by washing wells four times with PBS (300 μL/well).
35. In the following order, gently add 50 μL/well of each: peptide, negative or positive stimulants, APCs, and $CD4^+$ T cells (*see* **Notes 8** and **9**).
36. Incubate plate(s) for 24 h at 37 °C, 5% CO_2 (*see* **Note 10**).
37. At day 2, remove plates from the incubator and incubate at room temperature for 10 min.
38. Wash plate three times with PBS.
39. Wash plate four times with PBST.
40. Add 100 μL detection antibody to each well.
41. Incubate plate overnight at 4 °C, protected from light.
42. On day 3, wash plate four times with PBST.
43. Add 100 μL of S/AP conjugate solution to each well.
44. Incubate the plate for 2 h at room temperature, protected from light.
45. Wash plate four times with PBS.
46. Add 200 μL of pre-warmed BCIP/NBT substrate to each well at room temperature.
47. Observe spot development for 5–20 min.
48. Stop spot development by decanting substrate and rinsing plate five times with dH_2O (*see* **Note 11**).
49. Air dry plate under moderate air flow.
50. Scan plate with an ELISpot plate scanner.
51. Check that $CD4^+$ T cells isolated from both the adjuvant control mice and the vaccinated animals have comparable immunoreactivity. The ConA-stimulated wells (B1–3 and B4–6 in Fig. 2b) should have similar numbers of spots.
52. Determine the numbers of INF-γ producing cells (spots) per well as shown in Fig. 2b for each peptide using the following formula: $[(C_{4-6} - A_{4-6}) - (C_{1-3} - A_{1-3})]$.

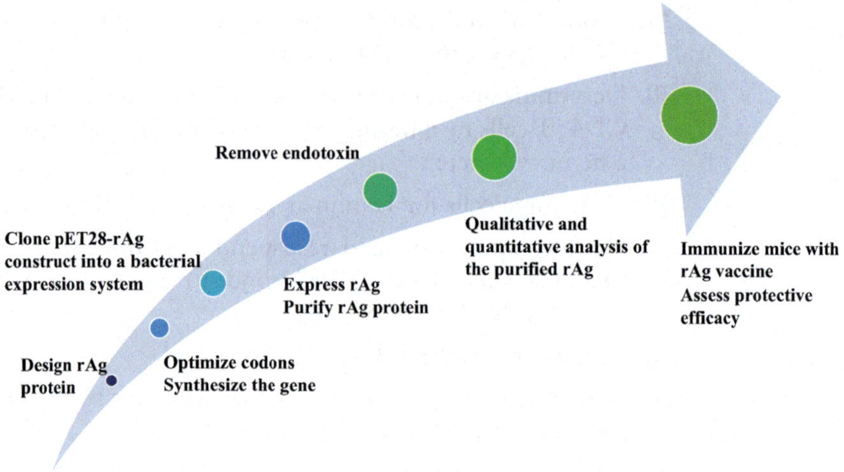

Fig. 3 Key steps in designing and producing rAg. With select candidate epitopes identified, the rAg amino acid sequence flanked with enhancing and spacer amino acids is designed, followed by DNA sequence design. The DNA fragment encoding the rAg is inserted into a bacterial expression vector (*pET28*) and transformed into *E. coli* for downstream expression and purification of rAg protein. Potential endotoxin copurified with the rAg is then removed using an ActiClean Etox affinity chromatography column. Residual endotoxin is quantified by the LAL assay. Purified rAg protein is then analyzed by SDS-PAGE for predicted molecular weight and contaminating proteins. The correct amino acid sequence is confirmed using LC-MS/MS. Concentration of rAg is quantified by the BCA assay. The vaccine is made of rAg and an adjuvant containing CpG plus IFA. HLA-DR4 transgenic mice are immunized with the rAg vaccine and intranasally challenged with *C. immitis* to assess protective efficacy

53. Rank the immunoreactive peptides by their capacity to stimulate the most INF-γ-producing CD4$^+$ T cells (*spots*) of the vaccinated mice. At this point in the epitope selection process, if a candidate epitope failed to produce a significant number of IFN-γ-producing cells after two independent experiments, eliminate the epitope from candidate pool.

3.3 Recombinant Antigen (rAg) Design, Production, and Purification

For a general overview of this process, *see* Fig. 3.

1. To design a multi-epitope driven vaccine, begin by adding an Ii key sequence (LRMKLPKS) to the N-terminus of each epitope amino acid sequence for enhanced antigen presentation [33] (*see* Fig. 4).
2. Separate each Ii key-epitope peptide sequence with a glycine-proline spacer (GPGPG) to disrupt junctional epitopes that are artificially created when epitopes are joined together [34].
3. Confirm the epitope arrangement within the rAg amino acid sequence continues to generate predicted promiscuous HLA-binders using the ProPred algorithm (*see* **Note 12**).

MGSSHHHHHHSSGLVPRGSHLRMKLPKSEPITOPEGPGPGLRMKL
PKSEPITOPEGPGPGLRMKLPKSEPITOPEGPGPGLRMKLPKSEP
ITOPEGPGPGLRMKLPKSEPITOPEGPGPGLRMKLPKSEPITOPE
GPGPGLRMKLPKSEPITOPEGPGPGLRMKLPKSEPITOPEGPGPG

Fig. 4 A representative rAg design. The rAg amino acid sequence incorporates multiple components that allow for purification and efficient antigen presentation. The rAg consists of a stretch of 20 amino acids (*blue*) derived from pET28 vector with a 6-histidine tag (*underlined*) allows for purification using a nickel-NTA resin affinity chromatography. The N-terminus of each HLA-DR binding epitope and flanking regions derived from the identified *Coccidioides* peptides (*red*) are connected to the Ii key sequence (LRMKLPKS). Each Ii key connected epitope is separated by a glycine-proline spacer (underlined GPGPG)

4. Use a commercial vendor to synthesize a codon-optimized DNA fragment that encodes rAg (*see* **Note 13**). The DNA fragment is cloned into a *pET28b* vector to generate the p*ET28-rAg* plasmid that is confirmed by DNA sequence analysis.
5. Transform p*ET28-rAg* into *E. coli* strain BL21(DE3) by standard cloning methodology [35].
6. A clone of the transformed bacterium is used to produce rAg using IPTG induction-based methodology as described elsewhere [35].
7. Grow the bacterial clone in 10 mL LB broth containing 50 μg/mL Kanamycin overnight.
8. Inoculate four bottles of LB broth (250 mL) with 2.5 mL overnight culture each.
9. Incubate the bacterial culture until the OD_{600} reaches above 1.2 (6–8 h).
10. Add IPTG to a final concentration of 1.5 mM and incubate for additional 4 h at 37 °C with vigorous shaking at 200 rpm.
11. Harvest bacterial cells by centrifugation at 5000 × *g*, 4 °C for 10 min.
12. Decant supernatant and store cell pellet overnight at −20 °C. Add bleach to a final concentration of 10% to sterilize the supernatant before discarding it into the sink.
13. Add desired amount of soluble protein extraction buffer (4 mL per gram of bacterial pellet) and thaw pellet on ice.
14. Transfer extraction buffer containing cell pellet to 50 mL centrifuge tubes.
15. Sonicate for 10–20 s and place the tube back on ice for 30 s. Repeat five times.
16. Centrifuge at 15,000 × *g*, 4 °C for 20 min.
17. Collect supernatant and store on ice (soluble fraction).

18. Repeat **steps 13–17** one more time. Combine both soluble fractions. Store the soluble fraction and pellet separately in −20 °C freezer until the solubility of rAg is determined as described below.
19. Check the soluble fraction for the presence or absence of rAg following the manufacturer's protocol using a His-Tag ELISA detection kit (*see* **Note 14).**
20. In the event that rAg is not extracted in the soluble fraction, continue to purify this recombinant protein using denaturing condition. Add desired amount of insoluble extraction buffer (4 mL per gram of bacteria) to cell pellet and repeat sonication as described in **step 15**.
21. Centrifuge and collect supernatant as described above to collect the insoluble fraction.
22. Follow manufacturer's affinity chromatography protocol to purify rAg using a gravity-flow nickel-NTA resin packed column under denaturing condition (*see* **Note 15).**
23. Dialyze rAg in the elution buffer containing 8 M urea and 250 mM imidazole by placing the protein solution in a Slide-A-Lyzer™ cassette submerged in 2 L of PBS containing 4 M urea. Place a magnetic stir bar in buffer and slowly mix overnight at 4 °C.
24. Dialyze protein for 8–12 h in PBS containing 2 M urea overnight.
25. Continue to dialyze the protein in PBS alone overnight. Retrieve the protein solution into a sterile 50 mL conical tube.
26. Remove endotoxin by passing protein solution through an ActiClean Etox column using gravity flow (*see* **Note 16**).
27. Quantify contaminating endotoxin using the Pyrochrome® LAL assay per the manufacturer's kinetic endpoint protocol and a 96-well microplate plate reader with temperature-control and kinetic endpoint capabilities.
28. Quantify rAg protein by BCA assay and confirm purity by standard SDS-PAGE and Coomassie Brilliant Blue staining protocols.
29. Confirm rAg protein sequence by liquid chromatography-tandem mass spectrometry (LC-MS/MS) analysis using a commercial service.

3.4 Evaluation of rAg-Induced Protective Efficacy in HLA Transgenic Mice

1. Prepare rAg vaccine. Each dose contains 10 μg rAg in 49 μL PBS, 10 μg CpG in 1 μL PBS, and 50 μL IFA. Scale up for the required doses. Vortex the mixture well until it does not separate into two phases.

2. Immunize HLA-DR4 transgenic mice with the rAg vaccine, as described in Subheading 3.2, **step 3**. HLA-DR4 mice vaccinated with IFA + CpG without the antigen are used as a negative control.
3. Confirm immunogenicity of rAg using an ELISpot assay as described in Subheading 3.2 using the incorporated peptides as stimulants (*see* **Note 17**).
4. After confirming rAg is immunogenic, immunize 6–10 weeks old, gender-matched HLA-DR4 mice with the rAg vaccine or the adjuvant control. At least ten mice per treatment group are necessary to obtain statistically significant data (*see* **Note 18**).
5. Inoculate *C. posadasii* (C735 isolate) culture on GYE agar plates on the day of booster immunization for use in downstream challenge inoculums. *Coccidioides* spores take 3–4 weeks to grow on GYE plates.
6. Mice are challenged with a potentially lethal dose of viable *Coccidioides* spores at 4 weeks after the last booster immunization. Three days before the scheduled challenge time, collect spores (arthroconidia) from 2 GYE agar plate cultures of *Coccidioides* (3–4 weeks old) by scraping the plates with a sterile cell lifter. Transfer the spore mat into an autoclaved Oak Ridge tube provided with a silicone gasket and screw cap. Add 10 mL PBS plus 15 autoclaved glass beads (5 mm diameter), screw the cap tightly, and shake vigorously by hand for 30 s.
7. Filter the suspension through a 40 μm sterile cell strainer to remove hyphal fragments. Collect the spores in a sterile Oak Ridge centrifuge tube.
8. Pellet the spores by centrifugation at 1200 × *g* for 10 min at room temperature, discard the supernatant into the disinfectant tank, and resuspend the spores in 5 mL PBS.
9. Determine the concentration of spores using a hemocytometer.
10. Dilute the spores to 10^7 spores/mL with PBS for long-term storage at 4 °C.
11. Plate inoculum to confirm dosage by preparing an aliquot of diluted spores to 10^3 spores/mL with PBS. Plate 5 GYE plates each with 100 μL of the diluted spores for testing viability (*see* **Note 19**).
12. Incubate the plates upside down in a 30 °C steady incubator for 3 days.
13. Count colony-forming units (CFUs) at the end of the 3 day incubation (*see* **Note 20**).
14. Prepare an aliquot of C735 spores at a concentration of 2.5×10^3 CFU/mL in PBS.

15. Vaccinated and control mice are anesthetized with isoflurane using a vaporizer and challenged with a potentially lethal dose of spores (75–90 spores in 35 μL) via an intranasal instillation method.
16. Plate 5 GYE plates, each with 35 μL of the spore solution to confirm the challenge dose.
17. Weigh each mouse daily and monitor prognosis of coccidioidomycosis (**see Notes 21** and **22**).
18. Evaluate survival over a period of 50 days and evaluate statistical significance of survivors of rAg-vaccinated mice versus control animals by the Kaplan-Meier test using log rank analysis.

4 Notes

1. CpG ODN is a class II sequence TCCATGACGTTCC TGACGTT (CpG region underlined) modified with phosphorothioate on all nucleotides to mitigate nucleases [36].
2. HLA-DR4 mice were genetically engineered from a C57BL/6 background and were backcrossed to MHC II-deficient mice lacking IAβ and IEα alleles to eliminate production of endogenous murine MHC II molecules [37, 38].
3. All culturing and preparatory procedures that involve live cells of *Coccidioides* are conducted in an annually certified biosafety cabinet located inside a biosafety level 3 laboratory. Prepare 1 L of freshly made 20% bleach in a 2 L beaker and an autoclaveable red bag inside the biosafety cabinet as a disinfectant station and a waste collection container, respectively. Discard all solution and used consumable supplies into the disinfectant tank immediately after usage.
4. Annotated genome databases of *C. posadasii* isolate C735 and *C. immitis* isolate RS are completed, while the other 12 available genomes are sequenced to 3–8× coverage.
5. From this point forward, conduct all work in a Class II biological safety cabinet and do not allow 96-well plate membranes to dry.
6. Only allow ethanol to rest on membrane for 60 s to allow for sufficient wetting. Extensive incubation may cause ethanol evaporation and membrane damage.
7. If necessary, add 10 μg/mL polymyxin-B to the peptide/antigen stimulants to mitigate LPS interference.
8. Gentle pipetting prevents swirling of well contents and prevents cells from concentrating at the edges of the wells.
9. If high spot numbers are detected for mice that are vaccinated with adjuvant alone, the following optional controls may be

included: wells contain APCs only to account for nonspecific IFN-γ production by APCs and scrambled peptide to control nonspecific stimulation.

10. To ensure uniform spot development and prevent spot-streaking, do not agitate, move, or bump plates during the incubation period.
11. A DI water faucet is sufficient, provided the water pressure is low enough to prevent damage to the plates. After the first wash, remove the bottom plastic backing and continue to carefully rinse both the top and the bottom of the membrane.
12. If an originally identified epitope included in the designed rAg does not sustain its promiscuous HLA binding property when tested by ProPed, it can be repositioned within the rAg to ensure its antigenic properties.
13. Ensure gene synthesis services include sequence optimization for codon usage, GC content, repeating DNA sequences, and secondary DNA structure for efficient protein expression in *E. coli*.
14. Most of *E. coli*-expressed recombinant antigens derived from *C. posadasii* are in bacterial inclusion bodies and insoluble in non-denaturing extraction buffer. They are purified using a denaturing condition with 6–8 M urea as a solubilization agent.
15. All Ni-NTA binding, washing, and elution buffers contain 8 M urea for purification of *Coccidioides* recombinant proteins under denaturing condition.
16. From this point forward, use pyrogen-free consumables to reduce endotoxin contamination.
17. If ELISpot shows that an epitope is processed with little efficiency or not at all, consider the following modifications: adjust the position of the epitope within the rAg vaccine, adjust the length of amino acids up and downstream of the core HLA-DR binding epitope, and consider further modifying flanking regions to promote epitope processing [39].
18. Both female and male HLA-DR4 mice are highly susceptible to *Coccidioides* infection. There is no detectable difference in susceptibility between male and female mice if a challenge dose higher than 30 spores is used.
19. Only *Coccidioides* spore preparation with cell viability over 90% can be used for vaccination and challenge.
20. *Coccidioides* spp. form a white to milky color, spider web-like colonies about 1–2 mm in diameter at the end of the 3 day incubation. Presence of smooth and big colonies on GYE plates is an indication of contamination.

21. Any mice that appear moribund prior to the scheduled endpoint will be euthanized. Moribund animals will be identified by the following criteria: (1) ruffled fur, (2) hunched posture, (3) weight loss greater than 20%, and (4) inability to eat or drink.

22. Vaccinated HLA-DR4 mice can display three distinct manifestations of coccidioidomycosis after an intranasal challenge with *Coccidioides* spores, including fatal acute, disseminated, and pulmonary disease conditions [13]. Mice with fatal acute disease will lose over 20% body weight and approach moribund condition by 12–20 days postchallenge, while protected animals with disseminated and pulmonary disease forms can survive to 50 days postchallenge.

Acknowledgment

This work was supported by a research grant from the National Institutes of Health, NIAID (R21 AI114762). Additional support was provided by *Coccidioides* research funds donated by the Valley Fever of the Americas Foundation and community supporters.

References

1. Brown J, Benedict K, Park BJ, Thompson GR 3rd (2013) Coccidioidomycosis: epidemiology. Clin Epidemiol 5:185–197
2. Abuodeh RO, Shubitz LF, Siegel E, Snyder S, Peng T, Orsborn KI, Brummer E, Stevens DA, Galgiani JN (1999) Resistance to *Coccidioides immitis* in mice after immunization with recombinant protein or a DNA vaccine of a proline-rich antigen. Infect Immun 67:2935–2940
3. Cole GT, Hurtgen BJ, Hung C-Y (2012) Progress toward a human vaccine against coccidioidomycosis. Curr Fungal Infect Rep 6: 235–244
4. Delgado N, Xue J, Yu J-J, Hung C-Y, Cole GT (2003) A recombinant beta-1,3-glucanosyltransferase homolog of *Coccidioides posadasii* protects mice against coccidioidomycosis. Infect Immun 71:3010–3019
5. Herr RA, Hung C-Y, Cole GT (2007) Evaluation of two homologous proline-rich proteins of *Coccidioides posadasii* as candidate vaccines against coccidioidomycosis. Infect Immun 75:5777–5787
6. Hurtgen BJ, Hung C-Y, Ostroff GR, Levitz SM, Cole GT (2012) Construction and evaluation of a novel recombinant T cell epitope-based vaccine against coccidioidomycosis. Infect Immun 80:3960–3974
7. Shubitz LF, Yu J-J, Hung CY, Kirkland TN, Peng T, Perrill R, Simons J, Xue J, Herr RA, Cole GT, Galgiani JN (2006) Improved protection of mice against lethal respiratory infection with *Coccidioides posadasii* using two recombinant antigens expressed as a single protein. Vaccine 24:5904–5911
8. Tarcha EJ, Basrur V, Hung C-Y, Gardner MJ, Cole GT (2006a) A recombinant aspartyl protease of *Coccidioides posadasii* induces protection against pulmonary coccidioidomycosis in mice. Infect Immun 74:516–527
9. Tarcha EJ, Basrur V, Hung C-Y, Gardner MJ, Cole GT (2006b) Multivalent recombinant protein vaccine against coccidioidomycosis. Infect Immun 74:5802–5813
10. Kirkland TN, Finley F, Orsborn KI, Galgiani JN (1998) Evaluation of the proline-rich antigen of *Coccidioides immitis* as a vaccine candidate in mice. Infect Immun 66: 3519–3522
11. Pappagianis D (1993) Evaluation of the protective efficacy of the killed *Coccidioides immitis* spherule vaccine in humans. The valley fever vaccine study group. Am Rev Respir Dis 148: 656–660
12. Edwards JE Jr (2012) Fungal cell wall vaccines: an update. J Med Microbiol 61:895–903

13. Hurtgen BJ, Castro-Lopez N, Jimenez-Alzate MD, Cole GT, Hung C-Y (2016) Preclinical identification of vaccine induced protective correlates in human leukocyte antigen expressing transgenic mice infected with Coccidioides posadasii. Vaccine 34:5336–5343
14. Allendorfer R, Brunner GD, Deepe GS Jr (1999) Complex requirements for nascent and memory immunity in pulmonary histoplasmosis. J Immunol 162:7389–7396
15. Wüthrich M, Warner T, Klein BS (2005) IL-12 is required for induction but not maintenance of protective, memory responses to *Blastomyces dermatitidis*: implications for vaccine development in immune-deficient hosts. J Immunol 175:5288–5297
16. Wüthrich M, Filutowicz HI, Warner T, Klein BS (2002) Requisite elements in vaccine immunity to *Blastomyces dermatitidis*: plasticity uncovers vaccine potential in immune-deficient hosts. J Immunol 169:6969–6976
17. Cox RA, Magee DM (1998) Protective immunity in coccidioidomycosis. Res Immunol 149: 417–428
18. Cox RA, Magee DM (2004) Coccidioidomycosis: host response and vaccine development. Clin Microbiol Rev 17:804–839
19. Cole GT, Xue JM, Okeke CN, Tarcha EJ, Basrur V, Schaller RA, Herr RA, Yu J-J, Hung C-Y (2004) A vaccine against coccidioidomycosis is justified and attainable. Med Mycol 42:189–216
20. Xue J, Hung C-Y, Yu J-J, Cole G-T (2005) Immune response of vaccinated and non-vaccinated mice to *Coccidioides posadasii* infection. Vaccine 23:3535–3544
21. Li K, Yu J-J, Hung C-Y, Lehmann PF, Cole GT (2001) Recombinant urease and urease DNA of *Coccidioides immitis* elicit an immunoprotective response against coccidioidomycosis in mice. Infect Immun 69:2878–2887
22. Shubitz LF, Dial SM, Perrill R, Casement R, Galgiani JN (2008) Vaccine-induced cellular immune responses differ from innate responses in susceptible and resistant strains of mice infected with *Coccidioides posadasii*. Infect Immun 76:5553–5564
23. Hung C-Y, Gonzalez A, Wuthrich M, Klein BS, Cole GT (2011) Vaccine immunity to coccidioidomycosis occurs by early activation of three signal pathways of T helper cell response (Th1, Th2, and Th17). Infect Immun 79: 4511–4522
24. Hung C-Y, Hurtgen BJ, Bellecourt M, Sanderson SD, Morgan EL, Cole GT (2012) An agonist of human complement fragment C5a enhances vaccine immunity against *Coccidioides* infection. Vaccine 30:4681–4690
25. Wuthrich M, Hung C-Y, Gern BH, Pick-Jacobs JC, Galles KJ, Filutowicz HI, Cole GT, Klein BS (2011) A TCR transgenic mouse reactive with multiple systemic dimorphic fungi. J Immunol 187:1421–1431
26. Orsborn KI, Shubitz LF, Peng T, Kellner EM, Orbach MJ, Haynes PA, Galgiani JN (2006) Protein expression profiling of *Coccidioides posadasii* by two-dimensional differential in-gel electrophoresis and evaluation of a newly recognized peroxisomal matrix protein as a recombinant vaccine candidate. Infect Immun 74:1865–1872
27. Rohrbough JG, Galgiani JN, Wysocki VH (2007) The application of proteomic techniques to fungal protein identification and quantification. Ann N Y Acad Sci 1111: 133–146
28. Salvat R, Moise L, Bailey-Kellogg C, Griswold KE (2014) A high throughput MHC II binding assay for quantitative analysis of peptide epitopes J Vis Exp 85:e51308
29. Neafsey DE, Barker BM, Sharpton TJ, Stajich JE, Park DJ, Whiston E, Hung C-Y, McMahan C, White J, Sykes S, Heiman D, Young S, Zeng Q, Abouelleil A, Aftuck L, Bessette D, Brown A, FitzGerald M, Lui A, Macdonald JP, Priest M, Orbach MJ, Galgiani JN, Kirkland TN, Cole GT, Birren BW, Henn MR, Taylor JW, Rounsley SD (2010) Population genomic sequencing of *Coccidioides* fungi reveals recent hybridization and transposon control. Genome Res 20:938–946
30. Sharpton TJ, Stajich JE, Rounsley SD, Gardner MJ, Wortman JR, Jordar VS, Maiti R, Kodira CD, Neafsey DE, Zeng Q, Hung C-Y, McMahan C, Muszewska A, Grynberg M, Mandel MA, Kellner EM, Barker BM, Galgiani JN, Orbach MJ, Kirkland TN, Cole GT, Henn MR, Birren BW, Taylor JW (2009) Comparative genomic analyses of the human fungal pathogens *Coccidioides* and their relatives. Genome Res 19:1722–1731
31. Singh H, Raghava GP (2001) ProPred: prediction of HLA-DR binding sites. Bioinformatics 17:1236–1237
32. Altshuler D, Pollara VJ, Cowles CR, Van Etten WJ, Baldwin J, Linton L, Lander ES (2000) An SNP map of the human genome generated by reduced representation shotgun sequencing. Nature 407:513–516
33. Humphreys RE, Adams S, Koldzic G, Nedelescu B, von Hofe E, Xu M (2000) Increasing the potency of MHC class II-presented epitopes by linkage to Ii-Key peptide. Vaccine 18:2693–2697
34. Livingston B, Crimi C, Newman M, Higashimoto Y, Appella E, Sidney J, Sette A

(2002) A rational strategy to design multiepitope immunogens based on multiple Th lymphocyte epitopes. J Immunol 168:5499–5506

35. Green MR, Sambrook J (2012) Molecular cloning: a laboratory manual. Cold Spring Harbor Laboratory Press, Cold Spring Habor, NY
36. Chu RS, Targoni OS, Krieg AM, Lehmann PV, Harding CV (1997) CpG oligodeoxynucleotides act as adjuvants that switch on T helper 1 (Th1) immunity. J Exp Med 186:1623–1631
37. Ito K, Bian HJ, Molina M, Han J, Magram J, Saar E, Belunis C, Bolin DR, Arceo R, Campbell R, Falcioni F, Vidovic D, Hammer J, Nagy ZA (1996) HLA-DR4-IE chimeric class II transgenic, murine class II-deficient mice are susceptible to experimental allergic encephalomyelitis. J Exp Med 183:2635–2644
38. Madsen LS, Andersson EC, Jansson L, Krogsgaard M, Andersen CB, Engberg J, Strominger JL, Svejgaard A, Hjorth JP, Holmdahl R, Wucherpfennig KW, Fugger L (1999) A humanized model for multiple sclerosis using HLA-DR2 and a human T-cell receptor. Nat Genet 23:343–347
39. Holland CJ, Cole DK, Godkin A (2013) Redirecting CD4(+) T cell responses with the flanking residues of MHC class II-bound peptides: the Core is not enough. Front Immunol 4:172

Chapter 5

Identification of Fungal T Cell Epitopes by Mass Spectrometry-Based Proteomics

Bernd Roschitzki and Salomé LeibundGut-Landmann

Abstract

CD4+ T cells play a key role in host defense against many fungal infections. T cells are also implicated in vaccine immunity to fungi. To date, only a small number of fungal antigens have been identified. Knowing the antigenic determinants of fungi-specific T cells greatly facilitates the detection, enumeration and characterizes the antifungal T cells and it constitutes an important step toward the design and development of vaccination strategies. This chapter describes a method of MHC-II ligand elution and mass spectrometric analysis to identify naturally processed and presented fungal peptide epitopes.

Key words Fungal antigens, T helper cells, Naturally processed and presented T cell epitopes, MHC-II ligand elution, Mass spectrometry

1 Introduction

The high morbidity and mortality associated with fungal infections constitutes an unmet need for better preventative and therapeutic approaches. Many fungal infections are not limited to immunocompromised hosts, but also affect otherwise healthy individuals, thus offering good prospects for active vaccination strategies. Multiple preclinical studies in mouse models demonstrate the feasibility of diverse vaccination strategies to induce immunity against clinically relevant fungal pathogens [1], and the successful completion of phase 1 trials with vaccines against *Candidaalbicans* has delivered promising results [2, 3].

Knowing the antigenic determinants that are recognized by fungus-specific T cells is a prerequisite for the development of fungal vaccines. Detailed knowledge on fungus-derived antigenic peptides is also the key for understanding T cell immunity against fungal infections. However, the genetic complexity of many fungi is impeding the rapid identification of T cell epitopes. A large number of peptides can theoretically be generated from the large and

Markus Kalkum and Margarita Semis (eds.), *Vaccines for Invasive Fungal Infections: Methods and Protocols*, Methods in Molecular Biology, vol. 1625, DOI 10.1007/978-1-4939-7104-6_5, © Springer Science+Business Media LLC 2017

complex fungal proteome. However, pathogen-specific T cell responses are generally limited to only a small number of different specificities.

Immunoproteomics approaches have proven useful for the identification of MHC-bound peptides in an unbiased manner [4]. They involve the purification of detergent-solubilized peptide-MHC complexes by immunoaffinity chromatography, the elution of MHC-bound peptides, and the application of liquid chromatography-mass spectrometry (LC-MS) for determining individual peptide sequences. Computational discrimination of host-derived sequences finally allows the identification of pathogen-derived peptides. Mass spectrometry (MS) is thus a core technology for the analysis of the MHC ligandome and allows gaining qualitative and quantitative insights into the MHC-presented peptide repertoire [5].

In this chapter, we describe an approach to identify putative $CD4^+$ T cell epitopes from the fungal pathogen *C. albicans* that are naturally processed and presented by murine antigen-presenting cells. The experimental strategy can be adapted for the identification of MHC-bound peptides from other fungal (and non-fungal) microbes, provided their (genome) sequence is known, and also in the context of other host species.

2 Materials

2.1 Mammalian Cells and Fungi

1. The DC line DC^{1940} [6] is grown in IMDM medium complete (*see* below). Cells should be kept at a density between 10^5 and 10^6 cells/ml (*see* **Note 1**).
2. *C. albicans* (strain SC5314) is stored in 30% glycerol at −80 °C. An aliquot of the frozen stock is grown on YPD agar (*see* below) at 30 °C overnight. A single colony is then transferred to 5 ml YPD liquid medium (*see* below) and grown for 6–10 h in a 12 ml round bottom tube in a shaking incubator at 180 rpm and 30 °C. From this preculture, a 20 ml culture of the YPD liquid medium is adjusted to $OD_{600} = 0.1$ and grown for 16–18 h in a 100 ml Erlenmeyer flask in a shaking incubator at 180 rpm and 30 °C.

2.2 Media, Buffers, and Other Reagents

1. YPD liquid medium: 20 g yeast extract, 10 g bactopeptone, and 20 g glucose in 1 L dH_2O. Autoclave prior to use. Store at room temperature.
2. YPD agar: 20 g yeast extract, 10 g bactopeptone, and 20 g glucose in 1 L dH_2O are mixed. 20 g agar are added before autoclaving. Pour into petri dishes once the agar has cooled down to 50 °C. Store at 4 °C.

3. IMDM medium complete: IMDM GlutaMAX™ Medium supplemented with 10% decomplemented fetal calf serum (FCS), 100 IU/ml Penicillin, 100 μg/ml Streptomycin, and 50 μM 2-Mercaptoethanol. Store at 4 °C.
4. PBS 1×.
5. Anti-MHC-II antibody (anit-I-A/I-E, clone M5/114, BioXCell,). Need 1 mg antibody per 1 ml pellet of infected DC^{1940} cells.
6. CNBr-activated Sepharose 4B (GE Healthcare).
7. 1 mM HCl.
8. Coupling buffer: 0.5 M NaCl, 0.1 M $NaHCO_3$, adjusted to pH 8.3.
9. Blocking buffer: 0.2 M Glycin.
10. Solubilization buffer (2×): dissolve 2.4 g CHAPS (Molecular biology grade, 1.2% w/v) and 6 complete™ protease inhibitor tablets in 200 ml PBS. Prepare fresh. A smaller volume can be prepared for smaller sample sizes.
11. Elution buffer: 0.2% Trifluoroacetic acid (TFA).
12. 10% Trifluoroacetic acid (TFA).
13. LC-MS-grade solvent A: 0.1% formic acid in water.
14. LC-MS-grade solvent B: 0.1% formic acid in acetonitrile.
15. LC-MS-Sample solution: 3% acetonitrile, 0.1% formic acid is prepared from solvent A and solvent B by mixing 97 parts solvent A and three parts solvent B.

2.3 Supplies

1. Table top centrifuge with swinging-out rotor for 5 ml round-bottom tubes and for 15 and 50 ml conical tubes.
2. CO_2 incubator adjusted to 37 °C with 5% CO_2.
3. Shaking incubator adjusted to 30 °C.
4. Rotating wheel for 50 ml conical tubes.
5. 300 cm^2 tissue culture flasks.
6. 50 ml conical tubes.
7. Petri dishes.
8. 12 ml round-bottom tube.
9. 100 ml Erlenmeyer flasks.
10. Econo-Pac® Disposable Chromatography columns.
11. Sonicator. Clean with alcohol and rinse with dH_2O prior to use. Use ear protection.
12. Beckmann ultracentrifuge with rotor Ti45/Ti70, ultracentrifuge tubes.
13. 1000 ml beaker.

14. Amicon Ultra-4 Centrifugal Filter Unit with Ultracel-10 membrane.
15. 1.5 ml Eppendorf tubes.
16. Vacuum concentrator.
17. Nano-HPLC-system equipped with a reverse-phase column (0.075 mm × 150 mm,) and coupled to a high-resolution MS system.

3 Methods

3.1 Infection of Dendritic Cells with *C. albicans*

Infection of approximately 10^{10} DC^{1940} cells is necessary to obtain sufficient MHC-II - peptide complexes for peptide elution. The infections can be done in batches with 3–5 × 10^9 cells each. Infected cells can be stored at −80 °C and pooled later for the preparation of the lysate.

1. Expand DC^{1940} cells to obtain the required cell number.
2. Seed 2 × 10^8 DC^{1940} cells in 50 ml IMDM medium complete per 300cm^2 tissue culture flask 1 day prior to the infection. Incubate overnight at 37 °C, 5% CO_2.
3. For infection, collect *C. albicans* yeast cells from an overnight culture in a YPD liquid medium. Wash three times in PBS. After each washing step, centrifuge for 5 min to pellet the cells. Determine the yeast cell concentration by measuring the OD_{600} with a photometer (1 OD_{600} ≈ 10^7 cells, *see* **Note 2**). Adjust the concentration to 1.5 × 10^8 yeast cells/ml in IMDM medium complete. Add 4 ml (= 6 × 108 yeast cells) to the DC^{1940} cells (without removing the medium from the dendritic cells). Swirl the flasks to distribute the yeast cells equally over the entire surface of the dendritic cells.
4. Incubate for 4 h at 37 °C, 5% CO_2 (*see* **Note 3**).
5. At the end of the infection period, collect the infected DC^{1940} cells from the flasks using a cell scraper and pool all cells in one conical 50 ml tube. Centrifuge for 5 min at 300 × *g*, 4 °C, to collect the cells.
6. Wash the infected DC^{1940} cells with PBS and centrifuge again for 5 min at 300 × *g*, 4 °C, to collect the cells. Remove the supernatant. Measure the volume of the cell pellet and calculate the overall volume of all cell pellets to be pooled in case the infection is done in batches.
7. Store the cell pellet in the conical 50 ml tube at −80 °C.

3.2 Peptide Elution

The elution of MHC-II-bound peptides is done over 2-days. On the first day, an affinity column consisting of an anti-MHCII antibody coupled to CNBr-activated Sepharose is prepared. Also on the first day, a lysate is prepared from the infected cells. The soluble fraction of the lysate, containing the MHC–peptide complexes, is then applied to the affinity column. On the second day, the peptide-loaded MHCII molecules are eluted with 0.2% TFA, and the peptides are separated from the MHCII molecules by size exclusion centrifugation.

3.2.1 Preparation of the CNBr-Sepharose Columns (Day 1)

1. Determine the amount of antibody and CNBr-Sepharose needed (1 mg antibody per 1 ml cell pellet; 37.5 mg CNBr Sepharose per 1 mg antibody. For an example: for a cell pellet of 4.5 ml, you need 4.5 mg antibody and 168.75 mg CNBr-Sepharose).
2. Weigh out the required amount of CNBr-Sepharose into a conical 50 ml tube.
3. For the activation of the CNBr-Sepharose, cover the CNBr-Sepharose with 1 mM HCl solution at room temperature, mix well, and incubate at room temperature for 30 min, with rotation.
4. Centrifuge the activated CNBr-Sepharose for 4 min at room temperature and 300 rpm without break. Remove the supernatant without touching the CNBr-Sepharose pellet.
5. Resuspend the anti-MHC-II antibody in coupling buffer at room temperature and add it to the CNBr-Sepharose pellet (the pellet should be covered with coupling buffer). Mix well and incubate at room temperature for 120 min, with rotation.
6. Determine the coupling efficiency:

   t_0: Remove 100 μl of the antibody-CNBr-Sepharose and put in an 1.5 ml conical tube, centrifuge for 2 min at 15,700 × *g*, transfer the supernatant in a new 1.5 ml conical tube, dissolve and measure the antibody concentration with a photometer, wavelength OD_{280} (1 OD_{280} = 0.7 mg/ml antibody).
   t_{end}: Remove 100 μl of the antibody-BrCN-sepharose, measure the antibody concentration as described for t_0.
   Coupling efficiency =100%—((antibody concentration at t_{end})/(antibody concentration at t_0) × 100%). The coupling efficiency should be ≥95%. Otherwise, incubate the CNBr-Sepharose with the antibody for a prolonged period of time.
7. Centrifuge the antibody-coupled CNBr-Sepharse for 4 min at room temperature and 300 rpm without break. Remove the supernatant without touching the CNBr-Sepharose pellet.
8. Add blocking buffer to cover the CNBr-Sepharose. Mix well by shaking and incubate at room temperature for 60 min, with rotation.
9. Centrifuge the antibody-coupled CNBr-Sepharse for 4 min at room temperature and 300 rpm without break. Remove the supernatant. Wash the pellet twice with PBS. Centrifuge as described.

10. Resuspend the CNBr-Sepharose in PBS and transfer to the column.
11. Wash the column with PBS for 30 min using gravity flow (flow rate 1–2 ml/min).

3.2.2 Preparation of the Cell Lysate (Day 1)

All the steps are done in the cold room. Precool the centrifuge including the rotor and the adaptors at 4 °C.

1. Thaw the cell pellet(s) and transfer into an Erlenmeyer flask. Pool pellets in case the infection was done in several batches (*see* Subheading 3.1, point 6).
2. Add 1 volume of freshly prepared solubilization buffer (2×). Stir slowly until the pellet is completely thawed.
3. Add 1 volume of solubilization buffer (1×). Stir for 60 min at 4 °C. Transfer the lysate into a 50 ml conical tube.
4. Homogenize by sonification: Place the 50 ml conical tube containing the lysate on ice in a 1000 ml beaker. Apply ultrasound for 3 x 20 s with breaks of 20 s in between.
5. Stir for 60 min at 4 °C.
6. Centrifuge the cell lysate for 20 min at 4 °C, 4000 rpm.
7. Transfer the supernatant to ultracentrifuge tubes. Fill the tubes until the very top and balance exactly with solubilization buffer (1×). Centrifuge for 60 min at 4 °C and 40,000 rpm.
8. Sterile filter the supernatant through a 0.2 μm filter.
9. Load the lysate of the CNBr-Sepharose column by running it over the column by gravity flow. Recover the flow through and run it over the column at least ten times. Collect the last flow through in a 50 ml conical tube and store at −20 °C (*see* **Note 4**).

3.2.3 Elution of MHC-II-Peptide Complexes from the CNBr- Column

1. Wash the column with PBS (flow rate 1–2 ml/min, $t \geq 30$ min).
2. Wash the column with dH_2O (flow rate 1–2 ml/min, $t \geq 30$ min) (*see* **Note 5**).
3. Let the column run dry prior to adding 0.2% TFA onto the column until the CNBr-Sepharose is covered.
4. At the first elution step, additionally add 10 μl 10% TFA per mg of antibody (*see* **Note 6**).
5. Close the column and shake gently for 15–30 min.
6. Elute the peptides into an Amicon tube that was washed with 0.2% TFA (*see* **Note 7**).
7. Repeat the elution with 0.2% TFA seven to nine times.
8. Centrifuge the Amicon tubes at 4 °C and 4,000 rpm until all eluate has passed through the filter.
9. Transfer the flow through in a 1.5 ml Eppendorf tube. Dry the peptides using a vacuum concentrator (*see* **Note 8**).
10. Store the samples at −80 °C until further use.

3.3 LC-MS/MS Analysis

Peptide identification is done using nano-HPLC-systems coupled to high-resolution and high-accuracy mass spectrometers. The usage of nano-scale HPLC and nano-scale ion sources coupled to MS enables a sensitive and comprehensive analysis of MHC bound peptides.

1. Dissolve the dried peptides in 15 μl LC-MS-Sample solution (*see* Subheading 2.2).
2. Load 4 μl of the peptide solution on a nano-LC-MS/MS system and elute the peptides using a linear gradient of increasing amount of acetonitrile (3–40%) in 50 min followed by a strong increase to 97% acetonitrile in 10 min using a constant flow rate of 300 nl/min (*see* **Note 9**).
3. Acquire high accuracy mass spectra with an Orbitrap Velos (Thermo Scientific) in a mass range of 300–2000 m/z and a resolution of 60,000@400 m/z FWHM (Full Width at Half Maximum). Operate the MS in data-dependent mode and record up to five MS/MS using collision-induced dissociation (CID) or up to three MS/MS using higher-energy collisional dissociation (HCD) of the most intense ions in the linear ion trap or in the Orbitrap, respectively. Enable charge state screening and acquire MS/MS only of doubly, triply, or quadruply charged ions. Exclude target ions already selected for MS/MS dynamically for 60 s (*see* **Note 10**).

3.4 Data Analysis

Recorded mass spectra are extracted to peak lists before the data can be analyzed with data base search algorithms such as Mascot. The statistical validation using peptide level FDR and Protein Prophet allows defining FDR thresholds for peptide spectrum matches (PSM) and proteins. Sequence alignments and text filtering provides a ranked overview of analyzed MHC binding peptides.

1. Generate peak lists by using Mascot Distiller software (Matrix Science).
2. Use a search engine (e.g., MASCOT) to analyze the recorded MS/MS spectra against a decoyed and concatenated Swiss-Prot database (*see* **Note 11**).
3. Set search parameters as follows: precursor tolerance 7 ppm, MS/MS tolerance 0.6 Da for ion trap spectra and 0.02 Da for Orbitrap spectra, specify oxidation of methionine as variable modification and enzyme specificity to none.
4. Validate data by using the Scaffold Local FDR algorithm for peptide assignments and for protein assignments the Protein Prophet algorithm [7] implemented in Scaffold (Proteome Software). Filter sequence assignments with a peptide FDR of 1% and a relaxed protein FDR of 10%.

5. Filter peptide by length (8–26 amino acids) and perform sequence alignment using online tools such as T-Coffee (www.tcoffee.org/).
6. Group peptides based on: (1) number of aligned overlapping sequences and (2) assigned protein, (3) assigned species.
7. Rank peptides with a high number of overlapping sequences and assignment to proteins of the pathogenic species.

3.5 Data Validation and Further Applications

In the following, possible approaches for initial validation of the identified peptides and further applications are outlined.

1. For peptide affinity predictions, the Immune Epitope Database (IEDB) Analysis Resource (http://tools.immuneepitope.org) provides a useful tool.
2. For assessing whether the identified MHC-II-bound peptides function indeed as $CD4^+$ T cell epitopes, the peptides should be synthesized synthetically and probed against pathogen-specific T cells. For this, activated or memory T cells from infected hosts (or T cells from TCR-transgenic mouse models, if available) are stimulated with antigen-presenting cells that are loaded with the peptides, and the response of the T cells is assessed by standard immunological methods that assess T cell activation, proliferation, and/or effector functions. The relative frequency of epitope-specific T cells within the repertoire of pathogen-specific can also be determined [6, 8].
3. Knowing the pathogen-derived T cell epitopes enables the generation of MHC-tetramers to investigate the endogenous repertoire of pathogen-specific T cells in immune hosts, but importantly also in pre-immune hosts where precursor frequencies are usually very low [9].
4. The protective capacity of the identified peptide antigens may initially be assessed in preclinical studies using experimental vaccination approaches in animal models [6, 8]. Protective potential is a prerequisite for a fungal antigen to serve as a vaccine candidate.
5. The identification of protective fungal T cell antigens is also an important step in the development of immunotherapeutic strategies against fungal infections, such as adoptive T cell therapy, which is explored in transplant recipients to restore the lacking T cell function [10–13].

4 Notes

1. DC^{1940} cells are $CD8\alpha^+$-like DC cell line derived from tumors of CD11c-SV40-eGFP transgenic mice [14]. They grow independently of any growth factor and express GFP in a constitutive

manner. Keep the cells at a density of 10^5–10^6 cells/ml. Detach the cells with 5 mM EDTA in PBS. After collecting the cells, wash them once in medium to remove traces of EDTA.

2. The yeast cell concentration corresponding to OD_{600} = 1 should be determined experimentally by counting the yeast cells under the microscope and by enumerating the colony-forming units on YPD agar.
3. The optimal duration of infection should be determined experimentally by assessing the peak of antigen presentation using T cell activation as a readout. Likewise, the infection dose may be modified to induce maximal antigen presentation.
4. The lysate may be run over the column cyclically using a pump (flow rate 1–2 ml/min, overnight). In this case, the first thing in the morning of day 2 is to run the lysate through the column linearly and to collect the flow through in a 50 ml conical tube. Store the flow through at −20 °C.
5. Washing first with PBS and afterward with H_2O is helpful to remove the detergent, which is very sticky.
6. Addition of 10% TFA for the first elution of the column helps to avoid any buffering effect of the sepharose and the bound proteins.
7. Fill the Amicon tube and filter with 0.2% TFA, incubate overnight. Empty the tube and centrifuge at 4,000 rpm.
8. Use high-quality Eppendorf tubes rather than low binding tubes at this step. Low binding tubes may leak the coating if they are used with acidic solutions.
9. Gradient length is optimized for medium complex peptide mixture. Longer and shallower gradients might be used for samples with higher complexity.
10. High accuracy precursor spectra are prerequisite and high accuracy fragment mass spectra are beneficial and accelerate database searches. The use of different fragmentation techniques (e.g., CID, HCD, ETD, EThCD, etc.) is providing additional sequence information [15]. Technical replicates in combination with time-dependent exclusion lists of already sequenced precursor signals can increase sequence coverage.
11. The usage of species-specific sequence databases could accelerate data analysis and increase the sensitivity.

Acknowledgments

We would like to thank Prof. Stefan Stevanović for technical advice and suggestions. Work in the LeibundGut-laboratory is supported by the Swiss National Science Foundation, the Gebert Rüf Foundation, the Promedica Foundation, and the University of Zürich.

References

1. Nanjappa SG, Heninger E, Wuthrich M, Gasper DJ, Klein BS (2012) Tc17 cells mediate vaccine immunity against lethal fungal pneumonia in immune deficient hosts lacking CD4+ T cells. PLoS Pathog 8:e1002771. doi:10.1371/journal.ppat.1002771
2. Cassone A, Casadevall A (2012) Recent progress in vaccines against fungal diseases. Curr Opin Microbiol 15:427–433. doi:10.1016/j.mib.2012.04.004
3. Schmidt CS, White CJ, Ibrahim AS, Filler SG, Fu Y, Yeaman MR et al (2012) NDV-3, a recombinant alum-adjuvanted vaccine for Candida and *Staphylococcus aureus*, is safe and immunogenic in healthy adults. Vaccine 30:7594–7600. doi:10.1016/j.vaccine.2012.10.038
4. Lemmel C, Stevanovic S (2003) The use of HPLC-MS in T-cell epitope identification. Methods 29:248–259
5. Hillen N, Stevanovic S (2006) Contribution of mass spectrometry-based proteomics to immunology. Expert Rev Proteomics 3:653–664. doi:10.1586/14789450.3.6.653
6. Bär E, Gladiator A, Bastidas S, Roschitzki B, Acha-Orbea H, Oxenius A et al (2012) A novel Th cell epitope of *Candida albicans* mediates protection from fungal infection. J Immunol 188:5636–5643. doi:10.4049/jimmunol.1200594
7. Nesvizhskii AI, Keller A, Kolker E, Aebersold R (2003) A statistical model for identifying proteins by tandem mass spectrometry. Anal Chem 75:4646–4658
8. Wuthrich M, Brandhorst TT, Sullivan TD, Filutowicz H, Sterkel A, Stewart D et al (2015) Calnexin induces expansion of antigen-specific CD4(+) T cells that confer immunity to fungal ascomycetes via conserved epitopes. Cell Host Microbe 17:452–465. doi:10.1016/j.chom.2015.02.009
9. Moon JJ, Chu HH, Pepper M, McSorley SJ, Jameson SC, Kedl RM et al (2007) Naive CD4(+) T cell frequency varies for different epitopes and predicts repertoire diversity and response magnitude. Immunity 27:203–213. doi:10.1016/j.immuni.2007.07.007
10. Perruccio K, Tosti A, Burchielli E, Topini F, Ruggeri L, Carotti A et al (2005) Transferring functional immune responses to pathogens after haploidentical hematopoietic transplantation. Blood 106:4397–4406. doi:10.1182/blood-2005-05-1775
11. Haque T, Wilkie GM, Taylor C, Amlot PL, Murad P, Iley A et al (2002) Treatment of Epstein-Barr-virus-positive post-transplantation lymphoproliferative disease with partly HLA-matched allogeneic cytotoxic T cells. Lancet 360:436–442. doi:10.1016/S0140-6736(02)09672-1
12. Papadopoulou A, Gerdemann U, Katari UL, Tzannou I, Liu H, Martinez C et al (2014) Activity of broad-spectrum T cells as treatment for AdV, EBV, CMV, BKV, and HHV6 infections after HSCT. Sci Transl Med 6:242ra83. doi:10.1126/scitranslmed.3008825
13. Peggs KS, Thomson K, Samuel E, Dyer G, Armoogum J, Chakraverty R et al (2011) Directly selected cytomegalovirus-reactive donor T cells confer rapid and safe systemic reconstitution of virus-specific immunity following stem cell transplantation. Clin Infect Dis 52:49–57. doi:10.1093/cid/ciq042
14. Steiner QG, Otten LA, Hicks MJ, Kaya G, Grosjean F, Saeuberli E et al (2008) In vivo transformation of mouse conventional CD8alpha+ dendritic cells leads to progressive multisystem histiocytosis. Blood 111:2073–2082. doi:10.1182/blood-2007-06-097576
15. Mommen GPM, Frese CK, Meiring HD, van Gaans-van den Brink J, de Jong APJM, van Els CACM et al (2014) Expanding the detectable HLA peptide repertoire using electron-transfer/higher-energy collision dissociation (EThcD). Proc Natl Acad Sci U S A 111:4507–4512. doi:10.1073/pnas.1321458111

Chapter 6

Intranasal Antifungal Vaccination Using DNA-Transfected Dendritic Cells

Shanjana Awasthi

Abstract

Dendritic cells are the most potent antigen-presenting cells, and are critical for the generation of an antigen-specific immune response and protective immunity. These unique features have been applied to dendritic cell-based immunization in a number of disease conditions. Our published results have demonstrated that the immunity induced by intranasal immunization with DNA-transfected dendritic cells results in reduced fungal burden, and alleviated lung tissue damage in a mouse model of pulmonary fungal infection. In this article, approaches for the preparation and characterization of DNA-transfected dendritic cells and intranasal immunization in mice are described.

Key words Dendritic cells, Genetic transfection, Antigen expression, Protective immunity, Fungal infection

1 Introduction

Dendritic cells are the most potent antigen-presenting cells, and play an important role in directing the immune responses against infectious stimuli and pathologic ligands [1, 2]. The unique features of dendritic cells have generated enormous recent interest in the field of immunology. Dendritic cells can take up pathogens and ligands, process them intracellularly, present the processed antigens on major histocompatibility complexes, migrate to lymphoid organs, and activate naive lymphocytes to generate antigen-specific immune responses. These properties have been utilized for the preparation of dendritic cell-based vaccines, immunization, and induction of an antigen-specific immune response. Dendritic cell-based immunization has shown efficacy in a number of disease conditions, including cancer (reviewed in [3–7]). Several preclinical, phase I, and phase II clinical trials have been conducted or are

Markus Kalkum and Margarita Semis (eds.), *Vaccines for Invasive Fungal Infections: Methods and Protocols*, Methods in Molecular Biology, vol. 1625, DOI 10.1007/978-1-4939-7104-6_6, © Springer Science+Business Media LLC 2017

underway [8–12]. As a result, Sipuleucel-T (trade name Provenge; Dendreon Corp, WA) was approved as the first autologous dendritic cell-based vaccine for the treatment of certain patients with advanced prostate cancer [13]. Dendritic cell-based approaches have also been tried against a number of infectious diseases for which an effective treatment or vaccine is not available, including fungal infections. The most recently published work describes the utility of dendritic cells for vaccination against *Cryptococcus gattii*, a fungal pathogen [14].

In our published studies, we utilized dendritic cells for vaccination in a mouse model of Coccidioidomycosis, a fungal infection caused by *Coccidioides spp.* A variety of factors, including the source of dendritic cells, pulsing or transfection of dendritic cells, route and dose of immunization, migration, antigen-presentation, and generation of immune responses, are important for the success of a dendritic cell-based vaccine. It is critical that the dendritic cells present the protective antigens or epitopes, and are capable of inducing an antigen-specific protective immune response. Many techniques, including the pulsing or genetic transfection of dendritic cells with isolated RNA, purified proteins, and DNA, have been employed. Using a commercially available nonviral transfection reagent, we transfected the dendritic cells with a plasmid DNA carrying a cDNA insert for *Coccidioides*-derived protective Antigen 2/proline-rich antigen (Ag2/PRA) [15–18]. After characterization of dendritic cells for their immunophenotype, viability, morphology, and presentation of the protective epitope, we prophylactically administered the DNA-transfected dendritic cells and challenged the mice with live arthroconidia of *Coccidioides* [19]. Our results demonstrated that the prophylactic administration of DNA-transfected dendritic cells encoding *Coccidioides*-Ag2/PRA can stimulate protective immune response, which results in suppression of fungal burden and alleviation of lung pathology [19, 20]. These approaches have been used or cited in published reports from other investigators [21–41]. This article provides procedure details of the transient transfection of dendritic cells with DNA, characterization of DNA-transfected dendritic cells, and intranasal immunization.

2 Materials

Prepare all solutions in sterile, commercially available endotoxin-free water or cell culture grade reagents. Store all reagents, solutions, and kits under the conditions recommended by the manufacturer, unless indicated otherwise. All animal procedures, safety precautions, and waste disposal regulations should be followed per the institutional guidelines.

2.1 Transient Transfection of Dendritic Cells with Plasmid DNA Carrying Coccidioides-Ag2/PRA-cDNA

1. Cells: Primary mouse bone marrow-derived dendritic cells or JAWS II dendritic cells are harvested and maintained, per the methods described elsewhere [16, 42]. Typical morphological characteristics of dendritic cells and viability (>95%) are determined by Diff Quik staining (Dade Behring, IL) of cytospin preparations of cells and trypan blue staining of cells, respectively.
2. Plasmid DNA: Plasmid DNAs are scaled up and purified using an endotoxin-free plasmid DNA extraction kit. Purified plasmid DNA is analyzed for the *Coccidioides*-Ag2/PRA-cDNA insert using restriction enzyme analysis. Any contamination with endotoxin is determined using the Limulus amebocyte lysate assay kit.
3. TransIT-TKO transfection reagent (Mirus Bio, WI).
4. Dulbecco's minimum essential medium (DMEM).
5. 24-well cell culture plate.
6. 5% CO_2 incubator at 37 °C.
7. 1.5 ml sterile microfuge tube.
8. Plasmid pHYG-EGFP (Clontech, CA) encoding enhanced green fluorescent protein (EGFP).
9. Complete culture medium for the maintenance of JAWS II dendritic cells: Alpha MEM containing ribonucleosides, deoxyribonucleosides, 4 mM L-glutamine, 5 ng/ml recombinant mouse granulocyte macrophage colony-stimulating factor, 20% fetal bovine serum, 1× penicillin-streptomycin mix (Invitrogen Thermo Fisher, MA), and 50 μg/ml gentamicin.
10. Complete culture medium for primary mouse bone marrow-derived dendritic cells: RPMI 1640 medium containing 10 mM *N*-2-hydroxyethylpiperazine-*N'*-2-ethanesulfonic acid, 1% MEM nonessential amino acids, 50 μM β-mercaptoethanol, 10 ng/ml recombinant mouse interleukin-4, 10 ng/ml recombinant mouse granulocyte macrophage colony-stimulating factor, 10% fetal bovine serum, 1× penicillin-streptomycin mix, and 50 μg/ml gentamicin.

2.2 Characterization of DNA-Transfected Dendritic Cells: Viability, Expression of Ag2/PRA Protein, and Immunophenotype

1. Cell culture grade Dulbecco's phosphate buffered saline (DPBS).
2. Centrifuge.
3. Cell lysis buffer: 1% Igepal CA-630, 0.1% sodium dodecyl sulfate, 1 mM ethylenediaminetetraacetic acid, and protease inhibitors (1.1 μM leupeptin, 1 μM pepstatin, and 0.2 mM phenylmethylsulfonyl fluoride).
4. Trypan blue stain.
5. Bicinchoninic acid (BCA) assay kit.

6. Tris-buffered saline (TBS): 20 mM Tris–HCl, pH 7.5, 150 mM NaCl.
7. Blocking buffer: 0.05% Tween 20 and 5% bovine serum albumin in TBS.
8. Ag2/PRA-specific antibody.
9. Alkaline phosphatase (AP)-conjugate substrate kit (Bio-Rad, CA).
10. Staining buffer: 1% heat-inactivated fetal bovine serum and 0.09% sodium azide in DPBS.
11. Fc block™.
12. Fluorescein isothiocyanate-, phycoerythrin-, or allophycocyanin-conjugated antibodies specific to the cell surface markers.

2.3 Intranasal Administration of DNA-Transfected Dendritic Cells in Mice

Age- and sex-matched, 5-to-6-week-old syngeneic mice.

3 Methods

3.1 Transient Transfection of Dendritic Cells with Plasmid DNA Carrying Coccidioides-Ag2/PRA-cDNA

1. Thaw endotoxin-free, characterized plasmid DNA on ice. Thaw TransIT-TKO transfection reagent at room temperature.
2. Harvest dendritic cells by gentle scraping and suspend the cells in DMEM. Seed 1×10^6 cells/100 µl per well in a 24-well cell culture plate and incubate at 37 °C for 30 min in a 5% CO_2 incubator.
3. Prepare the transfection reagent: DNA mix. Vortex the stock vial of transfection reagent. Aliquot 150 µl of DMEM in a 1.5 ml sterile microfuge tube, and add 4 µl of TransIT-TKO reagent. Vortex mix and incubate at room temperature for 5 min.
4. Add 2 µg of plasmid DNA to the diluted transfection reagent dropwise. Do not vortex at this stage. Invert mix the transfection reagent: DNA. Incubate the transfection reagent: DNA mix at room temperature for 5 min. Optimize the transfection reagent: DNA ratio at the same time (*see* **Note 1**).
5. Add transfection reagent: DNA mix to all corners and the centers of the wells with seeded cells for equal distribution. Incubate the cells at 37 °C for 4 h in a 5% CO_2 incubator.
6. Add an equal volume (250 µl) of complete culture medium containing antibiotics, growth factors, and fetal bovine

serum, used for the maintenance of dendritic cells, and continue with the incubation of cells at 37 °C in a 5% CO_2 incubator (*see* **Note 2**).

7. To analyze the transfection efficiency of a particular lot of transfection reagent, transfect one well of cells with plasmid pHYG-EGFP using the protocol described above, and monitor the green fluorescence with fluorescence microscopy daily (*see* **Note 3**).

3.2 Characterization of DNA-Transfected Dendritic Cells: Viability, Expression of Ag2/PRA Protein, and Immunophenotype

Before immunizing mice, determine the viability, expression of Ag2/PRA protein, and immunophenotype of DNA-transfected dendritic cells.

1. Collect nonadherent cells by pipetting and washing the wells with sterile, room temperature warmed, DPBS. Gently scrape the adherent cells with a pipette tip or other preferred methods, and pool with nonadherent cells. Wash the well with DPBS to collect remaining cells.
2. Centrifuge the pooled cell suspension of nonadherent and adherent cells at room temperature. Discard supernatant. Wash the cells twice with DPBS and prepare the cell lysate or suspension for further characterization or immunization (*see* **Note 4**).
3. Determine the viability using the trypan blue staining method. About 80–90% of the cells should be viable.
4. Prepare cell lysate in lysis buffer and store at −20 °C for the analysis of expression of *Coccidioides*-Ag2/PRA protein by dot immunoblotting.
5. Dot immunoblotting: Wash the cells with DPBS twice and scrape them using lysis buffer. Determine the protein concentration in cell lysates using a BCA assay kit. Load various amounts (0, 1.75, 2.5, 5.0, 10.0, and 20.0 μg) of cell lysate protein onto nitrocellulose membrane pre-wetted in TBS. Block the nonspecific sites in blocking buffer, and incubate with Ag2/PRA-specific antibody (1:1000), followed by secondary AP-labeled antibody (1:10,000) (*see* **Note 5**).
6. Determine the immunophenotype of cells by staining the cells with fluorochrome-conjugated antibodies specific to dendritic cell markers: Aliquot 0.5–1 × 10^6 cells per 100 μl of staining buffer. Add 1 μg Fc block™ to the cells and incubate on ice for 15 min in the dark. Add 1 μg each of fluorescein isothiocyanate-, phycoerythrin-, or allophycocyanin-conjugated antibodies specific to the cell surface markers. Incubate the cells for 30–45 min on ice in the dark, wash thrice with staining buffer, fix, and analyze using a flow cytometer. Use isotype control antibody-stained or unstained cells as controls (*see* **Notes 6** and **7**).

3.3 Intranasal Administration of DNA-Transfected Dendritic Cells in Mice

1. Acclimate the mice for 1 week prior to immunization. Anesthetize the mice at the time of immunization.
2. An aliquot of DNA-transfected dendritic cells (1–2.0 × 10^6 cells suspended in 30–40 μl) is prepared for intranasal immunization.
3. Gently hold the mice in an upright position. Use a 20–200 μl pipette tip to slowly instill the DNA-transfected dendritic cells alternately in each nostril.
4. Monitor the breathing in these mice during instillation.
5. Hold the mice upright for a few minutes, and lay them down at a 45° angle in their cages after the instillation procedure.
6. Monitor the mice for 30 min or until they are awake, before moving them to the animal housing area.

The procedures and steps described above are pertinent to the preparation and characterization of *Coccidioides*-Ag2/PRA-expressing dendritic cells and the immunization of mice. Refer to our published articles [16, 19] for additional procedures and downstream applications, such as in vivo SPECT/CT or PET imaging, an assessment of immune responses, and the efficacy of dendritic cell-based immunization against infectious challenge with live *Coccidioides* arthroconidia.

4 Notes

1. Use the transfection reagent: DNA ratio and duration of transfection that provide maximum expression of EGFP without a significant loss of cell viability.
2. Although the culture medium for the maintenance of JAWSII dendritic cells and primary mouse bone marrow-derived dendritic cells differs [15, 16, 19, 42], this transfection method has been used for both cell types.
3. Check each lot of commercially available transfection reagent for an assessment of transfection efficiency. This protocol has provided us with about 30–50% transfection efficiency among different experiments performed on separate occasions.
4. The number of cells to be used for immunization can be adjusted based on transfection efficiency between the experiments and with the use of different batches of transfection reagent.
5. Include a cell lysate of non-transfected cells as a control.
6. Determine the staining using the standard flow cytometric analysis method.
7. The functional ability of DNA-transfected dendritic cells can be tested by incubating the cells with lipopolysaccharide stimuli

and by studying the changes in immunophenotype and cytokine secretion with flow cytometry and commercially available ELISA kits, respectively.

Acknowledgments

The author acknowledges funding support from the San Antonio Area Foundation, San Antonio, TX (2003–2004) and Oklahoma Center for Advancement of Science and Technology, Oklahoma City, OK (2007–2010) for the research conducted on dendritic cell-based immunization for coccidioidomycosis. Editorial support from Ms. Kathy Kyler, Staff Editor at the University of Oklahoma Health Sciences Center, is appreciated.

References

1. Steinman RM (1991) The dendritic cell system and its role in immunogenicity. Annu Rev Immunol 9:271–296
2. Rescigno M, Winzler C, Delia D, Mutini C, Lutz M, Ricciardi-Castagnoli P (1997) Dendritic cell maturation is required for initiation of the immune response. J Leukoc Biol 61(4):415–421
3. Ahmed MS, Bae YS (2016) Dendritic cell-based immunotherapy for rheumatoid arthritis: from bench to bedside. Immune Netw 16(1):44–51
4. Constantino J, Gomes C, Falcao A, Cruz MT, Neves BM (2016) Antitumor dendritic cell-based vaccines: lessons from 20 years of clinical trials and future perspectives. Transl Res 168:74–95
5. Bagirova M, Allahverdiyev AM, Abamor ES, Ullah I, Cosar G, Aydogdu M, Senturk H, Ergenoglu B (2016) Overview of dendritic cell-based vaccine development for leishmaniasis. Parasite Immunol 38(11):651–662
6. Cockburn IA, Zavala F (2016) Dendritic cell function and antigen presentation in malaria. Curr Opin Immunol 40:1–6
7. Miller E, Bhardwaj N (2014) Advances in dendritic cell immunotherapies for HIV-1 infection. Expert Opin Biol Ther 14(11):1545–1549
8. Pyzer AR, Avigan DE, Rosenblatt J (2014) Clinical trials of dendritic cell-based cancer vaccines in hematologic malignancies. Hum Vaccin Immunother 10(11):3125–3131
9. Gursel DB, Schlaff CD, Boockvar JA (2012) Trials and tribulations of cancer immunotherapy: the dendritic cell vaccine shows promise in a phase I glioblastoma multiforme trial. Neurosurgery 71(6):N19–N21
10. Li S, Roberts S, Plebanski M, Gouillou M, Spelman T, Latour P, Jackson D, Brown L, Sparrow RL, Prince HM, Hart D, Loveland BE, Gowans EJ (2012) Induction of multi-functional T cells in a phase I clinical trial of dendritic cell immunotherapy in hepatitis C virus infected individuals. PLoS One 7(8):e39368
11. Curti A, Tosi P, Comoli P, Terragna C, Ferri E, Cellini C, Massaia M, D'Addio A, Giudice V, Di Bello C, Cavo M, Conte R, Gugliotta G, Baccarani M, Lemoli RM (2007) Phase I/II clinical trial of sequential subcutaneous and intravenous delivery of dendritic cell vaccination for refractory multiple myeloma using patient-specific tumour idiotype protein or idiotype (VDJ)-derived class I-restricted peptides. Br J Haematol 139(3):415–424
12. Baratelli F, Takedatsu H, Hazra S, Peebles K, Luo J, Kurimoto PS, Zeng G, Batra RK, Sharma S, Dubinett SM, Lee JM (2008) Pre-clinical characterization of GMP grade CCL21-gene modified dendritic cells for application in a phase I trial in non-small cell lung cancer. J Transl Med 6:38
13. Cheever MA, Higano CS (2011) PROVENGE (Sipuleucel-T) in prostate cancer: the first FDA-approved therapeutic cancer vaccine. Clin Cancer Res 17(11):3520–3526
14. Ueno K, Kinjo Y, Okubo Y, Aki K, Urai M, Kaneko Y, Shimizu K, Wang DN, Okawara A, Nara T, Ohkouchi K, Mizuguchi Y, Kawamoto S, Kamei K, Ohno H, Niki Y, Shibuya K, Miyazaki Y (2015) Dendritic cell-based immunization ameliorates pulmonary infection with

highly virulent *Cryptococcus gattii*. Infect Immun 83(4):1577–1586

15. Awasthi S, Cox RA (2003) Transfection of murine dendritic cell line (JAWS II) by a non-viral transfection reagent. BioTechniques 35(3):600–602, 604
16. Vilekar P, Awasthi V, Lagisetty P, King C, Shankar N, Awasthi S (2010) *In vivo* trafficking and immunostimulatory potential of an intranasally-administered primary dendritic cell-based vaccine. BMC Immunol 11:60
17. Zhu Y, Yang C, Magee DM, Cox RA (1996) Molecular cloning and characterization of *Coccidioides immitis* antigen 2 cDNA. Infect Immun 64(7):2695–2699
18. Peng T, Shubitz L, Simons J, Perrill R, Orsborn KI, Galgiani JN (2002) Localization within a proline-rich antigen (Ag2/PRA) of protective antigenicity against infection with *Coccidioides immitis* in mice. Infect Immun 70(7):3330–3335
19. Awasthi S, Awasthi V, Magee DM, Coalson JJ (2005) Efficacy of antigen 2/proline-rich antigen cDNA-transfected dendritic cells in immunization of mice against *Coccidioides posadasii*. J Immunol 175(6):3900–3906
20. Awasthi S (2007) Dendritic cell-based vaccine against *Coccidioides* infection. Ann N Y Acad Sci 1111:269–274
21. Hu B, Zhang Y, Zeng Q, Han Q, Zhang L, Liu M, Li X (2014) Intravitreal injection of ranibizumab and CTGF shRNA improves retinal gene expression and microvessel ultrastructure in a rodent model of diabetes. Int J Mol Sci 15(1):1606–1624
22. Banerjee P, Biswas A, Biswas T (2008) Porin-incorporated liposome induces toll-like receptors 2- and 6-dependent maturation and type 1 response of dendritic cell. Int Immunol 20(12):1551–1563
23. Hillyer L, Whitley C, Olver A, Webster M, Steevels T, Woodward B (2008) Adoptively transferred dendritic cells restore primary cell-mediated inflammatory competence to acutely malnourished weanling mice. Am J Pathol 172(2):378–385
24. Guo H, Hao J, Wu C, Shi Y, Zhao XY, Fang DC (2007) A novel peptide-nucleotide dual vaccine of human telomerase reverse transcriptase induces a potent cytotoxic T-cell response *in vivo*. Biochem Biophys Res Commun 357(4):1090–1095
25. Hu Y, Li M, Lu B, Wang X, Chen C, Zhang M (2016) Corticotropin-releasing factor augments LPS-induced immune/inflammatory responses in JAWSII cells. Immunol Res 64(2):540–547
26. Tang J, Yin R, Tian Y, Huang Z, Shi J, Fu X, Wang L, Wu Y, Hao F, Ni B (2012) A novel self-assembled nanoparticle vaccine with HIV-1 Tat_{49-57}/HPV16 $E7_{49-57}$ fusion peptide and GM-CSF DNA elicits potent and prolonged CD8(+) T cell-dependent anti-tumor immunity in mice. Vaccine 30(6):1071–1082
27. Chan YH, Chiang MF, Tsai YC, ST S, Chen MH, Hou MS, Lin KI (2009) Absence of the transcriptional repressor blimp-1 in hematopoietic lineages reveals its role in dendritic cell homeostatic development and function. J Immunol 183(11):7039–7046
28. Cutler JE, Deepe GS Jr, Klein BS (2007) Advances in combating fungal diseases: vaccines on the threshold. Nat Rev Microbiol 5(1):13–28
29. Capilla J, Clemons KV, Stevens DA (2007) Animal models: an important tool in mycology. Med Mycol 45(8):657–684
30. Jiang X, Shen C, Rey-Ladino J, Yu H, Brunham RC (2008) Characterization of murine dendritic cell line JAWS II and primary bone marrow-derived dendritic cells in *Chlamydia muridarum* antigen presentation and induction of protective immunity. Infect Immun 76(6):2392–2401
31. Tarcha EJ, Basrur V, Hung CY, Gardner MJ, Cole GT (2006) Multivalent recombinant protein vaccine against coccidioidomycosis. Infect Immun 74(10):5802–5813
32. Baumjohann D, Lutz MB (2006) Non-invasive imaging of dendritic cell migration *in vivo*. Immunobiology 211(6–8):587–597
33. Zhou H, Zhang D, Wang Y, Dai M, Zhang L, Liu W, Liu D, Tan H, Huang Z (2006) Induction of CML28-specific cytotoxic T cell responses using co-transfected dendritic cells with CML28 DNA vaccine and SOCS1 small interfering RNA expression vector. Biochem Biophys Res Commun 347(1):200–207
34. McCormick S, Santosuosso M, Small CL, Shaler CR, Zhang X, Jeyanathan M, Mu J, Takenaka S, Ngai P, Gauldie J, Wan Y, Xing Z (2008) Mucosally delivered dendritic cells activate T cells independently of IL-12 and endogenous APCs. J Immunol 181(4):2356–2367
35. Pham W, Kobukai S, Hotta C, Gore JC (2009) Dendritic cells: therapy and imaging. Expert Opin Biol Ther 9(5):539–564
36. Clemons KV, Capilla J, Stevens DA (2007) Experimental animal models of coccidioidomycosis. Ann N Y Acad Sci 1111:208–224
37. Dekaban GA, Hamilton AM, Fink CA, Au B, de Chickera SN, Ribot EJ, Foster PJ (2013) Tracking and evaluation of dendritic cell migra-

tion by cellular magnetic resonance imaging. Wiley Interdiscip Rev Nanomed Nanobiotechnol 5(5):469–483

38. Hung CY, Hurtgen BJ, Bellecourt M, Sanderson SD, Morgan EL, Cole GT (2012) An agonist of human complement fragment C5a enhances vaccine immunity against *Coccidioides* infection. Vaccine 30(31):4681–4690
39. Sagar D, Foss C, El Baz R, Pomper MG, Khan ZK, Jain P (2012) Mechanisms of dendritic cell trafficking across the blood-brain barrier. J Neuroimmune Pharmacol 7(1):74–94
40. Wang J, Tian M, Zhang H (2011) PET molecular imaging in stem cell therapy for neurological diseases. Eur J Nucl Med Mol Imaging 38(10):1926–1938
41. Pham GH, Iglesias BV, Gosselin EJ (2014) Fc receptor-targeting of immunogen as a strategy for enhanced antigen loading, vaccination, and protection using intranasally administered antigen-pulsed dendritic cells. Vaccine 32(40):5212–5220
42. Awasthi S, Magee DM (2004) Differences in expression of cell surface co-stimulatory molecules, toll-like receptor genes and secretion of IL-12 by bone marrow-derived dendritic cells from susceptible and resistant mouse strains in response to *Coccidioides posadasii*. Cell Immunol 231(1–2):49–55

Chapter 7

DNAhsp65 Vaccine as Therapy against Paracoccidioidomycosis

Alice M. Ribeiro, André C. Amaral, Maria Sueli S. Felipe, and Anamelia L. Bocca

Abstract

The conventional treatment for fungal diseases usually shows long periods of therapy and the high frequency of relapses and sequels. New strategies of the treatment are necessary. We have shown that the *Mycobacterium leprae* HSP65 gene can be successfully used as therapy against murine Paracoccidioidomycosis (PCM). Here, we described the methodology of DNAhsp65 immunotherapy in mice infected with the dimorphic fungus *Paracoccidioides brasiliensis*, one of PCM agent, evaluating cytokines levels, fungal burden, and lung injury. Our results provide a new prospective on the immunotherapy of mycosis.

Key words Paracoccidioidomycosis, DNA vaccine, HSP65, Systemic mycosis, Immunotherapy, *Paracoccioides brasiliensis*

1 Introduction

DNA vaccination is an encouraging alternative to traditional protein-based vaccines to induce efficient and protective immune responses, especially in diseases that involve the depression of cellular immune response. DNA vaccines offer several advantages over traditional vaccines, including better stability, rapid and low-cost production, and to elicit immune protection for a wide variety of infectious diseases [1, 2]. One molecule that has shown efficiency in inducing innate and adaptive immunity is the Heat-Shock Protein (HSP), conferring prophylaxis or immunotherapy against a great variety of illnesses, including tumors, autoimmune diseases, and tuberculosis [3, 4]. The DNAhsp65 vaccine from *Mycobacterium leprae* has conferred protection on mice against challenges from *M. tuberculosis* [5], *Leishmania major* [6], Paracoccidioidomycosis [7], and chromoblastomycosis [8]. Its effects are associated with a strong Th1 immune response and downregulation of Th2 cytokines.

Markus Kalkum and Margarita Semis (eds.), *Vaccines for Invasive Fungal Infections: Methods and Protocols*, Methods in Molecular Biology, vol. 1625, DOI 10.1007/978-1-4939-7104-6_7, © Springer Science+Business Media LLC 2017

Our research group demonstrated that hsp65 DNA vaccine induced a strong prophylactic response in mice experimentally infected with the dimorphic fungus *Paracoccidioides brasiliensis* (Pb) [7], showing Th1 polarization and efficient macrophage activation, which was able to contain fungal dissemination and disease progression.

P. brasiliensis infection, known as paracocciodiomycosis (PCM), is a chronic granulomatous disease and the most prevalent systemic endemic mycosis in South America, with a high incidence in Brazil, Colombia, Venezuela, and Argentina [9, 10]. As a result of inefficient cellular immune response the conventional therapy is long-term, which results in high toxicity, low efficiency, and relapses. Immunization of mice with DNAhsp65 vaccine before subsequent challenges with *P. brasiliensis* induced a reduction in fungal burden, modulation of the immune response toward a Th1 profile, cellular proliferation reestablishment, and the reduction of immunopathology in the lungs. These results provide a new prospect for the development of DNA-immunotherapy of PCM.

2 Materials (*See* Note 1)

2.1 Paracoccidioidomycosis Murine Model

The antifungal therapeutic activity of DNAhsp65 in fungal infection is determined in murine model.

1. Isogenic male Balb/c mice aged between 6 and 8 weeks. $n = 5$ animals per treatment group (*see* **Note 2**).
2. Yeast Peptone Dextrose (YPD) liquid medium: 2% peptone, 1% yeast extract, 2% glucose (w/v).
3. *Paracoccidioides brasiliensis* (Pb)18 fungal strain cultured for 5 days at 37 °C under 153 × *g* in 100 mL of sterile YPD liquid medium.
4. Phosphate Buffer Solution (PBS): NaCl 8 g, KCl 0.2 g, KH_2PO_4 0.122 g, $Na_2HPO_4.7H_2O$ 1.716 g, and distilled water 1 L.
5. Janus Green B vital dye.
6. Anesthetic solution: 80 mg/kg of ketamine and 10 mg/kg of xylazine (200 μL per animal).
7. Neubauer chamber.

2.2 DNAhsp65 Plasmid Construction

The DNAhsp65 vaccine is obtained as previously described by Farmacore Biotechnology Ltd. (Ribeirão Preto, S.P., Brazil) [11].

1. pVAX1 as vector (Invitrogen, Carlsbad, CA, USA).
2. The 3.3 kb fragment of *M. leprae* hsp65 subcloned into Bam HI and Not-I restriction sites in pVAX1 vector (Invitrogen, Carlsbad, CA, USA).

3. DH5α *E. coli* cultured in LB liquid medium containing kanamicin (50 μg/mL).
4. Endofree Plasmid Giga kit (Qiagen, Valencia, CA, USA).
5. Equipment to RNA/DNA quantification.
6. LPS quantification kit (QCL-1000® Chromogenic LAL Endpoint Assay Cambrex Corporation, Walkersville, MD, U.S.A.).

2.3 Evaluation of DNAhsp65 Treatment

Colony-forming units assay and histopathological analysis of lungs are used to investigate the antifungal effect of the DNAhsp65.

2.3.1 Fungal Burden Recovery

1. *P. brasiliensis* 192 (Pb192) filtrate [12] (*see* **Note 3**).
2. YPD liquid medium.
3. Petri dishes each containing 20 mL of Brain Heart Infusion solid culture medium supplemented with (v/v) 4% horse serum, 5% Pb192 filtrate, and gentamycin 40 mg/L (three Petri dishes for each animal).
4. Tissue grinder, Petri dish, and two pairs of sterile scissors and surgical pins for each group of treated animals.
5. PBS 1L, pH 7.0.

2.3.2 Histopathological Analysis

1. Surgical scissors, pins, and conical tubes to collect the lung tissue for each experimental group of animals.
2. Formalin neutral buffer 10%.
3. Paraffin, alcohol to dehydrate and tissue cassette.
4. Hematoxylin and eosin, silver and Masson's trichrome.

2.4 Lympho-proliferation Assay

The immune response activation after the DNAhsp65 treatment is performed by splenocyte culture to determine cytokine production, anti-specific HSP antibodies, and nitric oxide production.

1. Sterile surgical scissor and pin.
2. Petri dish containing 10 mL of RPMI supplemented medium prepared with 2 mM l-glutamine, 1 mM sodium pyruvate, 5% nonessential amino acids, 50μM 2 beta-mercaptoethanol, streptomycin (100 g/mL), and 5% fetal bovine serum.
3. 96-well plates v bottom.
4. Concanavalin A (Type IV–4 μg/mL).
5. F1 fraction of Pb18 yeast cells as described previously [13], *see* Subheading 3.5, **step 2**.
6. Sterile distilled water.

7. Solution of chloroform and methanol (2:1, v/v) at room temperature.
8. 1 N NaOH solution.
9. Ethanol p.a. grade.
10. Acetone.
11. Diethyl ether.
12. [H^3]-thymidine.
13. Incubator at 37 °C under 5% CO_2.
14. Liquid scintillation counter (Beckman Instruments Inc., Fullerton, CA, U.S.A.).

2.5 Cytokine Quantification Assay

The cytokines are quantified using commercial Enzyme Linked Immune Sorbent Assay (ELISA) kits.

1. Commercial kits to detect Th1, Th2, and Th17 cytokines.

2.6 Anti-HSP65-Specific Antibodies

Measure the specific IgG1 and IgG2a isotypes by ELISA.

1. 96-well high binding protein plate flat bottom.
2. rHSP65 protein (250 ng/100 μL well).
3. 1% bovine serum albumin in PBS.
4. PBS-T: 0.05%Tween 20 in PBS.
5. Peroxidase-labeled antibodies specific for mouse IgG1 or IgG2a isotypes.
6. o-phenylenediamine.
7. H_2SO_4 2N (stop solution).
8. Microplate ELISA reader at 490 nm.

2.7 Nitric Oxide (NO) Production Assays

NO_2 concentration in culture supernatants is used as an indicator of NO generation. The concentration of nitrite (NO_2^-) in spleen cell supernatants is measured by Griess assay, as described previously [14].

1. Solution 1: 1% sulfanilamide solution.
2. Solution 2: 0.1% naphthylethylene diamine dihydrochloride (NEED) in 5% H_3PO_4 solution.
3. Griess reagent prepared v/v (1:1 ratio) of solutions 1 and 2 (*see* **Note 4**).
4. Nitrite reductase buffer: 1 mM NADPH, 10 mM FAD, and 4 U/mL nitrate reductase in potassium phosphate 0.1 M pH 7.5.
5. Serial dilutions of $NaNO_2$ in PBS in a range of 1–200 μM.
6. Microplate ELISA reader at 540 nm.

3 Methods

3.1 DNAhsp65 Plasmid Construction

1. Digest the pVAX1 vector with BamHI and NotI and insert a fragment of the *Mycobacterium leprae* hsp65 gene. Use the pVAX1 vector without the hsp65 insert as a control.
2. Obtain the plasmids from transformed DH5a *Escherichia coli* and purify them using the Endofree Plasmid Mega kit.
3. Subject all samples to quantification of LPS using a commercial kit (*see* **Note 5**).

3.2 Paracoccidioidomycosis Murine Infection and Treatment Design

1. Anesthetize the mice intraperitoneally with 200 μL of anesthetic solution (prepared as described in Subheading 2.1, **item 6**). Ten minutes after injecting the anesthetic, hyperextend their necks and make a 0.5 mm cut to expose the trachea at the level of the thyroid (*see* **Note 6**).
2. Prepare the Pb18 fungal suspension to infect the mice, washing the 100 mL of culture of Pb18 in YPD by centrifuging in 1.015 × *g* for 3 min. Discard the supernatant. Add 10 mL of sterile PBS. After the third wash, add 3 mL of sterile PBS and count the cells in the Neubauer chamber. Adjust the fungal suspension for 6×10^6 viable cells/mL. Assess the fungal cells' viability by counting the fungal suspension mixed in equal volume with Janus Green B vital dye [15] and note that it must be higher than 80% (*see* **Note 7**).
3. Inject 50 μL of the Pb18 fungal suspension containing 3×10^5 viable fungal cells using a 26-gauge needle. The incisions must be immediately saturated using surgical thread and the animals should be kept in a warm place until the anesthetic effect passes (*see* **Note 8**).
4. Wait 30 days for the establishment of the infection. The animals should be kept in a 12 h dark/light cycle with water ad libitum (*see* **Note 9**).
5. Group five mice per treatment group in each polypropylene cage. To evaluate the therapeutic efficacy of DNAhsp65 vaccine, four groups should be formed: (a) Noninfected (noninfected animals, control receiving 50 μL of PBS as placebo); (b) Infected (infected animals, control receiving 50 μL of PBS as placebo); (c) Empty plasmid (infected animals, receiving 100 μL of plasmid containing DNAhsp65); (d) DNAhsp65 within plasmid (infected animals, receiving 100 μL of plasmid containing DNAhsp65).
6. All different treatments should be given by the intramuscular (i.m.) route. Initiate the treatment regimen after 30 days of infection with the Pb18 fungal strain and run it for 45 days using one dose of different treatments at day 30 and one dose

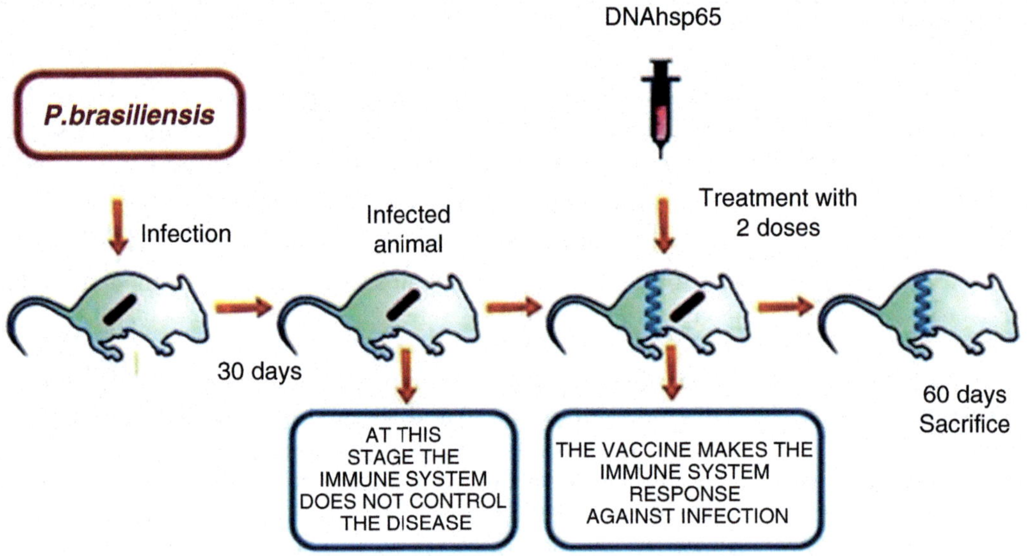

Fig. 1 Scheme of the experimental treatment design

at day 45. Then, 15 days after the administration of the last dose, euthanize the animals to evaluate the efficacy of the treatment. The scheme of the treatment is presented in Fig. 1.

3.3 Investigation of DNAhsp65 Treatment

3.3.1 Fungal Burden Determination in Lungs

The therapeutic efficacy of the DNAhsp65 treatment against PCM murine model is assessed by evaluating the fungal burden recovery from lungs by the Colony-Forming Units (CFU) assay. The lungs are chosen because they are the main organs affected during the PCM infection. The procedure must be conducted in sterile conditions to avoid contamination of the culture medium (Fig. 2b).

1. Anesthetize the mice as described in Subheading 3.2**step 1**. Collect the blood for immunological analysis and proceed to euthanasia as approved by Bioethical committee (*see* **Note 2**). Wash the mice by dipping in a container with ethanol 70% to minimize contamination. In a sterile chamber, lay the mice in dorsal position over a flexible surface (polystyrene sheet, for example) to expose the thoracic region in the sterile chamber. Fix each leg with pins to facilitate opening the abdomen using sterile surgical scissors and a sterile surgical tip to collect the entire lungs. Use another pair of scissors and tip to cut one part of the lung over a sterile Petri dish. Put it in a sterile recipient to weigh. Discard the animal carcass after collection in the appropriate place.
2. Put the weighed piece of lung in the tissue grinder and add 1 mL of sterile PBS (prepared as described in Subheading 2.1**item 3**). Proceed to macerate the organ until a homogenous suspension is obtained. Collect 100 μL of the suspension

and dispose of it into a Petri dish containing supplemented BHI agar media (prepared as described in Subheading 2.3.1). Spread the volume homogenously over the plate. Seal the plate with parafilm and maintain it at 37 °C for 14 days, counting the cells daily. This procedure must be repeated for each animal from each experimental group (*see* **Note 10**).

3. Present the data as a mean of the three Petri dishes from each animal as number of fungal cells per tissue gram.

3.3.2 Histopathological Analysis

1. Animals from each group should be euthanized at the scheduled times; remove lung fragments, fix in formalin 10% for 6 h, dehydrate in alcohol, and embed in paraffin.
2. Stain serial 5 μm sections with hematoxylin and eosin (H&E) and Masson's trichrome for lesion analysis and stain with silver for fungal counts.
3. Capture the histopathological images using a camera adapted to an optical microscope (Fig. 2c, d).

3.4 Lymphocyte Proliferation and Cytokine Quantification Assay

Total spleen cell proliferative responses are studied by $[H^3]$-thymidine incorporation, as previously described [16] (*see* **Note 11**) (Fig. 2e). The splenocytes are collected and cultured as follows.

1. Disrupt spleen cells in supplemented RPMI 1640 and wash them twice in RPMI medium; count, add to 96-well plates at a cell density of 3×10^5 cells/well, and subsequently stimulate with Concanavalin A (4 μg/mL) and F1 fraction of Pb18 yeast cells. Perform the experiments in triplicate at a final volume of 200 μL/well.
2. Obtain the F1 fraction of Pb18 yeast cells as described previously [13]. Disrupt the yeast cells by ultrasound and collect the walls, washing them three times with distilled water by centrifugation. Extract the lipids by soaking the walls in chloroform/methanol (2:1, v/v) at room temperature for 2 h. Re-extract the insoluble cell residue three more times; we named the resulting insoluble residue the cell wall fraction; fractionate this fraction by alkaline extraction with 1 N NaOH at room temperature for 1 h. Wash the alkali-insoluble sediment with water until a pH of 7.0 is obtained, wash with ethanol, and then wash with acetone and diethyl ether. The resulting white powder is referred to as F1 fraction.
3. Culture the spleen cells during 48 h at 37 °C under 5% CO_2.
4. Pulse the culture for 12 h with 1 μCie/well with H^3-labeled thymidine and then harvest. Incorporation of H^3-thymidine is measured using a liquid scintillation counter. Data are expressed as means ± SEM of counts per minute of H^3-thymidine incorporation. Supernatants of spleen cells cultured from experimental groups are used to perform cytokine production assays.

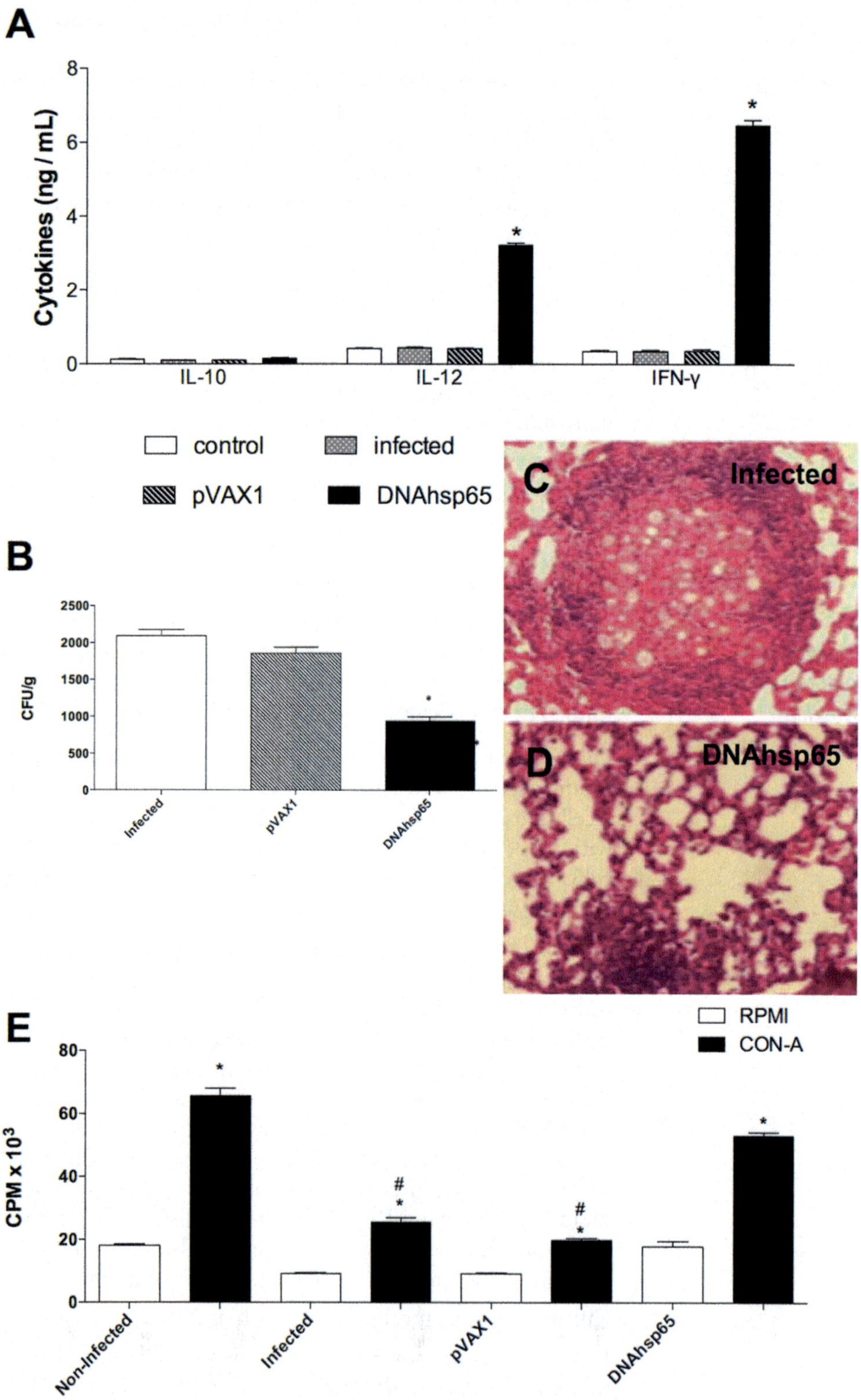

Fig. 2 Immune response evaluation after treatment of mice infected with *P. brasiliensis*. The mice experimentally infected with Pb18 were euthanized after 60 days post-infection. The spleen cells were cultured and assessed to (**a**) cytokines production and (**e**) splenocytes proliferation. The lungs were removed and assessed to (**b**) fungal burden and (**c, d**) histopathological analysis. Results are expressed as the mean ± SEM. $*p < 0.05$ in relation to control group or noninfected; # $p < 0.05$ in relation to noninfected stimulated with CON-A

5. Measure the cytokines using a commercial ELISA kit according to the guidelines established by the company. Calculate the cytokine level based on a standard curve provided by the commercial kit. Express the data as the mean (log10 ± SEM) (Fig. 2a).

3.5 Anti-HSP65-Specific Antibodies

The specific IgG1 and IgG2a isotypes are measured by ELISA (Fig. 3a, b).

1. Sensitize the 96-well plates with rhsp65 protein (250 ng/100uL well) overnight at 4 °C.
2. Plates are blocked with 1:100 dilution of mouse serum for 2 h at 37 °C. After washing with PBS-T, add the peroxidase-labeled antibodies specific for mouse IgG1 or IgG2a isotypes, diluted to 1:5000 for 2 h at 37 °C.
3. Wash the plates seven times with PBS-T and incubate with H_2O_2 and o-phenylenediamine for reaction development. Stop the reactions by the addition of stop solution.
4. Determine the optical densities at 490 nm in an ELISA reader.

3.6 Nitric Oxide (NO) Production Assays

3.6.1 Nitrite (NO_2^-) Measurement

The concentration of nitrite (NO_2^-) in total spleen cell supernatants is measured by a microplate Griess assay, as described previously [14] (Fig. 3c).

1. Add 100 μL of the culture supernatants to an equal volume (v/v) of Griess reagent and incubate at room temperature for 10 min. Determine the absorbance at 540 nm with a microplate reader. Determine the NO_2^- concentration using a standard curve of 1–200 μM of $NaNO_2$.
2. Perform the determinations in triplicate and express with mean ± SEM of μM of NO_2.

3.6.2 Nitrate (NO_3^-) Measurement

The concentration of nitrate (NO_3^-) of samples is determined by reduction of nitrate to nitrite as described previously [17] (Fig. 3d).

1. Add 50 μL of sample with 50 μL of nitrite reductase buffer during 12 h at 37 °C.
2. Determine the NO_3^- concentration using a standard curve of 1–200 μM of $NaNO_3$.
3. Determine the total amount of nitrite using the Griess method. The results are reported as M of NO_3.

4 Notes

1. All culture media, solutions, and materials used to infect the animals and to collect the organs to be processed must be sterilized.

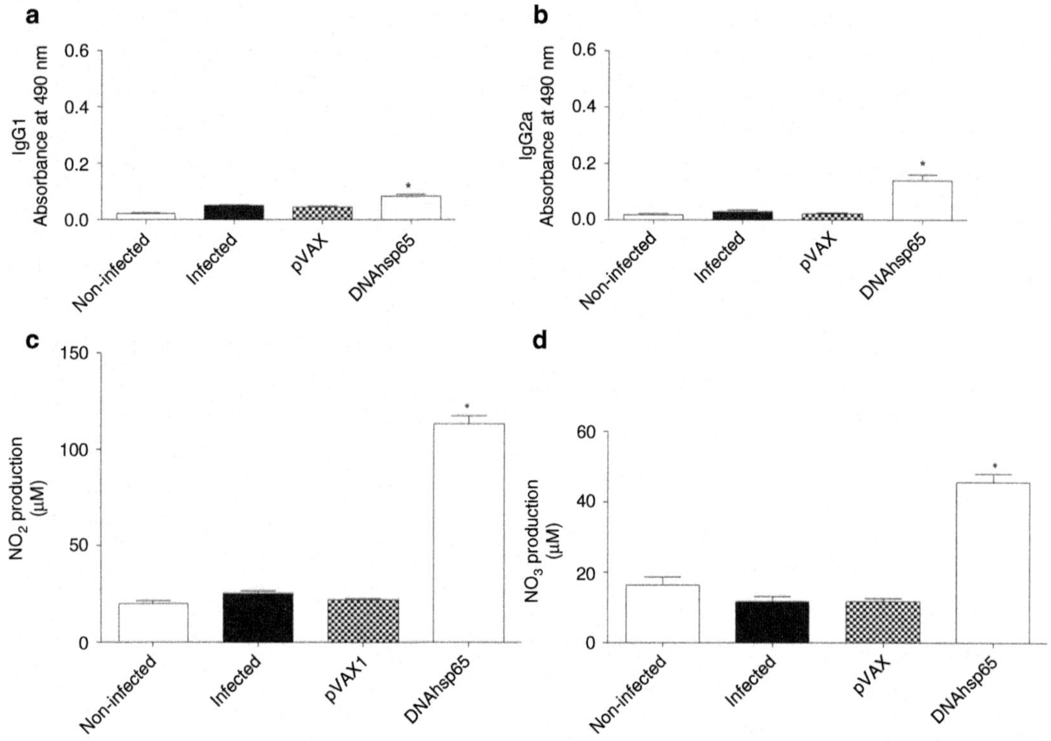

Fig. 3 Immune response evaluation after treatment of mice infected with *P. brasiliensis*. The mice experimentally infected with Pb18 were euthanized after 60 days post-infection. The spleen cells were cultured and assessed to (**a**) cytokines production and (**e**) splenocytes proliferation. The lungs were removed and assessed to (**b**) fungal burden and (**c**, **d**) histopathological analysis. Results are expressed as the mean ± SEM. *$p < 0.05$ in relation to control group or noninfected

2. All experiments have to be approved and conducted in accordance with the guidelines of the Bioethical Committee.
3. To obtain the Pb192 supernatant, cultivate 1×10^7 viable cells/mL of the *Paracoccidioides brasiliensis* Pb192 isolate in liquid BHI medium during 15 days. Then, centrifuge the total medium for 20 min and filter the supernatant in a 0.22 μm filter. Store at −8 °C.
4. The Griess reagent must be used until 6 h after its preparation.
5. The endotoxin amount for the sample must be below 0.1 endotoxin units/g.
6. To better expose the trachea, put a pen transversely under the animal's neck.
7. Put the suspension containing the Pb18 cells under vigorous shaking (vortexing) for 1 min to disperse the cells and facilitate counting.
8. After properly injecting the fungus suspension into the trachea, observe if the animal will be in apnea for about 5 s, returning to

normal breathing afterward. This is an indicative that Pb18 has reached the lungs.

9. To ensure that the infection has occurred properly, it is important to euthanize one or two animals after 30 days of infection and proceed to the fungal load recovery procedure (according Subheading 3.3.1 **step 1**). The growth of fungal cells from the macerate of the lungs is an indicative of the establishment of PCM and the experimental treatments could be safely started.
10. The material used in **steps 1** and **2** can be used for the same group of animals but not for processing the animals from the other treatment group to avoid contamination.
11. The T cell proliferation may be done by CSFE-based flow cytometric analysis too.

Acknowledgment

This work was supported by a grant from Coordenação de Aperfeiçoamento de Pessoal de Nível Superior (CAPES), Fundação de Apoio à Pesquisa do Distrito Federal (FAPDF), and Conselho Nacional de Desenvolvimento Científico e Tecnológico (CNPq).

References

1. Bolhassani A, Rafati S (2008) Heat-shock proteins as powerful weapons in vaccine development. Expert Rev Vaccines 7(8):1185–1199
2. Fioretti D, Iurescia S, Fazio VM et al (2010) DNA vaccines: developing new strategies against cancer. J Biomed Biotechnol 2010:174378
3. Wang XY, Kaneko Y, Repasky E et al (2000) Heat shock proteins and cancer immunotherapy. Immunol Investig 29(2):131–137
4. Doimo NT, Zárate-Bladés CR, Rodrigues RF et al (2014) Immunotherapy of tuberculosis with *Mycobacterium leprae* Hsp65 as a DNA vaccine triggers cross-reactive antibodies against mammalian Hsp60 but not pathological autoimmunity. Hum Vaccin Immunother 10(5):1238–1243
5. Lowrie DB (2006) DNA vaccines for therapy of tubercu losis: where are we now? Vaccine 24:1983–1989
6. Kumar A, Samant M (2016) DNA vaccine against visceral leishmaniasis: a promising approach for prevention and control. Parasite Immunol 38(5):273–281
7. Ribeiro AM, Bocca AL, Amaral AC et al (2010) HSP65 DNA as therapeutic strategy to treat experimental paracoccidioidomycosis. Vaccine 28(6):1528–1534
8. Siqueira IM, Ribeiro AM, Nóbrega YK et al (2013) DNA-hsp65 vaccine as therapeutic strategy to treat experimental chromoblastomycosis caused by *Fonsecaea pedrosoi*. Mycopathologia 175(5–6):463–475
9. Restrepo A (1985) The ecology of *Paracoccidioides brasiliensis*: a puzzle still unsolved. J Med Vet Mycol 23:323–334
10. Bocca AL, Amaral AC, Teixeira MM et al (2013) Paracoccidioidomycosis: eco-epidemiology, taxonomy and clinical and therapeutic issues. Future Microbiol 8(9):1177–1191
11. Rosada RS, de la Torre LG, Frantz FG et al (2008) Protection against tuberculosis by a single intranasal administration of DNA-hsp65 vaccine complexed with cationic liposomes. BMC Immunol 9:38
12. Singer-Vermes LM, Ciavaglia MC, Kashino SS et al (1992) The source of the growth-promoting factor affects the plating efficiency of *Paracoccidioides brasiliensis*. J Med Vet Mycol 30(3):261–264
13. Figueiredo F, Alves LMC, Silva CL (1993) Tumor necrosis factor production *in vivo* and *in vitro* in response to *Paracoccidioides brasiliensis* and the cell wall fractions thereof. Clin Exp Immunol 93:189

14. Green LC, Tannenbaum SR, Goldman P (1981) Nitrate synthesis in the germfree and conventional rat. Science 212:56–58
15. Dias MF, Mesquita J, Rodrigues N et al (2004) Viability of yeast form cells of *Paracoccidioides brasiliensis* after sonication. Med Mycol 42(1):43–49
16. Bocca AL, Hayashi EE, Pinheiro AG et al (1998) Treatment of *Paracoccidioides brasiliensis*-infected mice with a nitric oxide inhibitor prevents the failure of cell-mediated immune response. J Immunol 161(6): 3056–3063
17. Schmidt HH, Wilke P, Evers B et al (1989) Enzymatic formation of nitrogen oxides from L-arginine in bovine brain cytosol. Biochem Biophys Res Commun 165(1): 284–291

Chapter 8

Idiotypic Antifungal Vaccination: Immunoprotection by Antiidiotypic Antibiotic Antibodies

Luciano Polonelli, Walter Magliani, and Stefania Conti

Abstract

As implied by the idiotypic network theory, the interaction between the functional epitope of a microbicidal molecule (X) and its specific cell-wall receptor (RX) on sensitive microorganisms may be imaged by the bond between the idiotype (Id) of a neutralizing monoclonal antibody (anti-X Ab) and its anti-idiotype (anti-Id) X-like Ab (anti-anti-X Ab). Consequently, anti-X Ab Id may mimic RX acting as a vaccine (idiotypic vaccination) for the elicitation of protective anti-Id Abs with antibiotic activity (antibiobodies).

Key words Idiotype, Anti-idiotype, Fungi, Yeast killer toxin, Transphyletic vaccination

1 Introduction

Vaccines represent a powerful tool for control, elimination, and even eradication of infectious diseases worldwide [1]. The strategic importance of anti-infective immunization resulted in the definition of methodologically diverse but functionally homologous vaccinal approaches aiming at elicitation of protective antibodies (Abs) and establishment of immunological memory [2]. Among these, conventional vaccination relies on specific components or the entire etiological agent, recombinant vaccination employs the products of the gene coding for the antigen (Ag) able to induce protective Abs, reverse vaccinology makes use of bioinformatics to screen the entire genome of the pathogenic agent for the selection of suitable immunogenic proteins, and the antiidiotypic (anti-Id) vaccination exploits anti-Id Abs presenting the three-dimensional structure of the reference Ag [3–7]. In any case, specific elicited Abs exert classical protective functions. Conversely, idiotypic vaccination, based on the idiotypic network theory [8], is conceptually different from other immunization approaches, as elicited Abs display a direct microbicidal activity [9]. In idiotypic vaccination, in fact, protection is mediated by anti-Id Abs [10–12] which represent the internal image (i.e., mimic the biological activity) of an

Markus Kalkum and Margarita Semis (eds.), *Vaccines for Invasive Fungal Infections: Methods and Protocols*, Methods in Molecular Biology, vol. 1625, DOI 10.1007/978-1-4939-7104-6_8, © Springer Science+Business Media LLC 2017

exogenous molecule (X) (e.g., a killer toxin from the yeast *Wickerhamomyces anomalus*, former *Pichia anomala*, former *Hansenula anomala*, *Wa*KT), lethal to microorganisms (e.g., *Candidaalbicans*) presenting specific superficial receptors (RX) (e.g., β1,3 D-glucans) [13, 14], and are elicited by the idiotype (Id) of a X-neutralizing mAb (e.g., mAb KT4) [15] (Fig. 1). The protective anti-Id Abs behave, therefore, as X-like antibiotic Abs (antibiobodies) [16, 17]. Compared to other methods of immunization, idiotypic vaccination presents some peculiar features. In relation to the mode of action, protection mediated by antibiobodies is independent of the understanding of the mechanisms of pathogenicity of the infectious agent, and of the immune response required for protection; the same idiotypic vaccine administered through different routes can elicit protective antibiobodies recoverable in systemic and mucosal compartments [11, 12]. Idiotypic vaccination, moreover, may be effective against transphyletic microorganisms characterized by the same RX, e.g., β1,3 D-glucans. Accordingly, a β glucan preparation proved to be functionally homologous to the Id of the *Wa*KT-neutralizing mAb KT4 thus acting as a polyvalent, "universal" antifungal vaccine [18]. Furthermore, idiotypic vaccination is independent of the scarce or none immunogenicity of the RX molecule on sensitive microorganisms targeted by the elicited protective antibiobodies.

In its performance, idiotypic vaccination also provides for the possibility of obtaining, from animals immunized with anti-X mAb (e.g., mAb KT4), anti-anti-X mAb, or recombinant single chain fragment variable region (scFv), internal image of X (e.g., mAb

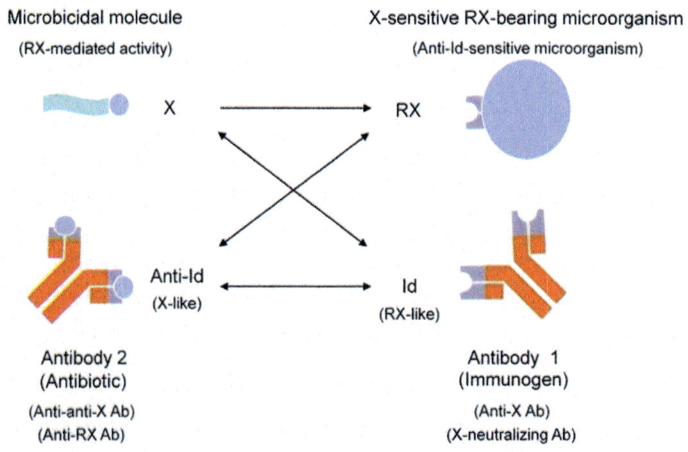

Fig. 1 Postulates of idiotypic vaccination. The interaction between the functional epitope of a microbicidal molecule (X) and its specific cell-wall receptor (RX) on X-sensitive microorganisms may be imaged by the bond between the idiotype (Id) of a X-neutralizing Ab and its anti-idiotype (anti-Id) Ab, postulating that Id can mimic RX acting as a vaccine (idiotypic vaccination) for the elicitation of protective anti-Id Abs with X-like antibiotic activity

K10 or scFv H6) [19, 20], to be used as potential therapeutic agents against infections caused by X-sensitive microorganisms belonging to different phyla or even kingdoms (*C. albicans*, *Pneumocystis carinii*, *Aspergillus fumigatus*, bacteria, protozoa) [19–21].

As a corollary, the concept of idiotypic vaccination may present a natural confirmation in the course of human infections. In serum or other biological fluids (e.g., vaginal secretion) of individuals infected by X-sensitive microorganisms (e.g., *C. albicans*), microbicidal X-like Abs (e.g., human natural yeast killer toxin-like Abs) elicited by superficial RX (e.g., β1,3 D-glucans) could be detected and purified by affinity chromatography with an anti-X mAb (e.g., mAb KT4), and proved to exert protective anti-infective activity [22–24].

2 Materials

The execution of the procedures described below requires the availability of an animal facility and laboratories furnished with common equipment (such as microscopes, laminar flow cabinets, incubators, centrifuges, refrigerators, freezers, etc.), and involves the use of sterile instruments and consumables (syringes, pipettes, test tubes, plates, tweezers, scissors, scalpels, etc.).

Prepare all the materials (media, reagents, solutions, etc.) according to the instructions of the manufacturers. Keep the materials and perform all the procedures at room temperature unless otherwise stated. Follow waste disposal rules for disposing each waste material.

2.1 Production of X

1. Microorganism (e.g., *W. anomalus* UCSC 25F) recognized to be a producer of X (e.g., *Wa*KT) [15].
2. Sterile distilled water.
3. Sabouraud dextrose broth.
4. Sabouraud dextrose agar (SDA).
5. Rotatory shaker.
6. 500 mL Erlenmeyer flasks.
7. Supplemented yeast extract–peptone–dextrose (YEPD) broth: YEPD broth added with 15% glycerol, buffered at pH 4.5 with 0.1 M citric acid and 0.2 M K_2HPO_4.
8. EDTA-free protease inhibitor cocktail (Complete, Roche, Mannheim, Germany).
9. Low protein-binding membrane filters, 0.45 μm pore size.
10. PM 10 membrane (Amicon, Merck Millipore Corporation, Darmst`adt, Germany).

11. Ultrafiltration unit under N_2 pressure.
12. HiPrep 16/60 Sephacryl S-200 High Resolution column (GE Healthcare, Little Chalfont, UK).
13. Elution buffer: 0.01 M citric acid–Na_2HPO_4 buffer, pH 4.5.
14. Amicon Ultra-15 (MW cutoff 10 kDa) centrifugal filter unit (Merck Millipore).

2.2 X Activity Assay

1. Microorganism of interest as a pathogen (e.g., *C. albicans*), proven to be sensitive to X (e.g., *Wa*KT) (*see* **Note 1**).
2. Sabouraud dextrose broth.
3. 96-well microtiter plates.
4. Microplate reader with 630 nm filter.

2.3 Characterization of X

1. Infrared spectroscope (Direct Detect® Infrared Spectrometer, Merck Millipore).
2. Protein electrophoresis equipment.
3. Reagents for electrophoresis:
   (a) polyacrylamide.
   (b) Tris–HCl buffers, pH 8.8 and 6.8.
   (c) 10% ammonium persulfate.
   (d) TEMED.
4. Coomassie blue stain.
5. Marker proteins (ColorBurst™ Electrophoresis Marker, Sigma-Aldrich).
6. Western blotting equipment.
7. Polyvinlymethylformamide (PVDF) membrane.
8. Ponceau S solution.
9. Automated microsequencer (Procise 492, Applied Biosystems, Palo Alto, CA, USA).
10. Acetonitrile.
11. Ammonium carbonate.
12. Endoproteinase Lys-C.
13. C18 reverse-phase HPLC column.

2.4 Characterization of RX

1. Various carbohydrate molecules linked to *p*-nitrophenyl and glucosidase.
2. Scanning electron microscope.

2.5 Production of Anti-X mAb

1. BALB/C mice.
2. Incomplete Freund's adjuvant.
3. NS1 myeloma cells.

4. Polyethylene glycol 1000.
5. Hypoxanthine–aminopterin–thymidine containing medium.
6. Microtiter plates and reagents for enzyme-linked immunosorbent assay (ELISA).
7. Mouse thymocytes.
8. SDS-PAGE and Western blot equipment and reagents.

2.6 Production of Anti-X mAb in Ascites Fluids

1. Pristane-treated syngeneic BALB/C mice.
2. Ammonium sulfate (50% of saturation).
3. Dialysis system.

2.7 Evaluation of the Neutralizing Properties of Anti-X mab Against X Activity

1. *C. albicans* culture.
2. Isotype-matched unrelated mAb.

2.8 Idiotypic Vaccination: Systemic Immunization of Animals

1. BALB/C mice.
2. Complete Freund's adjuvant.
3. Incomplete Freund's adjuvant.
4. Saline.
5. Isotype-matched unrelated mAb.

2.9 Idiotypic Vaccination: Mucosal Immunization of Animals

1. Oophorectomized female Wistar rats or female CD1 mice.
2. Estradiol benzoate.
3. Estradiol valerate.
4. Complete Freund's adjuvant.
5. Incomplete Freund's adjuvant.
6. Isotype-matched unrelated mAb.
7. Phosphate Buffered Saline (PBS).

2.10 Systemic Experimental Infection

1. *C. albicans* culture.

2.11 Mucosal Experimental Infection

1. *C. albicans* culture.
2. *Saccharomyces cerevisiae* culture.
3. Syringe equipped with a multipurpose calibrated tip (Combitip™).
4. Calibrated (1 μL) plastic loop.
5. PBS.
6. SDA plates containing 0.05% (w/v) chloramphenicol.

2.12 Detection of Anti-Id (Anti-anti-X) (X-like) Abs by Inhibition Competitive ELISA

1. Microtiter plates.
2. Bovine Serum Albumin (BSA, 1%)-carbonate buffer (pH 9.6).
3. Wash buffer: Tween 20 (0.5%) in PBS.
4. Humid chamber with a cover.
5. Peroxidase-conjugated rabbit Abs to mouse immunoglobulins.
6. Citrate buffer.
7. Hydrogen peroxide.
8. Tetramethylbenzidine.
9. 1 N sulfate acid.
10. Microplate reader.

2.13 Affinity Chromatography Purification of Anti-Id (Anti-anti-X) (X-like) Abs

1. Affigel 10 (Bio-Rad Laboratories Inc.).
2. Buchner funnel.
3. Wathman filter paper number 2.
4. Deionized water.
5. 1 M ethanolamine–HCl (pH 8).
6. Affinity chromatography empty column (30 mL).
7. 0.05 M potassium phosphate (pH 7.1).
8. 2 M sodium chloride in 0.05 M sodium phosphate (pH 7.1).
9. Spectrophotometer.
10. Dialysis system.
11. PBS.
12. Microtiter plates and reagents for ELISA.

2.14 Evaluation of In Vitro Activity of Affinity Chromatography Purified Anti-Id (Anti-anti-X) (X-like) Abs by Colony-Forming Units (CFU) Assay

1. *C. albicans* culture.
2. SDA plates.
3. Sterile distilled water.
4. Microtiter plates round bottom.

2.15 Neutralization of Anti-Id (Anti-anti-X) (X-like) Abs by Anti-X mAb

1. *C. albicans* culture.
2. Tools and reagents for CFU assay.

2.16 Passive Transfer of Immunity Mediated by Anti-Id (Anti-anti-X) (X-like) Abs

1. BALB/C mice or oophorectomized estradiol-treated female rats.
2. *C. albicans* culture.

3 Methods

3.1 Production of X

1. Maintain the X-producing microorganism (e.g., *W. anomalus* UCSC 25F) in the culture collection in sterile distilled water and subculture on Sabouraud dextrose agar (SDA) (*see* **Note 2**).
2. Inoculate 5 mL of an appropriate medium (e.g., Sabouraud broth) with a loopful of a 48-h-old culture and incubate at 20 °C overnight at 150 rpm on a rotatory shaker.
3. Fill five 500 mL Erlenmeyer flasks with 100 mL of supplemented YEPD broth. Inoculate each flask with 1 mL of the overnight culture and aerobically incubate by shaking (150 rpm) at 20 °C for 72 h.
4. After this period, centrifuge at 5000 × *g*, 5 min at 4 °C, add one tablet of EDTA-free protease inhibitor cocktail, then filtrate the supernatant through low protein binding membranes, and concentrate to a volume of 3 mL with a PM 10 membrane in an ultrafiltration unit under N_2 pressure.
5. Apply the concentrated supernatant to an HiPrep 16/60 Sephacryl S-200 High Resolution column and elute using elution buffer (flow rate 0.6 mL/min).
6. After evaluation of biological activity in collected fractions as described below (*see* Subheading 3.2, X activity assay), combine active fractions and concentrate by filtration through an Amicon Ultra-15 centrifugal filter unit at 4000 × *g*, 4 °C.

3.2 X Activity Assay

1. Maintain the X-sensitive microorganism (e.g., *C. albicans*) in the culture collection in sterile distilled water and subculture on SDA.
2. Mix a 50 μL aliquot of concentrated supernatant or eluted fraction with 200 μL of Sabouraud broth containing 5×10^4 cells of the microorganism (e.g., *C. albicans*) sensitive to X (e.g., *Wa*KT) and seed into the wells of 96-well microtiter plates.
3. Incubate the plates at 26 °C for 18–20 h and follow the growth of the indicator strain by measuring the optical density at 630 nm (OD_{630}) using a microplate reader.
4. Perform each assay in triplicate and evaluate the results as the mean of OD_{630} ± S.D.
5. Detect X activity by calculating the growth inhibition of the indicator strain, using the OD_{630} values in X-free wells as a control (*see* **Note 3**).

3.3 Characterization of X

1. Determine purified X (e.g., *Wa*KT) concentration by infrared spectroscopy.
2. Analyze the purified X in sodium dodecyl sulfate polyacrylamide gel electrophoresis (SDS-PAGE) [25] using 7% resolving gel and 4% polyacrylamide stacking gel.

3. To determine the mass of the purified X, stain the gel with Coomassie blue and compare X electrophoretic mobility with that of marker proteins.
4. To determine N-terminal sequence, electroblot the band of the purified X obtained on SDS-PAGE onto a PVDF membrane. Stain the membrane with Ponceau S solution to visualize the protein. Excise the band from the membrane and submit directly to sequencing using an automated microsequencer.
5. To obtain internal amino acid sequences, excise the band of the purified X obtained on SDS-PAGE and treat with acetonitrile and ammonium carbonate to remove impurities. After dehydration, digest the protein with endoproteinase Lys-C for 18 h at 37 °C.
6. Purify the resulting peptides by reverse-phase HPLC and submit to N-terminal microsequencing [26].

3.4 Characterization of RX

1. Investigate X (e.g., *Wa*KT) activity using spheroplasts derived from cells of a X-sensitive microorganism (e.g., *C. albicans*).
2. Study the potential hydrolytic activity of X (e.g., *Wa*KT) using various molecules (e.g., sugars) covalently linked to *p*-nitrophenyl as substrates as well as specific inhibitors (e.g., glucosidase).
3. Assess the ultrastructural modifications induced by X (e.g., *Wa*KT) activity on X-sensitive microorganisms (e.g., *C. albicans*) by scanning electron microscopy [14].

3.5 Production of Anti-X mAb

1. Inject intraperitoneally BALB/C mice, 3 weeks old, 18 g body weight, with 50 μg of purified X (e.g., *Wa*KT), mixed with 0.1 mL of incomplete Freund's adjuvant, once a week for 1 month.
2. Give a booster injection of X (e.g., *Wa*KT) alone intraperitoneally three days before the scheduled fusion to be carried out according to established protocols briefly summarized thereafter.
3. Three days after the booster injection, sacrifice the mice, remove the spleens, and carefully collect spleen cells.
4. After centrifugation and counting, fuse the spleen cells with a proper number of NS1 myeloma cells (ratio 4:1) by using polyethylene glycol 1000.
5. Subject the cells to a 1-month-long selection regime by culturing in the hypoxanthine–aminopterin–thymidine containing medium.
6. Screen for the hybrids producing the desired anti-X Ab by testing the hybrid supernatant through an ELISA in microtiter plates coated with the concentrated target antigen X diluted 1:1000 in carbonate buffer (pH 9.6).

7. Propagate and clone twice by limiting dilution, in the presence of mouse thymocytes (10^5/well) or proper growth factors, hybridoma cultures secreting anti-X Abs (e.g., mAb KT4) that react only with the reference antigen X (e.g., *Wa*KT).
8. Expand the clones that continue to produce the desired anti-X mAb (e.g., mAb KT4).
9. Ascertain the isotype of the produced mAb (e.g., mAb KT4) by ELISA (capture, indirect, or antigen-mediated) or double immunodiffusion procedures using specific rabbit or goat Abs against mouse immunoglobulins (IgG1, IgG2a, IgG2b, IgG3, IGM, IgA) [15].
10. Verify anti-X mAb (e.g., mAb KT4) reactivity against the reference antigen X (e.g., *Wa*KT) through Western blot analysis. Electroblot the band of the purified X obtained by SDS-PAGE (15 mA for 18 h) to nitrocellulose sheets at 60 V for 3 h. Cut the nitrocellulose sheets into strips and incubate with 5% horse serum for 30 min in PBS, then incubate the strips at 37 °C with 2 mL of a 1:10 dilution of hybridoma culture fluid containing anti-X Ab (e.g., mab KT4) in a rotatory shaker for 30 min. Wash the strips for 10 min with PBS, block them with 5% horse serum in PBS, and incubate for 30 min at 37 °C in a shaker with 3 mL of horseradish peroxidase-coupled rabbit anti-mouse immunoglobulins. Wash the strips for 30 min with two changes of PBS and stain them with 4-chloro-1-naphthol and hydrogen peroxide [15].

3.6 Production of Anti-X mAb in Ascites Fluids

1. Inject hybridoma cells (10^7) producing anti-X mAb (e.g., mAb KT4) intraperitoneally into pristane-treated syngeneic BALB/C mice [15].
2. After a reasonable period of time, in which an abdominal ascites in mice is observed, repeatedly and successively withdraw the ascites fluid by a syringe.
3. Purify the recovered ascites fluid by precipitation with ammonium sulfate and dialyze against PBS.
4. Determine the protein concentration by the Lowry method [27] or by spectroscopy or spectrophotometry, and store in aliquots (20 mg/mL) at −20 °C.

3.7 Evaluation of the Neutralizing Properties of Anti-X mab Against X Activity

1. Add graduated amounts of anti-X mAb (e.g., mAb KT4) ascites fluid to 1 mL of X (e.g., *Wa*KT) for 24 h at 4 °C [15].
2. Discard the sediment, if any, and test the supernatants for activity against the recognized X-sensitive microorganism (e.g., *C. albicans*), in comparison to X (e.g., *Wa*KT) alone, according to appropriate in vitro procedures (*see* Subheadings 3.2 and 3.14).
3. Consider using ascites fluid containing an isotype-matched unrelated mAb as a negative control [15].

3.8 Idiotypic Vaccination: Systemic Immunization of Animals (See Notes 4–9)

1. Divide a suitable number of animals (BALB/C mice, 3 weeks old, 18 g body weight) into groups (at least 12 animals/group) to be immunized with various doses of anti-X mAb (e.g., mAb KT4), in order to compare the effect of different immunogen amounts, or to be used for controls (a group to be immunized with an isotype-matched unrelated mAb and a group of non-immunized animals, to control eventual nonspecific protective effects).
2. Inject subcutaneously the animals with 50 μg of anti-X mAb (e.g., mAb KT4) emulsified with 0.5 mL of complete Freund's adjuvant.
3. Two weeks later boost subcutaneously each animal with 50 μg of anti-X mAb (e.g., mAb KT4) in incomplete Freund's adjuvant.
4. After 1 week, divide the immunized animals into three groups and inject by the intravenous (iv) route with equal volumes of different amounts of anti-X mAb (e.g., mAb KT4): 25, 100 or 400 μg in 0.2 mL saline.
5. Repeat, after 2 weeks, the iv immunization with the same amounts of anti-X mAb (e.g., mAb KT4).
6. At the same time, immunize a group of animals twice subcutaneously (50 μg) and then boost twice (100 μg) with an isotype-matched unrelated mAb according to the described schedule of immunization.
7. To verify the elicitation of protective anti-Id (anti-anti-X) (X-like) Abs, collect by eye bleeding, at regular time intervals, serum samples from at least three animals of each group (i.e., the three immunization groups as well as the animals non-immunized and immunized with the isotype-matched unrelated mAb [11]).

3.9 Idiotypic Vaccination: Mucosal Immunization of Animals

1. Divide a suitable number of animals into groups (oophorectomized female Wistar rats, 80–100 g body weight, treated by subcutaneous injections of 0.5 mg of estradiol benzoate [12] or female CD1 mice maintained under pseudoestrus condition by subcutaneous injection of 0.2 mg of estradiol valerate [28], at least six animals/group) to be immunized with anti-X mAb (e.g., mAb KT4) or to be used for controls (a group to be immunized with an isotype-matched unrelated mAb and a group of non-immunized animals).
2. Immunize the animals by the intravaginal route with 100 μg of anti-X mAb (e.g., mAb KT4) emulsified in 0.1 mL of complete Freund's adjuvant on days 0 and 7.
3. Administer the same amount of anti-X mAb (e.g., mAb KT4) in incomplete Freund's adjuvant (0.1 mL) on days 14 and 21.

4. Use the same schedule to immunize the animals with the same amount of an isotype matched irrelevant mAb as a control. Give also complete and incomplete Freund's adjuvant to a group of control non-immunized animals.
5. To verify the elicitation of protective anti-Id (anti-anti-X) (X-like) Abs, collect samples of vaginal fluids at regular time intervals from each animal. Wash the vaginal cavity by gentle injection and aspiration of 0.5 mL PBS, and repeat three times always by the same operator. Collect the final fluid, centrifuge at 3500 × *g*, 15 min at 4 °C, and store the supernatant at −20 °C until use [12].

3.10 Systemic Experimental Infection

1. 52 days after the beginning of immunization, infect the animals (immunized and control groups) with a suitable inoculum of a pathogenic microorganism recognized to be sensitive to X (e.g., *C. albicans*). Inject iv two different inocula (e.g., 1×10^6 and 5×10^6 cells/0.2 mL saline) in two groups (six animals each) of animals immunized iv with different doses (25, 100, and 400 μg) of anti-X mAb (e.g., mAb KT4) as well as control animals (non-immunized and immunized with the isotype-matched unrelated mAb).
2. Maintain the animals until death occurs and register the date [11].
3. Compare the survival curves of anti-X mAb-immunized and control animals by the Mantel-Cox log rank test, and the differences in the median survival time (in days) by the Mann-Whitney U test.

3.11 Mucosal Experimental Infection

1. Nine days after the fourth administration of anti-X mAb (e.g., mAb KT4), irrelevant mAb, or adjuvant only (day 30), infect intravaginally the animals with a vaginopathic X-sensitive microorganism (e.g., *C. albicans*) (10^7 cells in 0.1 mL of PBS) and challenge a group of non-immunized rats also with an identical number of cells of a non-vaginopathic strain of an X-sensitive microorganism (e.g., *Saccharomyces cerevisiae*) for control.
2. Inject yeast cells into the vaginal cavity through a syringe equipped with Combitip™ [12].
3. Take samples of vaginal fluids at regular time intervals after the intravaginal challenge with the X-sensitive microorganisms for colony-forming units (CFU) enumeration using a calibrated plastic loop.
4. After intravaginal insertion and tampering, vigorously suspend the content of each loop in 0.1 mL of PBS, streak aliquots over SDA plates, then incubate at 28 °C for 48–72 h.
5. Evaluate one vaginal sample per animal and consider the animal infected when at least one CFU is present in one loop of vaginal fluid, i.e., >10^3 CFU/mL [12].

6. Compare the differences in CFU numbers between anti-X mAb-immunized and control animals by Student's *t*-test, and the differences in the number of infected animals over total by the Fisher's exact test.

3.12 Detection of Anti-Id (Anti-anti-X) (X-like) Abs by Inhibition Competitive ELISA

1. Determine the anti-anti-X (anti-Id) Ab concentrations in animal sera, or vaginal fluids, by an inhibition competitive ELISA [11, 12].
2. Fill the wells of microtiter plates with 0.2 mL of X (e.g., *Wa*KT) previously diluted 1:1000 in Bovine Serum Albumin (BSA)-carbonate buffer (pH 9.6) and hold the plates overnight at 4 °C.
3. In the same time, prepare a mixture (100 μL) of a predetermined optimal concentration of anti-X mAb (e.g., mAb KT4) (50 μL) and samples (50 μL), i.e., mouse sera diluted 1:250 in 0.03% BSA–PBS or vaginal fluids diluted 1:10 in BSA–PBS, from the animals immunized with anti-X mAb, immunized with the isotype-matched unrelated mAb, and non-immunized. A mixture of anti-X mAb (e.g., mAb KT4) (50 μL) and diluent alone (BSA–PBS, 50 μL) serve as a control of the assay. Keep the mixtures overnight at 4 °C.
4. After this time period, aspirate the excess of X (e.g., *Wa*KT) from the wells of the microtiter plates and rinse each well five times with 0.3 mL of the wash buffer.
5. Dispense into the wells of the sensitized plates, together with proper controls, the previously prepared mixtures. Perform each assay at least in duplicate.
6. Incubate the plates for 1 h at 37 °C in a humid chamber with a cover to prevent evaporation. At the end of the incubation period, wash the plates five times with the wash buffer.
7. Dispense in each well 100 μL of a solution of peroxidase-conjugated rabbit Abs to mouse immunoglobulins, diluted 1:100 in Tween 20-PBS.
8. Reincubate the plates for 1 h at 37 °C under the above-described conditions and repeat washing five times.
9. Reveal the bound peroxidase by adding 100 μL of a 0.005% citrate buffer solution of hydrogen peroxide together with a 1:50 solution of tetramethylbenzidine.
10. Incubate the plates for 30 min in the dark and stop the reaction by adding 200 μL of 1 N sulfate acid.
11. Read the absorbance of the specimens at 450 nm in the bichromatic mode and calculate the average of the absorbance values of the serum or vaginal fluid samples belonging to each group/day. Evaluate the inhibiting activity of the anti-Id (anti-anti-X) (X-like) Abs eventually present by comparison with the absorbance values obtained in the reaction with anti-X mAb and diluent alone [11, 12].

3.13 Affinity Chromatography Purification of Anti-Id (Anti-anti-X) (X-like) Abs

1. Perform purification of anti-Id (anti-anti-X) (X-like) Abs from the sera, or vaginal fluids, of animals immunized with anti-X mAb (e.g., mAb KT4) by affinity chromatography, using immobilized anti-X mAb (e.g., mAb KT4) as ligand.
2. Lodge 13 mL of Affigel 10 in a Buchner funnel containing a Wathman filter paper and wash the resin with 100 mL of deionized water at 4 °C.
3. After washing, place the resin into a beaker and add 1.5 mL of anti-X mAb (e.g., mAb KT4) obtained from ascites fluid.
4. Hold the beaker at 4 °C for 2–4 h gently shaking every 20 min, then stop the reaction with 1.2 mL of 1 M ethanolamine–HCl (pH 8) and maintain 1 h at 4 °C.
5. Pack the resin into a column plugged with cotton wool and elute the unbound anti-X mAb (e.g., mAb KT4) with 0.05 M potassium phosphate.
6. Equilibrate the resin with 2 M sodium chloride in 0.05 M sodium phosphate (pH 7.1), followed by 0.05 M sodium phosphate at the same pH.
7. For chromatography, adsorb anti-Id (anti-anti-X) (X-like) Abs by slow introduction into the column of sera (100 μL) or vaginal fluids (1 mL) from animals immunized with anti-X mAb and allow the sample to remain in contact with the resin for 2 h at 4 °C.
8. Elute the unbound material with 0.05 M sodium phosphate buffer until the absorbance at 276 nm reaches the baseline.
9. Elute the bound material by 2 M sodium chloride in 0.05 M sodium phosphate and immediately dialyze against PBS at pH 7.2 (three changes at 4 °C) [11, 12].
10. Isotype evaluation of affinity chromatography-purified anti-Id (anti-anti-X) (X-like) Abs could be performed by a conventional ELISA procedure using the purified Abs diluted 1:4 in BSA carbonate buffer as coating Ag and peroxidase-conjugated or alkaline phosphatase-conjugated anti-mouse or anti-rat Abs as a probe.

3.14 Evaluation of In Vitro Activity of Affinity Chromatography Purified Anti-Id (Anti-anti-X) (X-like) Abs by CFU Assay

1. Grow the cells of the X-sensitive microorganism (e.g., *C. albicans*) on SDA plates for 24 h at 30 °C.
2. After incubation, collect the cells from isolated colonies, suspend in sterile distilled water and number by microscopic counting. Properly dilute the cell suspension to obtain approximately 5×10^4 viable cells/mL.
3. Add 10 μL of the prepared cell suspension to microtiter plate wells (round bottom) containing 90 μL of anti-Id (anti-anti-X) (X-like) Abs purified by affinity chromatography or 90 μL of PBS (growth control). Perform each assay in triplicate.

4. After incubation for 6 h at 37 °C, dispense and streak the entire content of each microwell on the surface of SDA plates, and incubate at 30 °C up to the colony growth.
5. Enumerate the colonies and evaluate the activity of purified anti-Id Abs by calculating the percentual reduction of CFU average number in comparison to the growth control [11, 12].

3.15 Neutralization of Anti-Id (Anti-anti-X) (X-like) Abs by Anti-X mAb

1. Mix affinity chromatography purified anti-Id Abs with an equal volume of anti-X mAb (e.g., mAb KT4) purified from ascites fluid or an equal volume of an isotype-matched unrelated mAb and keep the mixtures overnight at 4 °C [11].
2. Perform a CFU assay (*see* Subheading 3.14) by adding 10 μL of the proper suspension of the X-sensitive microorganism (e.g., *C. albicans*) to 90 μL of the mixture of anti-Id Abs and anti-X mAb (e.g., mAb KT4) ascitic fluid, 90 μL of the mixture of anti-Id Abs and an isotype-matched unrelated mAb, or 90 μL of PBS (growth control). Perform each assay in triplicate. Proceed as previously described for the evaluation of anti-Id Abs activity (*see also* **Note 9**).

3.16 Passive Transfer of Immunity Mediated by Anti-Id (Anti-anti-X) (X-like) Abs

1. Collect the sera, or vaginal fluids, from animals immunized with anti-X mAb (e.g., mAb KT4), or used as controls (immunized with an isotype-matched unrelated mAb or non-immunized animals) following the last immunization.
2. Inject 0.5 mL of the serum, or vaginal fluid (pooled from at least three animals), intraperitoneally, or intravaginally, to naive, nonimmunized animals (e.g., BALB/C mice or oophorectomized estradiol-treated female rats).
3. After 30 min, inoculate each recipient animal with the usual challenge of X-sensitive microorganism (e.g., *C. albicans*) and monitor systemic or mucosal experimental infection as previously described (*see* Subheadings 3.10 and 3.11).

4 Notes

1. It can be presumed a wide spectrum activity of X (e.g., *Wa*KT) against strains of microorganisms belonging to different species, genera, and even kingdoms. For evaluation, adapt the procedure (*see* Subheadings 2.2 and 3.2, X activity assay) to the growth requirements of potential X-sensitive microorganisms [29–32].
2. It can be presumed a production of X from strains of microorganisms belonging to different species or genera. For evaluation, adapt the growth requirements of potential X-producer microorganisms [13].

3. In alternative, the activity of X (e.g., *Wa*KT) can be determined by a colony forming unit assay against the X-sensitive microorganism (e.g., *C. albicans*) (*see* Subheading 3.14).
4. An X-like mAb (e.g., *Wa*KT-like mAb K10) can be produced in Fischer-344 rats by immunization with a X-neutralizing mAb (e.g., *Wa*KT-neutralizing mAb KT4) bearing the internal image of RX (e.g., β1-3 D-glucans) of X-sensitive microorganisms (e.g., *C. albicans*) [19].
5. An anti-anti-anti-anti-X mAb (e.g., mAb K20), functionally mimicking X (e.g., *Wa*KT), can be produced from BALB/C mice presenting anti-anti-anti-X Abs (e.g., anti-*Wa*KT, mAb KT4-like Abs) following immunization with an anti-anti-X rat mAb (e.g., *Wa*KT-like mAb K10) [33].
6. X-like (e.g., *Wa*KT-like) anti-anti-X mAb (e.g., mAb K10) and anti-anti-anti-anti-X mAb (e.g., mAb K20) can kill in vitro X-sensitive microorganisms (e.g., *C. albicans*), an activity that can be neutralized by anti-X mAb (e.g., mAb KT4), and are capable of competing with each other and with X (e.g., *Wa*KT) for binding to RX (e.g., β1,3 D-glucans) of X-sensitive microorganisms (e.g., *C. albicans*) [33, 34].
7. X-like (e.g., *Wa*KT-like) anti-anti-anti-anti-X mAb (e.g., mAb K20) can be used to select peptide mimics of RX (e.g., β1,3 D-glucans) from random peptide phage display libraries [33].
8. Peptide mimics of RX can be used as immunogens in BALB/C mice in the form of either keyhole limpet hemocyanin (KLH)-conjugates or peptide-encoding minigenes (DNA immunization) for the elicitation of X (e.g., *Wa*KT)-like serum Abs characterized by microbicidal activity against X-sensitive microorganisms (e.g., *C. albicans*) [33].
9. X-like (e.g., *Wa*KT-like) Abs can be inhibited by a RX-like transphyletic molecule (e.g., laminarin, a soluble algal β1,3 D-glucan preparation) [33].

References

1. World Health Organization (2012) Global Vaccine Action Plan 2011–2020. World Health Organization, Geneva
2. Arnon R, Ben-Yedidia T (2003) Old and new vaccine approaches. Int Immunopharmacol 3(8):1195–1204
3. U.S. Department of Health and Human Services, National Institutes of Health, National Institute of Allergy and Infectious Diseases (2008). NIH publication no. 08-4219 Understanding vaccines what they are how they work. www.niaid.nih.gov/topics/vaccines/documents/undvacc.pdf
4. Nascimento IP, Leite LC (2012) Recombinant vaccines and the development of new vaccine strategies. Braz J Med Biol Res 45(12): 1102–1111
5. Rappuoli R (2000) Reverse vaccinology. Curr Opin Microbiol 3(5):445–450
6. Nisonoff A (1991) Idiotypes: concepts and applications. J Immunol 147(8):2429–2438
7. Sollner J (2016) Systems vaccinology: applications, trends, and perspectives. Methods Mol Biol1403:107–130.doi:10.1007/978-1-4939-3387-7_5

8. Jerne NK (1974) Towards a network theory of the immune system. Ann Immunol (Paris) 125C(1–2):373–389
9. Casadevall A, Pirofski L-A (2012) A new synthesis for antibody-mediated immunity. Nat Immunol 13(1):21–28. doi:10.1038/ni.2184
10. Polonelli L, Morace G (1988) Yeast killer toxin-like anti-idiotypic antibodies. J Clin Microbiol 26(3):602–604
11. Polonelli L, Lorenzini R, De Bernardis F et al (1993) Idiotypic vaccination: immunoprotection mediated by anti-idiotypic antibodies with antibiotic activity. Scand J Immunol 37(1):105–110
12. Polonelli L, De Bernardis F, Conti S et al (1994) Idiotypic intravaginal vaccination to protect against candidal vaginitis by secretory, yeast killer toxin-like antiidiotypic antibodies. J Immunol 152(6):3175–3182
13. Guyard C, Evrard P, Corbisier-Colson AM et al (2001) Immuno-crossreactivity of an anti-*Pichia anomala* killer toxin monoclonal antibody with a *Williopsis saturnus* var. *mrakii* killer toxin. Med Mycol 39(5):395–400
14. Guyard C, Dehecq E, Tissier JP et al (2002) Involvement of β-glucans in the wide-spectrum antimicrobial activity of *Williopsis saturnus* var. *mrakii* MUCL 41968 killer toxin. Mol Med 8(11):686–694
15. Polonelli L, Morace G (1987) Production and characterization of yeast killer toxin monoclonal antibodies. J Clin Microbiol 25(2):460–462
16. Polonelli L, Conti S, Gerloni M et al (1991) "Antibiobodies": antibiotic-like antiidiotypic antibodies. J Med Vet Mycol 29(4):235–242
17. Cassone A, Conti S, De Bernardis F, Polonelli L (1997) Antibodies, killer toxins and antifungal immunoprotection: a lesson from nature? Immunol Today 18(4):164–169
18. Torosantucci A, Bromuro C, Chiani P et al (2005) A novel glyco-conjugate vaccine against fungal pathogens. J Exp Med 202(5):597–606
19. Polonelli L, Séguy N, Conti S et al (1997) Monoclonal yeast killer toxin-like candidacidal anti-idiotypic antibodies. Clin Diagn Lab Immunol 4(2):142–146
20. Magliani W, Conti S, De Bernardis F et al (1997) Therapeutic potential of antiidiotypic single chain antibodies with yeast killer toxin activity. Nat Biotechnol 15(2):155–158
21. Magliani W, Conti S, Frazzi R et al (2005) Protective antifungal yeast killer toxin-like antibodies. Curr Mol Med 5:443–452
22. Polonelli L, De Bernardis F, Conti S et al (1996) Human natural yeast killer toxin-like candidacidal antibodies. J Immunol 156(5):1880–1885
23. Conti S, Fanti F, Magliani W et al (1998) Mycobactericidal activity of human natural, monoclonal, and recombinant yeast killer toxin-like antibodies. J Infect Dis 177(3):807–811
24. Séguy N, Cailliez JC, Delcourt P et al (1997) Inhibitory effect of human natural yeast killer toxin-like candidacidal antibodies on *Pneumocystis carinii*. Mol Med 3(8):544–552
25. Laemmli UK (1970) Cleavage of structural proteins during assembly of head of bacteriophage T4. Nature 227(5259):680–685
26. Guyard C, Séguy N, Cailliez JC et al (2002) Characterization of a *Williopsis saturnus* var. *mrakii* high molecular weight secreted killer toxin with broad-spectrum antimicrobial activity. J Antimicrob Chemother 49(6):961–971
27. Lowry OH, Rosebrough NJ, Farr AL, Randall RJ (1951) Protein measurement with the Folin phenol reagent. J Biol Chem 193(1):265–275
28. Pericolini E, Gabrielli E, Ballet N et al (2016) Therapeutic activity of a *Saccharomyces cerevisiae*-based probiotic and inactivated whole yeast on vaginal candidiasis. Virulence. doi:10.1080/21505594.2016.1213937
29. Polonelli L, Morace G (1986) Reevaluation of the yeast killer phenomenon. J Clin Microbiol 24(5):866–869
30. Polonelli L, Dettori G, Cattel C, Morace G (1987) Biotyping of mycelial fungus cultures by the killer system. Eur J Epidemiol 3(3):237–242
31. Morace G, Dettori G, Sanguinetti M et al (1988) Biotyping of aerobic actinomycetes by modified killer system. Eur J Epidemiol 4(1):99–103
32. Polonelli L, Menozzi MG, Campani L et al (1992) Anaerobic yeast killer system. Eur J Epidemiol 8(3):471–476
33. Polonelli L, Beninati C, Teti G et al (2014) Yeast killer toxin-like candidacidal Ab6 antibodies elicited through the manipulation of the idiotypic cascade. PLoS One 9(8):e105727. doi:10.1371/journal.pone.0105727
34. Polonelli L, Fanti F, Conti S et al (1990) Detection by immunofluorescent anti-idiotypic antibodies of yeast killer toxin cell wall receptors of *Candida albicans*. J Immunol Methods 132(2):205–209

Chapter 9

Peptide Vaccine Against Paracoccidioidomycosis

Carlos P. Taborda and Luiz R. Travassos

Abstract

The chapter reviews methods utilized for the isolation and characterization of a promising immunogen candidate, aiming at a human vaccine against paracoccidioidomycosis. Peptide P10 carries a T-CD4+ epitope and was identified as an internal sequence of the major diagnostic antigen known as gp43 glycoprotein. It successfully treated massive intratracheal infections by virulent *Paracoccidioides brasiliensis* in combination with chemotherapy.

An introduction about the systemic mycosis was found essential to understand the various options that were considered to design prophylactic and therapeutic vaccine protocols using peptide P10.

Key words *Paracoccidioides* spp., *Paracoccidioides brasiliensis*, Vaccine, Peptide, Protection

1 Introduction

Paracoccidioidomycosis (PCM) is a systemic mycosis, caused by the thermally dimorphic fungus *Paracoccidioides* spp. Currently, the genus *Paracoccidioides* is recognized as phylogenetically divided into two species named *P. brasiliensis* (cryptic species S1, PS2, PS3, PS4) and *P. lutzii* (recently discovered species that includes the isolated "Pb01-like" group) [1–3]. These pathogenic fungi are endemic in the Americas, from Mexico to Argentina, with the largest number of reported cases in Brazil, Colombia, and Venezuela [4]. In the 1996–2006 period, 517,058 deaths by infectious and parasitic diseases were documented in Brazil. Systemic fungal infections were responsible for 3583 deaths and paracoccidioidomycosis, cited in 51.2% of these deaths occupied the tenth position among the infectious and parasitic diseases of high mortality [5].

Conidia/spores, probably present in the soil, are considered the infective forms. The host infection most often occurs by inhalation of conidia which reach the bronchioles and terminal alveoli, where they transform into yeast forms, that initiate an infection that can spread to other tissues through the hematogenous and lymphatic systems [6, 7].

Markus Kalkum and Margarita Semis (eds.), *Vaccines for Invasive Fungal Infections: Methods and Protocols*, Methods in Molecular Biology, vol. 1625, DOI 10.1007/978-1-4939-7104-6_9,

The disease is characterized by pulmonary involvement and eventual spread to other organs and systems, mainly the oral mucosa and skin. It is classically associated with residents of rural areas, mainly man-workers between 30 and 50 years of age [6, 8]. Women are protected by hormones that prevent the mycelium-to-yeast transition during the first phase of infection [9, 10].

PCM can be clinically classified, according to disease manifestations, into different categories: (1) subclinical infection, detected only by a positive skin test; (2) acute or subacute forms (usually young patients of both sexes, with fungus infection of the reticulo-endothelial system) and chronic (typical of male adults, can be unifocal when a single organ is affected, usually the lungs, or multifocal, involving more than one site, especially the lungs and oral mucosa) [11, 12]. The occurrence of sequelae after clinical manifestation of the disease is common. They are characterized by chronic obstructive pulmonary fibrosis, dysphonia, and scars in the larynx [13]. It was shown that more than half the patients in the chronic form had lung radiological lesions after treatment [14].

The onset of the disease, its spread and severity depend on factors inherent to the fungus, as its virulence, antigenic composition, environmental conditions but, predominantly, on factors related to the host's ability to develop an effective immune response [15, 16]. Smoking and excessive alcohol consumption are pre-existing risk conditions that may play a role in the transformation of infection in an active disease, since they interfere with the host defense mechanisms and have implications in the granuloma formation [17].

The treatment of paracoccidioidomycosis is complex, requiring prolonged administration (over one or 2 years) of antifungals, even after clinical improvements to avoid the appearance of relapses. Frequently, the prolonged treatment leads to interruption of chemotherapy. Useful drugs in PCM treatment are itraconazole, the best option in mild to moderate clinical forms [18, 19]. The combination of trimethoprim-sulfamethoxazole is the alternative most widely used for outpatient PCM treatment [12].

The implementation of immune strategies that can be applied in conjunction with drug therapy is being studied aiming to reduce the time of treatment, reestablish an effective immune response, and prevent posttreatment sequelae [20]. Earlier, it was generally believed that antibodies had no ability to protect against systemic fungal diseases. The presence, however, of high titers of antibodies in PCM is associated with acute and more aggressive disease [12]. The study developed by Dr. Arturo Casadevall (John Hopkins University, USA) on the modulation of the immune response with monoclonal antibodies in experimental cryptococcosis completely changed the former concepts on the role of antibodies in fungal diseases [21–25]. In PCM, passive transference of monoclonal and polyclonal antibodies has been described as being able to increase the phagocytosis and the survival of animals infected with *P. brasiliensis* [26–28] and *P. lutzii* [29].

Peptides can be adequately synthetized and used for vaccine development. They can induce B cell and T cell responses and in many cases a combined response of Th-1 and Th-2 lymphocytes is most effective. There are cases in which immunosuppression or immunological imbalance with a predominant Th-1 response should be stimulated for host protection against fungal infection [30, 31].

Peptides used in vaccine protocols may show instability, degradation susceptibility, modification after injection, rapid renal filtration, and can be restricted by the genetic background of the human recipient [30]. Prior definition of cell target (dendritic cells, macrophages, lymphocytes, etc.), site of inoculation (intradermal, subcutaneous, intravenous, etc.), or type of delivery complex (liposomes, virosomes, microspheres, nanoparticles, etc.) is essential for the success of vaccination [30, 32–36].

In contrast to monoclonal antibodies, there is no licensed peptide vaccine for humans, although in experimental models, the use of peptides and fungal antigens has been effective in therapeutic vaccination protocols [30]. In addition to vaccines, passive transfer of specific monoclonal antibodies can increase the immune response and enhance the protective effect of chemotherapy [26, 30].

The major antigenic molecule for vaccine development against PCM is the 43,000-Da glycoprotein (gp43) that was first described in 1986 by Puccia et al. [37]. A high frequency of patients with PCM has antibodies against the gp43, and decreased titers of IgG, IgA, and IgM anti-gp43 correlated with clinical improvement [38, 39]. The gp43 is found in intracellular vacuoles and then accumulates throughout the cell wall and is secreted in the supernatant where it represents almost 80% of the exoantigenic protein [40, 41]. The gene of the gp43 was cloned, sequenced, and expressed in *Escherichia coli* [42]. The recombinant protein has 416 amino acids with a leader sequence of 35 residues [42]. The mature glycoprotein has a single *N*-glycosylation site with a high-mannose $Hex_{13}GlcNAc_2$ oligosaccharide [43]. A peptide of 15-mer (QTLIAIHTLAIRYAN) denominated P10, was identified in the gp43, mediating delayed-type hypersensitivity reactions and sensitizing T-$CD4^+$ lymphocytes, adjacent to the *N*-glycosylation site [44]. A C-terminal amidated synthetic P10 peptide when administered subcutaneally in complete Freund adjuvant was able to reduce the lung fungal burden in BALB/C mice intratracheally infected with yeasts of *P. brasiliensis.* The antifungal response was characterized by a predominant Th-1 response rich in IFN-γ and IL-12 (44). Later, the combination of antifungal drugs and P10 immunization was tested in different protocols with high efficiency in both immunocompetent [45] and immunosuppressed animals [46].

We describe next the essential methods used for peptide vaccine tests against a fungal infection. Experimental paracoccidioidomycosis was used as a model for vaccine development.

2 Materials

2.1 Culture Media

1. *Sabouraud glucose medium (supplemented with asparagine and thiamine)*: Sabouraud glucose (broth or agar) see manufacturer's instructions, 0.14% of L-asparagine, 0.01% of thiamine, 1.5% agar.
2. *Medium UBA*: 6.1 g Yeast extract, 16.1 g dextrose, 15 g of casein peptone, 0.31 g K_2HPO_4, 0.12 g $MgSO_4.7H_2O$, 0.006 g $MnSO_4.H_2O$, 0.006 g NaCl, 0.006 g of $FeSO_4$ to 1000 ml of distilled H_2O.
3. *Brain Heart Infusion (BHI)- Medium supplemented*: Brain Heart Infusion (BHI) see manufacturer's instructions, 4% (vol/vol) fetal bovine serum, 0.5% D(+)glucose, EDTA 300 μM final concentration, 5% of filtered culture supernatant from *Paracoccidioides brasiliensis* Pb192, yeast culture (grown in BHI for 15 days at 37 ° C and constant agitation at 150 rpm), Streptomycin/penicillin 10 IU/ml, 1.5% Agar.
4. *Mycosel medium (per liter) to maintain the shape of the mold*: Dextrose 10 g, Agar 15.5 g, Cycloheximide 0.4 g, Chloramphenicol 0.05 g, Papain digest of soybean meal 10 g, pH 6.9.
5. *Chemically defined MMcM (Morton-Modified Synthetic McVeigth) (per liter) to maintain the shape of the mold*: Dextrose 10 g, KH_2PO_4 1.5 g, $MgSO_4$ 0.5 g, $CaCl_2$ 0.15 g, $(NH_4)_2SO_4$ 2 g, L-asparagine 2 g, L-cystine 0.2 g (previously dissolved in NaOH 1 N), adjust to pH 7.0 with HCl 1 N. After sterilization, add: Trace elements 1.0 ml (*see* **Note 1**), Vitamins 10.0 ml (*see* **Note 2**), Penicillin 20 U/ml or Gentamicine 50 μg/ml.

2.2 Immuno chemistry

1. Sabouraud Dextrose agar.
2. Erlenmeyer flask.
3. UBA medium (same as Subheading 2.1, **item 2**).
4. Fernbach flask.
5. Thimerosal (0.2 g/l).
6. Filter paper.
7. Amicon concentrator.
8. N2 gas supply.
9. Y-10 filtration membrane.
10. SDS-PAGE system.
11. Silver staining for proteins.
12. Bradford reagent.
13. Bovine serum albumin.

14. Centrifuge.
15. CNBr-activated Sepharose-4B column (Sigma, St. Louis, USA) bound to anti-gp43 17c monoclonal antibody (Rosana Puccia, unpublished method) [26, 27, 41].
16. Phosphate buffered saline pH 7.4 (PBS).
17. 0.1 M glycine-HCl, pH 2.8.
18. Tris 2 M, pH 9.0.
19. Spectrophotometer at 280 nm.
20. Amicon cell (Amicon Stirred Ultra Filtration Cells, Millipore, USA).

2.3 Proteomics

1. Gel filtration column: (0.1 × 30 cm) Superose 6 10/300 GL column.
2. 50 mM ammonium acetate.
3. Internal size-markers: thyroglobulin (M_r 669,000, 5 mg/ml); ferritin (M_r 440,000, 0.4 mg/ml); BSA (M_r 67,000, 8 mg/ml); ribonuclease A (M_r 13,700, 1 mg/ml).
4. Speed-vac.
5. 0.4 M ammonium bicarbonate.
6. 8 M urea.
7. 0.045 M (dithiothreitol) DTT.
8. 0.1 M iodoacetamide.
9. Trypsin: Prepare trypsin in 1 mM HCl at 1 mg/ml (20 μl of 1 mM HCl for a 20 μg vial). This results in a solution containing 1 mg/ml trypsin, pH 3.0.
10. Ultra-pure water.
11. C-18 microcolumn with 10 μl tip.
12. 50% acetonitrile/H2O with 0.1% formic acid.
13. LTQ Orbitrap XL™ ETD Hybrid Ion Trap-Orbitrap Mass Spectrometer (Thermo)—nano LC ultra 1D plus (Ekisgent).
14. 50 μl microsyringe (Hamilton, Reno, NV, USA).
15. MaxEnt3 tool (available on MaxLynx 4.1 software).
16. MASCOT software (www.matrixscience.com).
17. Protean program (protein sequence analysis) of Lasergene biocomputing software for Windows, 1994 (DNASTAR Inc., Madison, Wis.) [44, 47].

2.4 Animals

1. *Specific Pathogen-Free mice*: mouse haplotypes [BALB/c (*H-2d*), A/Sn (*H-2a*), and C57BL (*H-2b*)] (*see* **Note 3**).
2. *Animal room*: Adequate animal room must be used—Biosafety categories II (yeast) and III (mold) for *Paracoccidioides* spp.

3. *Dexamethasone phosphate solution for immunosuppression of mice*: The corticoid is added to the drinking water of animals 20 days before infection and remained until the day of sacrifice 60 days post infection. Assuming an average water intake of 5 ml per day for 30 days, the daily dexamethasone phosphate dose was calculated as 0.15 mg/kg.

2.5 Intratracheal Infection

1. Ketamine/xylazine (80 mg/kg and 10 mg/kg) solution for anesthesia of mice (intraperitoneal injection).
2. *Paracoccidioides brasiliensis* strains: Pb18 and Pb339 (*see* **Note 4**).
3. Sterile PBS (per liter): NaCl 8 g, KCl 0.2 g, KH_2PO_4 0.2 g, Na_2HPO_4 1.16 g.
4. Surgical scissors.
5. Gauge-needle (26 G × 1/2″).
6. Silk (5.0) or surgical glue.
7. Tubes for blood collection.
8. Centrifuge.

2.6 Therapeutic Vaccine and Antifungal Drugs

1. 0.1 mM cationic lipid dioctadecyldimethylammonium bromide (DODAB).
2. 1 mM NaCl.
3. Ketoconazole 8 mg/kg (Janssen-Cilag®, Brazil), itraconazole 10 mg/kg (Janssen-Cilag®, Brazil), and fluconazole 10 mg/kg (Pfizer®, USA) must be kept at room temperature. The drugs are solubilized in 2% DMSO, before being diluted in PBS or culture medium. Fluconazole is directly soluble in water.
4. Amphotericin B 1.5 mg/kg (fungizon® Bristol Mayers Squibb, Brazil) was solubilized in sterile water and shortly afterward stored at 4 ° C and protected from light.
5. Sulfamethoxazole 15 mg/kg (Sigma, St. Louis, MO) was presolubilized in 2% DMSO.
6. Sulfamethoxazole/trimethoprim 15 mg/3 mg/kg (Bacsulfitrin Ducto, Brazil) was diluted in PBS with 2% of DMSO.

2.7 Colony-Forming Units (CFU)

1. Sterile PBS.
2. Sample dissociator gentleMACS™.
3. Supplemented BHI-agar medium (same as Subheading 2.1, **item 3**).
4. Incubator 37 ° C in 5% CO_2 and 95% humidity.

2.8 Cytokine Analysis

1. Protease inhibitors: benzamidine HCl (4 mM), EDTA disodium salt (1 mM), *N*-ethylmaleimide (1 mM), and pepstatin (1.5 mM) (Sigma).
2. Cytokine detection kits.

3 Methods

3.1 Biosafety and Culture Conditions

Paracoccidioides spp., are designated by the "*health and safety document from the Advisory Committee on Dangerous Pathogens, Categorization of pathogens According to hazard and categories of containment*" (Executive, 2013 # 9187) as a pathogen of categories II (yeast) and III (mold), and must be manipulated in class III containment laboratory for microbiological safety stream class II.

1. Maintain the isolates in the yeast phase at 37 °C in Sabouraud glucose medium (supplemented with asparagine and thiamine).
2. Maintain the shape of the mold at Mycosel medium and chemically defined MMcm at 18 °C.
3. Isolate, clone, and sequence the gp43 from Pb339 [42].

3.2 Immuno chemistry: Crude Antigen Preparation

1. After 5–10 days of culture on Sabouraud Dextrose agar at 37° C, transfer the yeast forms to an Erlenmeyer flask containing 50 ml of medium UBA.
2. Keep the suspension under stirring for 3 days at 37 ° C. Then transfer to a Fernbach flask containing 500 ml of the same medium and incubate for additional 7–10 days, under the same conditions.
3. After this period, kill the cells with thimerosal (0.2 g/l) and collect the supernatant (crude exoantigen) after paper filtration.
4. Concentrate the exoantigen in an Amicon concentrator under N_2, using Y-10 filtration membrane.
5. Perform dosage and monitoring of proteins by SDS-PAGE followed by silver staining and Bradford method [48].

3.3 Immuno chemistry: Glycoprotein of 43 kDa Purification

1. Starting from the culture supernatant of *P. brasiliensis* Pb339 (crude exoantigen after centrifugation at 20,000 × *g* [rotor radius 20 cm] for 20 min to remove precipitated material), purify the gp43 by affinity chromatography on CNBr-activated Sepharose-4B column bound to anti-gp43 17c monoclonal antibody.
2. Apply the exoantigen slowly to the affinity column, and after passing through the material to be purified, wash the column with PBS in fast flow to remove unwanted substances.
3. Elute the gp43 with 5 ml of 0.1 M glycine-HCl, pH 2.8, and immediately neutralize with 100 μl of Tris 2 M, pH 9.0.
4. Collect 1 ml fractions and read the absorbance in a spectrophotometer at 280 nm. Pool the fractions with the highest absorbance.
5. Dialyze the resulting volume with 0.15 M PBS (pH 7.4), and then concentrate under N_2, at 4 °C in the Amicon cell using Y-10 membrane.

6. Determine protein concentration by Bradford method, using bovine serum albumin as default protein, monitor on SDS-PAGE gel, stain with Silver staining to assess the actual purity of the sample [37].

3.4 Proteomics: Gel Filtration Chromatography

1. Apply an aliquot of 300 μl of exoantigen along with the internal size-markers to a gel filtration column pre-equilibrated with 50 mM ammonium acetate. This technique aims at the separation of molecules according to size by passing them through a chromatographic matrix. Use the flow rate of 1 ml/min.
2. Collect 1 ml fractions and test in dot-blots, with sera of mice infected with *P. brasiliensis* Pb18.

3.5 Proteomics: Preparation of Samples for Mass Spectrometry

Prepare the fractions derived from gel filtration that were positive in dot-blotting for mass spectrometry as follows.

1. Concentrate a fraction volume of 50 μl in speed-vac and resuspend in 20 μl of 0.4 M ammonium bicarbonate and 8 M urea.
2. Thereafter, add 5 μl of 0.045 M DTT and incubate for 15 min at 50 °C. After cooling to room temperature, add 5 μl 0.1 M iodoacetamide.
3. Incubate for 15 min at room temperature, protect from light.
4. Add 2 μl trypsin, and 130 μl of ultra-pure water to dilute the urea to 1 M. Incubate the solution for 24 h, and then desalt in a C-18 microcolumn in a 10 μl tip according to the manufacturer's instructions.

3.6 Proteomics: Analysis of Peptides by Mass Spectrometry

1. Resuspend peptides in 20 μl 50% acetonitrile/H_2O with 0.1% formic acid and directly infuse into a LTQ Orbitrap XL™ ETD Hybrid Ion Trap-Orbitrap Mass Spectrometer—nano LC ultra 1D plus, at a flow rate of 0.5 μl/min, using a 50 μl microsyringe.
2. Perform the fragmentation of doubly or singly charged ions under different collision energies, using argon as a collision gas, to determine the best fragmentation spectra to be used for sequencing.
3. Acquire the fragmentation spectra every 0.5 s, and obtain the final spectrum by combining 1.5 min of spectrum acquisition. Deconvolute collision-induced dissociation (CID) spectra using MaxEnt3 tool, to convert doubly charged into singly charged ions.
4. Identify proteins by searching the database using MASCOT software [49], with the following search parameters: 0.08 isotopic mass tolerance; 0.02 Da fragment mass tolerance; methionine oxidation as variable modification; carbamidomethylation of cysteine residues as fixed modification; one missed tryptic cleavage allowed.

3.7 In Silico Analysis

Bioinformatics is a very powerful tool for the analysis of possible epitope candidates for a vaccine. In addition, there are several sites/programs available for the analysis of proteins of immunological interest. Predictions or possible epitopes should be confirmed with the proper immunological mediators. In the case of gp43 we used several parameters to map the P10 peptide sequence. The Jameson-Wolff antigenic index, the Kyte-Doolittle hydrophilicity plot, Eisenberg's alpha helix amphipathic regions, Emini's surface probability plot, and the Alessandro Sette major histocompatibility complex (MHC II) motif method (H-2^d mice) were used to analyze the gp43, by the Protean program of Lasergene biocomputing software for Windows.

3.8 Validation of the Peptide Vaccine

The P10 sequence is conserved in most isolates of *P. brasiliensis*, moreover, three mouse haplotypes [BALB/c (*H-2d*), A/Sn (*H-2a*), and C57BL (*H-2b*)], presented the synthetic P10 as inferred from its protective effects against experimental PCM [20, 44]. Also, using the TEPITOPE algorithm covering 25 Caucasian HLD-DR types, P10 and neighboring peptides in the gp43 were predicted to bind to 90% of these molecules. This was indeed shown examining primary peripheral blood mononuclear cell responses from sensitized individuals [50]. The promiscuous nature of P10 in its presentation by human MHC-II molecules is thus a fundamental feature in the validation of this peptide as a vaccine [20, 51].

3.9 Animal Model

Most experiments on the immune protection by the P10 peptide were run in BALB/c mice, susceptible to *P. brasiliensis* infection. It is possible that adjustments in the protocols have to be made when using other mouse haplotypes that may exhibit different intensities of pro-inflammatory responses [20]. Different strains of mice as well as route of infection can lead to unparalleled results. Intraperitoneal, intravenous, intranasal, and intratracheal routes of infection have been used. In our model, that mimics the subacute or chronic disease model, the intratracheal route has been used as a standard method of infection.

1. Collect the yeast cells and wash three times with phosphate buffer (pH 7.2).
2. After the last wash, let the suspension still for a few minutes, for sedimentation of cell clumps.
3. Collect the upper suspension, containing single or few budding cells and count the yeast cells in a Neubauer chamber. Analyze the yeast viability by trypan blue exclusion staining and consider it appropriate for use with more than 95% of viability.
4. Anesthetize BALB/c mice (6–8 week-old males) intraperitoneally with 200 μl of a solution containing 80 mg/kg ketamine and 10 mg/kg of xylazine.

5. Five to ten minutes after anesthesia, fix the mice to the "surgical table," hyperextend the necks and incise just to expose the trachea at the level of the thyroid with surgical scissors.
6. Each animal was injected with 3×10^5 viable yeasts of *P. brasiliensis* Pb18 in 50 μl PBS using a gauge-needle [44, 46] (*see* **Notes 5** and **6**).
7. Suture the incisions with 5–0 silk or surgical glue.

3.10 Polyclonal Serum from Infected Mice

1. Sacrifice the intratracheally infected mice after 30 days, and collect the blood by cardiac puncture.
2. Separate the plasma by keeping the tubes at 4 °C for 1 h and then centrifuge for 10 min at low rotation to avoid cell lysis.
3. Keep the serum frozen at −70°C.

3.11 Peptide Delivery and Adjuvants

P10 peptide with amidated C-terminal can be synthesized by commercial companies. HPLC and MS peptide analyses performed by the manufacturer must indicate 98% purity. Early experiments associated P10 with complete Freund's adjuvant which is not accepted for human or animal use [20]. Alternative ways of delivering P10 and using other adjuvants were investigated: incomplete Freund's adjuvant, FliC flagellin, alum, cationic lipid [52], P10-minigene in plasmid DNA accompanied or not by a plasmid carrying IL-12 insert [53, 54], nanoparticles [55] and dendritic cells [33]. A multiple truncated antigen peptide (MAP) construction with a branched lysine was also studied; however, the complexity of the technique is not suitable for large-scale use [56].

3.12 Therapeutic Vaccine

1. Initiate vaccination consisting of the peptide P10 associated with the DODAB as an adjuvant, 30 days after infection [57].
2. Administer the formulation subcutaneously in the dorsal region of the neck on days 30, 37, and 42 post-infection, total of three doses. Each dose consisted of 20 μg of P10 and 0.1 mM DODAB, solubilized in 1 mM NaCl.
3. Use a therapeutic vaccine with P10 simultaneously with chemotherapy. Mice received doses of 10 mg/kg itraconazole (ITC), or 15 mg sulfamethoxazole plus 3 mg trimethoprim/kg (SMT/TMP), or Sulfamethoxazole 15 mg/kg, or 8 mg/kg ketoconazole, or 10 mg/kg fluconozole every 24 h, or Amphotericin B 1.5 mg/kg every 48 h for 30 days (until day 60, post-infection).

3.13 Published P10-Vaccination Results

1. *Additive protection activity of P10*: The protective effect of peptideo P10 is associated with cellular immune, IFN-γ-dependent, Th1 response [30]. We observed significant improvement of animal health submitted to experimental PCM when the intratracheally infected mice were treated with

an antifungal drug and immunized with P10. The combined drug treatment with peptide immunization achieved maximum protection, with significant reduction in the lung CFUs, preservation of pulmonary alveolar structure, and prevention of fungal dissemination [45, 46, 58].

2. *Fibrosis*: The primarily affected organ in PCM is the lung and fibrosis is detected in 90% of patients in the chronic form and in 10% of patients with acute/subacute PCM [14]. Fibrosis is an important problem during the healing process [59]. We observed that the therapeutic vaccine using peptide P10 or passive transfer of monoclonal antibodies induce cellular immune responses in addition to the protective effect of chemotherapy with possibly controlling relapses and reducing fibrosis sequels [26, 45, 52]. One of our most important results using different adjuvants showed that the immunization with P10 and cationic lipid resulted in a lung tissue with no collagen fibers of Type 1 and no detectable fungal cells [52].
3. *DNA vaccine*: A vaccine using plasmid DNA carrying the full gene of the gp43 was tested with partial protection in BALB/c mice infected with *P. brasiliensis* [60]. Rittner et al. (2012) [53] tested a new protocol using DNA vaccine encoding P10 with or without a plasmid encoding IL-12, which is administered without adjuvant. We found that DNA vaccine with the P10 insert with or without co-vaccination with the IL-12 plasmid, if given prior to or 1 month after infection, significantly reduced the fungal burden [53, 54]. Most significantly, in a long-term infection model the combined DNA vaccine (plasmids carrying P10 and murine IL-12) achieved virtual sterilization after 6 months with histologically normal lungs and undetectable fungal burden [53].
4. *Final considerations*: The protective effects of P10 vaccine (peptide or DNA encoding P10) are very significant in intratracheally infected mice. In humans, the routine PCM treatment with antifungal drugs, itraconazole, sulfamethoxazole/trimethoprim, amphotericin B, and even voriconazole should be efficient to control systemic PCM as an attack treatment to avoid patients' death. Since the treatment takes several years and some patients interrupt medication after improvement of clinical signs but without complete elimination of the fungus, relapses and sequels are frequently observed. A therapeutic vaccine could improve the present situation by stimulation of the immune response for fungal clearance, reduction of treatment time, thus, hopefully avoiding treatment interruption, and possible reduction or elimination of severe relapses and fibrotic sequels.

3.14 Immuno suppression of Mice to Mimic (Chemically) the Acute Form

1. Immunosuppress the animals with daily doses of 0.15 mg/kg of dexamethasone phosphate for a period of 20 days, added to the drinking water to be consumed *ad líbitum*, and changed once a week.
2. Accommodate the animals in isolators to maintain appropriate sterile environment, with autoclaved shaving woods, food, and water delivered to the animals.
3. Perform the cage changes in a laminar flow hood twice a week.

3.15 Determination of Fungal Load in the Lungs and Other Organs

1. Use supplemented BHI solid medium to determine the fungal loads in experimentally infected mice.
2. After sacrificing the mice using accepted procedures [44, 58], remove the organs (lung, liver, and spleen), weigh and homogenize in sterile PBS 1× with the aid of a sample dissociator gentleMACS™.
3. After steeping, streak-plate 100 μl of homogenized tissue on Petri dishes containing supplemented BHI-agar medium and incubate the plates at 37 °C in 5% CO_2 and 95% humidity for 4 weeks.
4. During this period, inspect the plates daily and count the number of colony-forming units (CFU).
5. Plot the fungal load as CFU per gram of tissue.

3.16 Histology

1. A good histological preparation depends on the techniques to obtain the specimen. The cardiac perfusion usually results in good slides with preserved tissue. In case of no interference, administration of heparin diluted 1:50, 10 min before animal euthanasia, can prevent blood clots formation. A neutral pH solution followed by formalin 10% was injected into aortic arch employing a thin silicone tubing connected to a peristaltic pump (or alternatively a syringe can substitute peristaltic pump). The tissue fixation by immersion in the formalin 10% solution instead perfusion is an option.
2. Once the material was included in paraffin, cut by microtome and fixed in the slide, there are several available staining methods. In medical mycology hematoxylin and eosin staining (good for tissue structural characteristics, but do not reveal all cellular components) and Silver staining as the Grocott-Gomori's methenamine silver stain, mainly detecting fungal elements, are the most used staining methods. For fibrosis evaluation, tissues sections are stained with Gomori's silver reticulin–stain to assess the changes occurring in the organization of reticulin fibers (collagen III), and with Masson's trichrome–stain to identify collagen I type fibers. The histological result of one P10-adjuvant vaccination experiment is shown in Fig. 1.

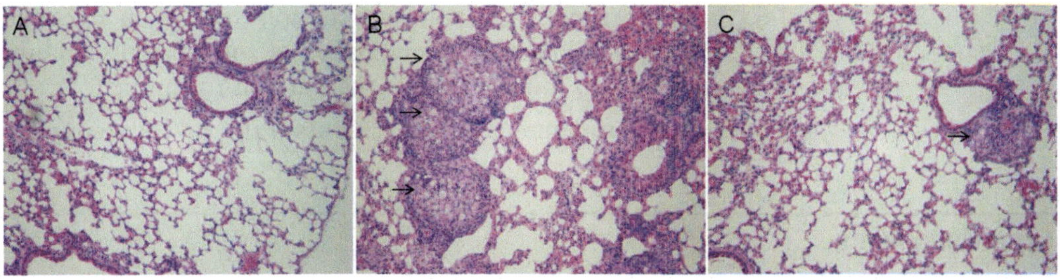

Fig. 1 Histological sections of murine lungs from BALB/c mice immunized with P10-cationic lipid after 30 days of infection. (**a**) Uninfected and non-immunized control mice; (**b**) large granulomas in infected mice; (**c**) infected and immunized with P10-cationic lipid. 40× magnification. Hematoxylin and eosin staining; arrows indicate granulomas

3.17 Cytokine Detection

1. Quantification of cytokines helps to understand the immunological profile during infection by *P. brasiliensis*. Cytokine profile of Th-1, Th-2, Th-17, and Treg lymphocytes present in supernatant of macerated organs such as lung, liver, spleen, are important to understand the vaccine modulation and results must be analyzed together with CFU and histology.
2. The procedure is similar to that for the determination of fungal load in the organs (3.14); however, tissues were homogenized in 2 ml of PBS in the presence of protease inhibitors: benzamidine HCl (4 mM), EDTA disodium salt (1 mM), *N*-ethylmaleimide (1 mM), and pepstatin (1.5 mM). There are several manufacturers of cytokine detection kits.
3. Express the results as cytokine mass/per gram of tissue.

4 Notes

1. Trace elements composition (100 ml): H_3BO_3 0.0057 g, $CuSO_4.5H_2O$ 0.0157 g, $Fe(NH_4)_2(SO_4)_2.6H2O$ 0.1404 g, $MnSO_4.14H_2O$ 0.0081 g, $(NH_4)_6Mo_7O_{24}.4H_2O$ 0.0036 g, $ZnSO_4.7H_2O$ 0.0792 g. Sterilize with 0.22 μm filter and keep to −20 °C.
2. Vitamin composition (100 ml): Thiamine 0.006 g, Niacin 0.006 g, calcium 0.006 g, Inositol 0.003 g, Biotin 0.0001 g, Riboflavin 0.001 g, Folic acid 0.01 g, Choline 0.01 g, Pyrodoxine 0.01 g. Sterilize with 0.22 μm filter and keep to −20 °C.
3. Be sure that the local Ethics Committee approved all procedures involving experimental animals.
4. Two isolates of *Paracoccidioides brasiliensis* were used, Pb18 (traditionally used in experimental models in Brazil, characterized as a high-virulence isolate) [61] and *P. brasiliensis* Pb339, traditionally being used for antigen production [62].

5. Each experiment must include all controls (sham infection, animals only infected, animals infected and treated with antifungal drugs, animals immunized only with adjuvant).
6. Each experimental group must contain at least eight animals.

Acknowledgments

The authors thank Fundação de Amparo a Pesquisa do Estado de São Paulo (Fapesp) for research grants and the National Research Council (CNPq) for career fellowships.

References

1. Theodoro RC, Teixeira MM, Felipe MSS et al (2012) Genus *Paracoccidioides*: species recognition and biogeographic aspects. PLoS One 7(5):e37694
2. Teixeira MM, Theodoro RC, Nino-Vega G et al (2014) *Paracoccidioides* species complex: ecology, phylogeny, sexual reproduction, and virulence. PLoS Pathog 10(10):e1004397
3. Bocca AL, Amaral AC, Teixeira MM et al (2013) Paracoccidioidomycosis: eco-epidemiology, taxonomy and clinical and therapeutic issues. Future Microbiol 8(9):1177–1191
4. Taborda CP, Urán ME, Nosanchuk JD et al (2015) Paracoccidioidomycosis: challenges in the development of a vaccine against an endemic mycosis in the Americas. Rev do Inst Med Trop São Paulo 57(Suppl 19):21–24
5. Prado M, Silva MB, Laurenti R et al (2009) Mortality due to systemic mycoses as a primary cause of death or in association with AIDS in Brazil: a review from 1996 to 2006. Mem Inst Oswaldo Cruz 104(3):513–521
6. Restrepo AM (1985) The ecology of *Paracoccidioides brasiliensis*: a puzzle still unsolved. Sabouraudia 23(5):323–334
7. Oliveira HC, Assato PA, Marcos CM et al (2015) *Paracoccidioides*-host interaction: an overview on recent advances in the paracoccidioidomycosis. Front Microbiol 6:1319
8. Wanke B, Aidê MA (2009) Chapter 6 - paracoccidioidomycosis. J Bras Pneumol 35(12):1245–1249
9. Stover EP, Schar G, Clemons KV et al (1986) Estradiol-binding proteins from mycelial and yeast-form cultures of *Paracoccidioides brasiliensis*. Infect Immun 51(1):199–203
10. Loose DS, Stover EP, Restrepo A et al (1983) Estradiol binds to a receptor-like cytosol binding protein and initiates a biological response in *Paracoccidioides brasiliensis*. Proc Natl Acad Sci U S A 80(24):7659–7663
11. Franco M (1987) Host-parasite relationships in paracoccidioidomycosis. J Med Vet Mycol 25(1):5–18
12. Shikanai-Yasuda MA, Telles Filho FDQ, Mendes RP et al (2006) Consenso em paracoccidioidomicose. Rev Soc Bras Med Trop 39(3):297–310
13. Shikanai-Yasuda MA (2015) Paracoccidioidomycosis treatment. Rev Inst Med Trop São Paulo 57(Suppl 19):31–37
14. Tobón AM, Agudelo CA, Osorio ML et al (2003) Residual pulmonary abnormalities in adult patients with chronic paracoccidioidomycosis: prolonged follow-up after itraconazole therapy. Clin Infect Dis 37(7):898–904
15. MJS M-G, Monteiro da Silva JL, Fátima da Silva J et al (2008) Interactions of *Paracoccidioides brasiliensis* with host cells: recent advances. Mycopathologia 165(4–5):237–248
16. Benard G (2008) An overview of the immunopathology of human paracoccidioidomycosis. Mycopathologia 165(4–5):209–221
17. Camargo ZP, Franco MF (2000) Current knowledge on pathogenesis and immunodiagnosis of paracoccidioidomycosis. Rev Iberoam Micol 17(2):41–48
18. Marques SA (2012) Paracoccidioidomycosis. Clin Dermatol 30(6):610–615
19. Martinez R (2015) Epidemiology of paracoccidioidomycosis. Rev Inst Med Trop São Paulo 57(Suppl 19):11–20
20. Travassos LR, Taborda CP, Colombo AL (2008) Treatment options for paracoccidioidomycosis and new strategies investigated. Expert Rev Anti-Infect Ther 6(2):251–262
21. Fries BC, Taborda CP, Serfass E et al (2001) Phenotypic switching of *Cryptococcus neoformans*

occurs *in vivo* and influences the outcome of infection. J Clin Invest 108(11):1639–1648
22. Taborda CP, Rivera J, Zaragoza O et al (2003) More is not necessarily better: prozone-like effects in passive immunization with IgG. J Immunol 170(7):3621–3630
23. Taborda CP, Casadevall A (2001) Immunoglobulin M efficacy against *Cryptococcus neoformans*: mechanism, dose dependence, and prozone-like effects in passive protection experiments. J Immunol 166(3):2100–2107
24. Casadevall A, Pirofski L (2011) A new synthesis for antibody-mediated immunity. Nat Immunol 13(1):21–28
25. Albuquerque P, Casadevall A (2012) Quorum sensing in fungi – a review. Med Mycol 50(4):337–345
26. Buissa-Filho R, Puccia R, Marques AF et al (2008) The monoclonal antibody against the major diagnostic antigen of *Paracoccidioides brasiliensis* mediates immune protection in infected BALB/c mice challenged intratracheally with the fungus. Infect Immun 76(7):3321–3328
27. Gesztesi JL, Puccia R, Travassos LR et al (1996) Monoclonal antibodies against the 43,000 Da glycoprotein from *Paracoccidioides brasiliensis* modulate laminin-mediated fungal adhesion to epithelial cells and pathogenesis. Hybridoma 15(6):415–422
28. de Mattos Grosso D, de Almeida SR, Mariano M et al (2003) Characterization of gp70 and anti-gp70 monoclonal antibodies in *Paracoccidioides brasiliensis* pathogenesis. Infect Immun 71(11):6534–6542
29. Thomaz L, Nosanchuk JD, Rossi DCP et al (2014) Monoclonal antibodies to heat shock protein 60 induce a protective immune response against experimental *Paracoccidioides lutzii*. Microbes Infect 16(9):788–795
30. Travassos LR, Rodrigues EG, Iwai LK et al (2008) Attempts at a peptide vaccine against paracoccidioidomycosis, adjuvant to chemotherapy. Mycopathologia 165(4–5):341–352
31. Benard G, Patzina RL, Schwab JB et al (2012) Fatal septic shock due to a disseminated chronic form of paracoccidioidomycosis in an aged woman. Med Mycol 50(4):407–411
32. Thind SK, Taborda CP, Nosanchuk JD (2015) Dendritic cell interactions with *Histoplasma* and *Paracoccidioides*. Virulence 6(5):424–432
33. Magalhães A, Ferreira KS, Almeida SR et al (2012) Prophylactic and therapeutic vaccination using dendritic cells primed with peptide 10 derived from the 43-kilodalton glycoprotein of *Paracoccidioides brasiliensis*. Clin Vaccine Immunol 19(1):23–29
34. Braga CJ, Rittner GMG, Henao JEM et al (2009) *Paracoccidioides brasiliensis* vaccine formulations based on the gp43-derived P10 sequence and the Salmonella enterica FliC flagellin. Infect Immun 77(4):1700–1707
35. Arnon R (1986) Synthetic peptides as the basis for future vaccines. Trends Biochem Sci 11(12):521–524
36. Jiang S, Song R, Popov S et al (2006) Overlapping synthetic peptides as vaccines. Vaccine 24(37–39):6356–6365
37. Puccia R, Schenkman S, Gorin PAJ et al (1986) Exocellular components of *Paracoccidioides brasiliensis*: identification of a specific antigen. Infect Immun 53(1):199–206
38. Taborda CP, Camargo ZP (1993) Diagnosis of paracoccidioidomycosis by passive haemagglutination assay of antibody using a purified and specific antigen-gp43. J Med Vet Mycol 31(2):155–160
39. Taborda CP, Camargo ZP (1994) Diagnosis of paracoccidioidomycosis by dot immunobinding assay for antibody detection using the purified and specific antigen gp43. J Clin Microbiol 32(2):554–556
40. Travassos LR, Puccia R, Cisalpino P et al (1995) Biochemistry and molecular biology of the main diagnostic antigen of *Paracoccidioides brasiliensis*. Arch Med Res 26(3):297–304
41. Puccia R, Takaoka DT, Travassos LR (1991) Purification of the 43 kDa glycoprotein from exocellular components excreted by *Paracoccidioides brasiliensis* in liquid culture (TOM medium). J Med Vet Mycol 29(1):57–60
42. Cisalpino PS, Puccia R, Yamauchi LM et al (1996) Cloning, characterization, and epitope expression of the major diagnostic antigen of *Paracoccidioides brasiliensis*. J Biol Chem 271(8):4553–4560
43. Almeida IC, Neville DCA, Mehlert A et al (1996) Structure of the N-linked oligosaccharide of the main diagnostic antigen of the pathogenic fungus *Paracoccidioides brasiliensis*. Glycobiology 6(5):507–515
44. Taborda CP, Juliano MA, Puccia R et al (1998) Mapping of the T-cell epitope in the major 43-kilodalton glycoprotein of *Paracoccidioides brasiliensis* which induces a Th-1 response protective against fungal infection in BALB/c mice. Infect Immun 66(2):786–793
45. Marques AF, da Silva MB, Juliano MAP et al (2006) Peptide immunization as an adjuvant to chemotherapy in mice challenged intratracheally with virulent yeast cells of *Paracoccidioides brasiliensis*. Antimicrob Agents Chemother 50(8):2814–2819

46. Muñoz JE, Luft VD, Amorim J et al (2014) Immunization with P10 peptide increases specific immunity and protects immunosuppressed BALB/c mice infected with virulent yeasts of *Paracoccidioides brasiliensis*. Mycopathologia 178(3–4):177–188
47. Perez-Riverol Y, Sanchez A, Ramos Y et al (2011) In silico analysis of accurate proteomics, complemented by selective isolation of peptides. J Proteome 74(10):2071–2082
48. National Science Foundation (2006) Bradford protein assay protocol. 1–3
49. Perkins DN, Pappin DJ, Creasy DM et al (1999) Probability-based protein identification by searching sequence databases using mass spectrometry data. Electrophoresis 20(18):3551–3567
50. Iwai LK, Yoshida M, Sidney J et al (2003) In silico prediction of peptides binding to multiple HLA-DR molecules accurately identifies immunodominant epitopes from gp43 of *Paracoccidioides brasiliensis* frequently recognized in primary peripheral blood mononuclear cell responses from sensitized individuals. Mol Med 9(9–12):209–219
51. Leo KI, Yoshida M, Sadahiro A et al (2007) T-cell recognition of *Paracoccidioides brasiliensis* gp43-derived peptides in patients with paracoccidioidomycosis and healthy individuals. Clin Vaccine Immunol 14(4):474–476
52. Mayorga O, Muñoz JE, Lincopan N et al (2012) The role of adjuvants in therapeutic protection against paracoccidioidomycosis after immunization with the P10 peptide. Front Microbiol 3:154
53. GMG R, Muñoz JE, Marques AF et al (2012) Therapeutic DNA vaccine encoding peptide P10 against experimental paracoccidioidomycosis. PLoS Negl Trop Dis 6(2):1–9
54. de Amorim J, Magalhães A, Muñoz JE et al (2013) DNA vaccine encoding peptide P10 against experimental paracoccidioidomycosis induces long-term protection in presence of regulatory T cells. Microbes Infect 15(3):181–191
55. Amaral AC, Marques AF, Muñoz JE et al (2010) Poly-lactic acid-glycolic acid nanoparticles markedly improve immunological protection provided by peptide P10 against murine paracoccidioidomycosis. Br J Pharmacol 159(5):1126–1132
56. Taborda CP, Nakaie CR, Cilli EM et al (2004) Synthesis and immunological activity of a branched peptide carrying the T-cell epitope of gp43, the major exocellular antigen of *Paracoccidioides brasiliensis*. Scand J Immunol 59(1):58–65
57. Lincopan N, Espíndola NM, Vaz AJ et al (2009) Novel immunoadjuvants based on cationic lipid: preparation, characterization and activity in vivo. Vaccine 27(42):5760–5771
58. Marques AF, da Silva MB, Juliano MAP et al (2008) Additive effect of P10 immunization and chemotherapy in anergic mice challenged intratracheally with virulent yeasts of *Paracoccidioides brasiliensis*. Microbes Infect 10(12–13):1251–1258
59. Franco L, Najvar L, Gomez BL et al (1998) Experimental pulmonary fibrosis induced by *Paracoccidioides brasiliensis* conidia: measurement of local host responses. AmJTrop Med Hyg 58(4):424–430
60. Pinto AR, Puccia R, Diniz SN et al (2000) DNA-based vaccination against murine paracoccidioidomycosis using the gp43 gene from *Paracoccidioides brasiliensis*. Vaccine 18:3050–3058
61. Kurokawa CS, Lopes CR, Sugizaki MF et al (2005) Virulence profile of ten *Paracoccidioides brasiliensis* isolates. Association with morphologic and genetic patterns. Rev Inst Med Trop São Paulo 47(5):257–262
62. Camargo ZP, Taborda CP, Rodrigues EG et al (1991) The use of cell-free antigens of *Paracoccidioides brasiliensis* in serological tests. J Med Vet Mycol 29(1):31–38

Chapter 10

Methodology for Anti-Cryptococcal Vaccine Development

Ashok K. Chaturvedi and Floyd L. Wormley Jr

Abstract

Cryptococcus neoformans and *Cryptococcus gattii*, the predominant etiological agents of cryptococcosis, are fungal pathogens that cause disease ranging from a mild pneumonia to life-threatening infections of the central nervous system (CNS). *C. neoformans* is widely considered an opportunistic fungal pathogen which targets individuals with impaired immune systems, while *C. gattii* is predominantly associated with fungal infections in immunocompetent individuals. However, *C. neoformans* and *C. gattii* have certainly been identified as the causative agent of cryptococcosis in both immune compromised and immune competent individuals. Cell-mediated immunity (CMI) by T-helper (Th) 1-type $CD4^+$ T cells is the predominant host defense mechanism against cryptococcosis. Consequently, there has been great interest in identifying cryptococcal antigens that elicit protective CMI against *Cryptococcus* infection. Although many different cryptococcal proteins have been shown to stimulate potent cellular responses, there remains no standardized vaccine available for the prevention of cryptococcal infections in humans. Several studies have identified immunodominant antigens that may serve as attractive candidates for the development of novel subunit vaccines for the treatment and/or the prevention of cryptococcosis. The purpose of this chapter is to describe one methodology to screen and isolate cryptocococcal proteins that induce protective immune responses against cryptococossis.

Key words *Cryptococcus*, Cryptococcosis, Proteomics, Meningoencephalitis, Antibodies, Gel electrophoresis and fractionation

1 Introduction

Cryptococcusneoformans and Cryptococcus gattii, the predominant causative agents of cryptococcosis, are encapsulated fungal pathogens that can cause life-threatening infections of the central nervous system (CNS) in immune compromised and immune competent individuals [1]. Cryptococcal meningoencephalitis is the most common disseminated fungal infection in AIDS patients [2]. Global estimates suggest that one million cases of cryptococcal meningitis occur each year resulting in approximately 620,000 deaths [3]. Those who are successfully treated for AIDS-associated cryptococcal meningitis oftentimes require life-long maintenance anti-fungal therapy due to a high relapse rate [2, 4]. Additionally, the incidence

Markus Kalkum and Margarita Semis (eds.), *Vaccines for Invasive Fungal Infections: Methods and Protocols*, Methods in Molecular Biology, vol. 1625, DOI 10.1007/978-1-4939-7104-6_10, © Springer Science+Business Media LLC 2017

of *C. gatti* has been notable within animal and human populations on Vancouver Island, British Columbia, Canada, the Pacific Northwest, Southwest, Southeast, and Northeast regions of the US and in Mediterranean Europe [5–12], thus underscoring the potential of cryptococcal disease to emerge as a significant problem in unique clinical settings and patient populations. The increase in cryptococcosis, combined with reduced efficacy of the currently available drugs, highlights the need for new antifungal drugs, immunotherapeutics, and/or vaccines to protect at-risk populations (i.e., patients with compromised immune systems and immune competent persons residing in areas observed to contain *C. gattii*). Proteomic tools have been used to identify an array of proteins that are highly prevalent during disease and have the potential to induce protective immune responses against cryptococcosis. Potentially immunogenic cryptococcal antigens are usually preselected for analysis based on their serological activity [13–16]. However, proteins that are immune dominant for B cells may not necessarily be immune dominant for T cells. Therefore, where immune recognition and protection are mediated predominantly by T cells, strategies should be implemented to identify proteins that induce antigen-specific T cell responses. In our previous studies, we elected to use a combined proteomic and immunological approach to screen complex mixtures of *C. neoformans* and *C. gattii* proteins for those proteins that were immune dominant based on serologic reactivity and efficacy to elicit pro-inflammatory and Th1-type cytokine responses against *C. neoformans* and *C. gattii* antigens [17, 18]. We also evaluated the efficacy of selected protein fractions to induce protective immune responses in a murine model of pulmonary cryptococcosis. Herein, we provide a detailed methodology for the isolation and testing of cryptococcal proteins as candidates for the development of novel subunit vaccines for the treatment and/or the prevention of cryptococcosis.

2 Materials

Prepare all buffers using ultrapure water and analytical grade reagents. Store all reagents at room temperature unless otherwise indicated. Carefully follow all guidelines and regulations when disposing biohazardous waste materials.

2.1 Mice

Female BALB/c (H-2^{d}) mice (*see* **Note 1**).

2.2 Strains and Media

1. *C. neoformans* strain H99 (serotype A, Mat α).
2. H99γ (an IFN-γ producing *C. neofromans* strain derived from H99; ATCC® 208821™) [19].
3. *C. gattii* strain R265 (serotype B; ATCC® MYA-4093™).

4. Yeast extract peptone dextrose (YPD) agar: 1% yeast extract, 2% peptone, 2% dextrose, and 2% bacto agar.
5. YPD broth: 1% yeast extract, 2% peptone, 2% dextrose.
6. RPMI complete media (*see* **Note 2**).

2.3 Protein Extraction

1. Ammonium carbonate buffer, pH 8.4: 20 mM ammonium carbonate, 1% (v/v) beta-mercaptoethanol (β-ME), and protease inhibitors cocktail (*see* **Note 3**).
2. YeastBuster™ Protein Extraction Reagent: tris(hydroxypropy) phosphine (THP) and protease inhibitors cocktail (*see* **Note 3**).
3. Amicon Ultrafree-15 centrifugal filter device.
4. RC DC Protein Assay Kit (Bio-Rad, Hercules, CA).
5. ReadyPrep 2-D Cleanup Kit (Bio-Rad, Hercules, CA; *see* **Note 4**).
6. Syringe and 0.45 μM filter.
7. Centrifuge.

2.4 Gel-Free Fractionation and One-Dimensional Gel Electrophoresis

1. GELFREE™ 8100 Fractionation System.
2. Pre-formulated GELFREE™ 8100 HEPES running buffer.
3. GELFREE™ 8100 Tris Acetate sample buffer.
4. GELFREE™ 8100 8% Tris Acetate Cartridge.
5. Criterion electrophoresis equipment.
6. 12.5% SDS-PAGE Criterion Precast Gels.
7. Tris/glycine/SDS (TGS) running buffer.
8. SYPRO Ruby protein gel stain.
9. Gel documentation system.

2.5 Two-Dimensional Gel Electrophoresis

1. Immobilized pH gradient (IPG) strips (ReadyStrip IPG, 11 cm, pH 4–7).
2. Rehydration buffer: 8 M urea, 2% CHAPS, 50 mM dithiothreitol (DTT) DTT, 0.2% w/v Bio-lite 3/10 ampholytes, and trace bromophenol blue.
3. Equilibration buffer: 6 M urea, 2% SDS, 375 mM Tris–HCl pH 8.8, 20% glycerol, 2% DTT, 2.5% w/v iodacetamide.
4. ReadyPrep ™ 2-D Starter Kit.
5. Isoelectric focusing (IEF) by PROTEAN IEF (Bio-Rad, Hercules, CA).
6. ReadyPrep Overlay agarose (Bio-Rad, Hercules, CA).
7. 12.5% SDS-PAGE Criterion Precast Gels for second dimension.

2.6 Immunoblot Analysis

1. Hybond-P PVDF membranes.
2. Semi-Dry Electrophoretic Transfer Cell.

3. Tris-buffered saline with Tween-20 (TBS-T): 20 mM Tris, 500 mM NaCl, and 1% Tween 20.
4. Blocking solution: 5% nonfat milk in TBS-T.
5. The immune sera derived from mice immunized with *C. neoformans* strain H99γ or heat-killed *C. neoformans* on day 14 post-secondary challenge with wild-type (WT) *C. neoformans* strain H99. For *C. gattii* use immune sera collected on day 14 post infection from mice immunized with a cell wall associated (CW) and/or cytoplasmic (CP) protein preparation.
6. Goat anti-mouse IgG HRP-conjugated antibody (Pierce Biotechnology Inc., Rockford, IL).
7. SuperSignal West Dura Extended Duration Substrate (Pierce Biotechnology Inc., Rockford, IL).

2.7 Cytokines Analyses

1. Tissue homogenizer.
2. 1× PBS with protease inhibitors cocktail (Roche Diagnostics GmbH, Mannheim, Germany).
3. Bio-Plex Protein Array system (Luminex-based technology; Bio-Rad Laboratories, Hercules, CA).

2.8 Cytokine Recall Analyses

1. RPMI complete media: RPMI media supplemented with 10% heat-inactivated fetal bovine serum, 2 mM L-glutamine, 100 U penicillin/ml, 100 μg of streptomycin/ml, and 50 mM 2-mercaptoethanol.
2. Nylon filters 70 μm.
3. Hen egg lysozyme (HEL; 1 μg/ml).
4. Concanavalin A (Con A; 1 μg/ml).
5. Standard 96-well round-bottom culture plates.
6. Limulus amebocyte lysate kit for the detection of endotoxin in isolated proteins.

2.9 Excision, Trypsinization, and Identification of Protein Bands by HPLC-ESI-MS/MS

1. Protein destaining: 40 mM NH_4CO_3/50% acetonitrile, dehydrate in acetonitrile.
2. Protein digestion: trypsin (sequencing grade) in 40 mM NH_4CO_3/10% acetonitrile.
3. Protein extraction: 0.1% trifluoroacetic acid (TFA) followed by 0.1% TFA/50% acetonitrile.
4. Capillary HPLC-electrospray ionization tandem mass spectra (HPLC-ESI-MS/MS) is performed using a Thermo Fisher LTQ linear ion trap mass spectrometer fitted with a New Objective PicoView 550 nanospray interface.
5. Eksigent NanoLC micro HPLC: column, PicoFrit™ (New Objective; 75 μm i.d.) packed to 10 cm with C18 adsorbent (Vydac; 218MS 5 μm, 300 A); mobile phase A, 0.5% acetic acid (HAc)/0.005% trifluoroacetic acid (TFA); mobile phase

B, 90% acetonitrile/0.5% HAc/0.005% TFA; gradient 2–42% B in 30 min; flow rate, 0.4 μl/min. MS conditions: ESI voltage, 2.9 kV; isolation window for MS/MS, 3; relative collision energy, 35%; scan strategy.

6. For database search, NCBInr database [NCBInr 20,130,102 (22,378,659 sequences; 7,688,401,091 residues)] by means of Mascot (version 2.4.1), Scaffold™ 4.0.

2.10 Vaccination with Protein and/or Protein Fractions

1. 2% isoflurane for anesthesia.
2. Rodent anesthesia device (Eagle Eye Anesthesia, Jacksonville, FL).
3. Cryptococcal proteins solubilized in sterile endotoxin-free PBS (HyClone Lab. Inc., Logan, UT).
4. Pipette and endotoxin-free tips for intranasal inhalation.

2.11 Statistical Analysis

GraphPad Prism version 5.00 for Windows.

3 Methods

Carry out all the experiments at room temperature unless otherwise specified.

3.1 Protein Extraction

1. Grow *C. neoformans or C. gattii* yeast in YPD broth for approximately 16–18 h at 30 °C with constant shaking. Wash fungal cells twice in sterile PBS followed by centrifugation and divide into two parts for the extraction of cell wall (CW) or cytoplasmic (CP) proteins, as previously described [12–14].
2. For the isolation of CW proteins, suspend cell pellets in ammonium carbonate buffer, pH 8.4 containing 1% (v/v) β-mercaptoethanol (ME) and protease inhibitor cocktail and incubate for 45 min at 37 °C with gentle agitation. After incubation, remove the cells by centrifugation and collect and filter-sterilize supernatant fluid containing CW proteins using a 0.45-μM filter (*see* **Note 5**).
3. For the isolation of CP proteins, add YeastBuster™ Protein Extraction Reagent containing a protease inhibitor cocktail and tris (hydroxypropy)phosphine (THP) and incubate for 45 min at 30 °C with gentle agitation. After incubation, remove the cells by centrifugation, collect and filter-sterilize supernatant fluid containing CP proteins using a 0.45-μM filter (*see* **Note 5**).
4. Desalt the supernatants individually and concentrate them by centrifugation through an Amicon Ultrafree-15 centrifugal filter device according to manufacturer's instructions (*see* **Note 6**).

5. Determine protein concentration using RC DC Protein Assay Kit following manufacturer's instructions.
6. Further concentrate the proteins and remove nonprotein contaminants using the ReadyPrep 2-D Cleanup Kit according to the manufacturer's instructions.

3.2 Gel-Free Fractionation and One-Dimensional Gel Electrophoresis

1. Dissolve *Cryptococcus* CW and CP proteins in sample buffer (included in the fractionation buffer kit) to a total volume of 150 μl. We have previously used 50 to 100 μg of individual protein preparations [13, 14] (*see* **Note 7**).
2. Proteins can be separated into 12 fractions based on their molecular weight using the GELFREE™ 8100 Fractionation System containing HEPES running and Tris Acetate sample buffers. Load 150 μl of proteins in sample buffer into individual loading chambers of an 8% Tris-Acetate Cartridge designed to separate proteins in the mass range 3.5–150 kDa, with resolution between 35 kDa and 150 kDa. Follow the instructions provided with the device to separate protein preparation into 12 fractions (*see* **Note 8**).
3. After collection of all 12 individual CW and CP fractions, run standard 1-D gel electrophoresis using 12.5% SDS-PAGE Criterion Precast Gels. Separate the proteins for 55 min at 200 V in Tris/glycine/SDS (TGS) running buffer using Criterion electrophoresis equipment. Following gel electrophoresis, stain the proteins in the gels using SYPRO Ruby protein gel stain (Fig.1).

3.3 Two-Dimensional Gel Electrophoresis

1. Rehydrate immobilized pH gradient (IPG) strips (ReadyStrip IPG, 11 cm, pH 4–7) in 200 μl of rehydration/sample buffer containing 200 μg of the *Cryptococcus* CW or CP proteins (*see* **Note 9**).
2. Carry out isoelectric focusing (IEF) using PROTEAN IEF under the following conditions: step 1, 250 V for 20 min; step 2, ramped to 8000 V over 2.5 h, and step 3, 8000 for a total of 30,000 V/h.
3. After IEF, place gel strips into equilibration buffer for 15 min.
4. Alkylate disulfide groups using equilibration buffer of the same composition substituting 2.5% w/v iodacetamide instead of DTT.
5. Drain equilibrated IPG strips and place on the top of 12.5% SDS-PAGE Criterion Precast Gels and seal it using hot ReadyPrep Overlay agarose.
6. Separate proteins in the second dimension using Criterion electrophoresis equipment for 55 min at 200 V in Tris/glycine/SDS (TGS) running buffer.

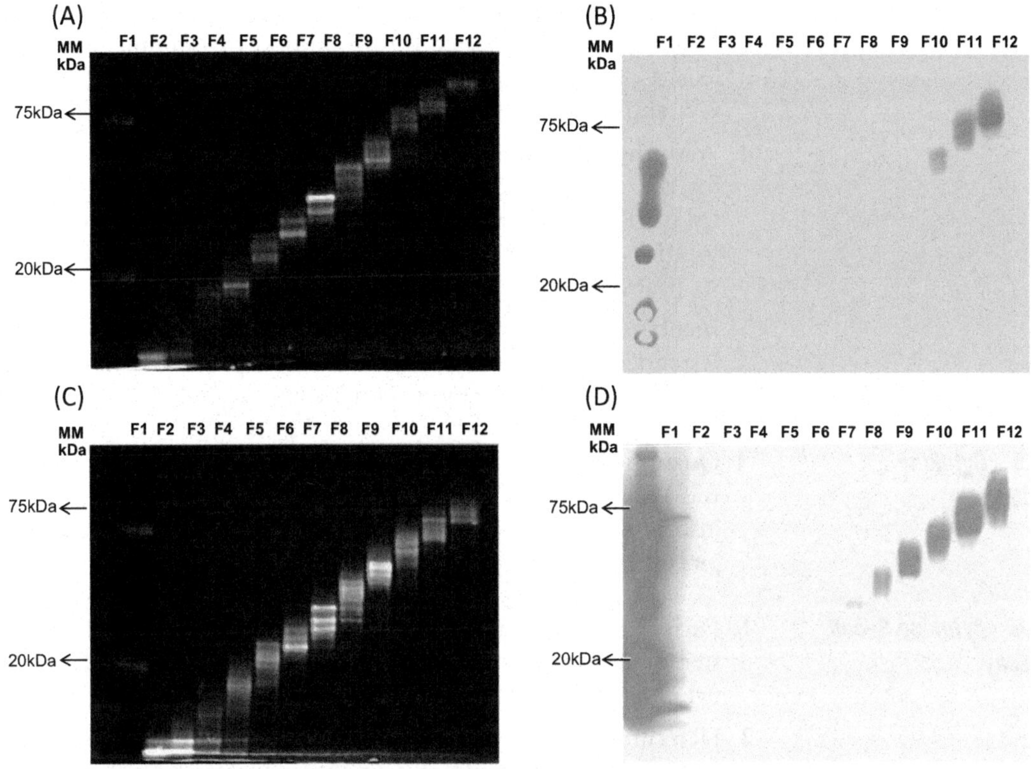

Fig. 1 Fractionation of *C. gattii* cell wall associated proteins (**a**) and Cytoplasmic proteins (**c**). 500 μg of *C. gattii* cell wall associated proteins and cytoplasmic proteins were fractionated into 12 fractions ranging in molecular weight from 3.5 to 150 kDa. The fractions were visualized using 1-D gel electrophoresis, followed by Sypro staining. Immunoblot analysis of *C. gattii* cell wall associated protein fractions (**b**) and cytoplasmic protein fractions (**d**). Protein fractions were separated by 1-D gel electrophoresis. Protein fractions were transferred to PVDF membranes and incubated with pooled serum taken on day 14 post-secondary infection of mice immunized using *C gattii* cell wall and cytoplasmic proteins. In case of cell wall proteins, fractions F10, F11, and F12 contain immunogenic proteins (**b**), while fractions F8–F12 were found to be immunogenic in cytoplasmic fractions (**d**)

7. Stain proteins in the gel using Sypro Ruby Red or, alternatively, transfer to polyvinylidene difluoride (PVDF) membranes for immunoblot analysis.

3.4 Immunoblot Analysis

1. Transfer the resolved proteins to Hybond-P PVDF membranes using a Semi-Dry Electrophoretic Transfer Cell according to manufacturer's instructions (*see* **Note 10**).
2. Subsequently, block the membranes in blocking solution for 1 h at room temperature.
3. Discard the blocking solution and incubate the membranes overnight at 4 °C with a 1:200 dilution of banked immune sera collected on day 14 post-secondary challenge from mice immunized with *C. neofomans* strain H99γ or heat-killed *C. neoformans* if probing for immune dominant *C. neoformans*

CW and CP proteins [12]. If probing for immune-dominant *C. gattii* proteins, use a 1:200 dilution of immune sera collected on day 14 post infection from mice immunized with CW and CP proteins [14].

4. Wash the membrane six times in TBS-T (5 min per wash) and, for the detection of antibody binding, add goat anti-mouse IgG HRP-conjugated antibody diluted 1:1000 in blocking solution for 1 h at room temperature. Wash membrane again six times in TBS-T.
5. Incubate the membrane briefly with SuperSignal West Dura Extended Duration Substrate and detect protein spots using a ChemiDoc XRS camera or similar camera (*see* **Note 11**).

3.5 Cytokine Analyses

1 Quantification of cytokines can be accomplished using the Bio-Plex Protein Array system according to manufacturer's instructions. Multiple assays are available for single or multiplexed analysis of cytokines.

3.6 Cytokine Recall Assay

1. Excise spleens from BALB/c mice vaccinated with H99γ or sterile PBS on day 60 post-immunization and press through nylon filters 70 μm to obtain single-cell splenocyte population.
2. Determine the endotoxin content of the CW and CP proteins fractions by using a Limulus amebocyte lysate kit prior to use. Endotoxin content should be less than 1 EU/50 μg protein.
3. Culture the splenocytes (1×10^6/well in 100 μl) in RPMI complete media with individual protein fractions (50 μg each), hen egg lysozyme (HEL; 1 μg/ml), or concanavalin A (Con A; 1 μg/ml) as negative and positive controls, respectively, at 37 °C and 5% CO_2 in 96-well round-bottom culture plates.
4. After 24 h collect the culture supernatants and use the Bio-Plex Protein Array System to determine the cytokine levels within the supernatants.

3.7 Excision, Trypsinization, and Identification of Protein Bands by HPLC-ESI-MS/MS

1. Protein spots excision and identification was accomplished at the Institutional Mass Spectrometry Laboratory, The University of Texas Health Science Center at San Antonio.
2. Manually excise the protein spots of interest from gel using a sterile scalpel after 2-D gel electrophoresis (*see* **Note 12**).
3. Destain the excised spots in 40 mM NH_4CO_3/50% acetonitrile, dehydrate in acetonitrile, and digest overnight at 37 °C with trypsin in 40 mM NH_4CO_3/10% acetonitrile. Extract tryptic digests with 0.1% TFA followed by 0.1% TFA/50% acetonitrile.
4. Vacuum dry combined extracts by vacuum centrifugation and resuspend in 0.5% TFA. Analyze the digests by capillary HPLC-ESI-MS/MS using a Thermo Fisher LTQ linear ion

trap mass spectrometer fitted with a New Objective PicoView 550 nanospray interface.

5. Complete, online HPLC separation of the digests with an Eksigent NanoLC micro HPLC. Survey scan followed by acquisition of data-dependent collision-induced dissociation (CID) spectra of the seven most intense ions in the survey scan above a set threshold.
6. Search MS datasets against the NCBInr database by means of Mascot. Also consider methionine oxidation and cysteine carbamidomethylation as variable modifications for all searches. Use Scaffold™ 4.0 to conduct an X! Tandem subset search of the Mascot data followed by cross-correlation of the results of both searches. Consider 95% and 99%, respectively, scaffold confidence levels for acceptance of peptide assignments and protein identifications.

3.8 Vaccination and Survival

1. Immunize mice with individual protein fractions or fractions of interest via intranasal inhalation as this mimics the most likely route of introduction of *Cryptococcus* into humans. To do this, BALB/c mice are anesthetized with 2% isoflurane using a rodent anesthesia device. Dissolve 50–100 μg of protein in 50 μl of sterile endotoxin-free PBS for inoculation via intranasal inhalation. Determine endotoxin content of the protein preparations to be minimal (less than 1 EU/μg protein) prior to use. Immunizations or inoculations with *Cryptococcus* yeast are done using a yeast inoculum of 1×10^4 CFU of *Cryptococcus* in 50 μl of sterile endotoxin-free PBS. Mice are mock immunized with 50 μl of sterile endotoxin-free PBS. Immunize mice three times, with 4 week intervals between each immunization. Ten days following the final immunization, infect mice with 1×10^4 *Cryptococcus* by nasal inhalation as previously described [12, 13].
2. Monitor survival twice a day and sacrifice mice that appear moribund or not maintaining normal habits (grooming).

4 Notes

1. All animal experiments should be performed following NIH guidelines and in accordance with the Institutional Animal Care and Use Committee in, preferably, an AAALAC-certified facility. Animals are typically allowed a 1 week acclimatization period in the facility before experiments are started.
2. Always prepare fresh culture of *C. neoformans* and *C. gattii* strains. YPD media can be stored at room temperature but store RPMI at 4 °C.

3. Ammonium carbonate buffer and YeastBuster™ Protein Extraction Reagent can be stored at 4 °C. Bring them to the room temperature prior to using and add (β-ME) plus protease inhibitor cocktail to ammonium carbonate and tris(hydroxypropy) phosphine (THP) (included in the kit) and protease inhibitor cocktail to YeastBuster™ Protein Extraction Reagent.
4. Prechill nanopure water and wash buffer prior to use.
5. According to the size of cell pellets add extraction buffer, for example if pellet volume is 5 ml then add 10 ml of ammonium carbonate buffer for cell wall protein extraction and/or 10 ml of YeastBuster™ Protein Extraction Reagent containing a protease inhibitor cocktail and THP for cytoplasmic protein extraction. Do not put excessive pressure on syringe filter while sterile-filtering samples through 0.45-μM filters. Instead, change the filter to avoid failure of filter and loss of sample.
6. Keep Amicon Ultrafree-15 centrifugal filter device containing sample at 4 °C or on ice during use. Also, maintain centrifuge temperature at 4 °C to limit protein degradation. Use fixed angle centrifuge while filtering through Amicon filters and use according to manufacturer's instructions.
7. Always maintain a total volume of protein sample buffer at 150 μl. Dissolve the protein pellet obtained after cleanup in the sample buffer by vortexing vigorously. Some of the sample volume may be reduced below 150 μl which can be made up after solubilization of protein pellet. Warm the sample at 50 °C for 10 min and then cool the sample to room temperature. Quick spin the sample to avoid loading any insoluble debris before applying to the loading chamber of cartridge. Protein concentration for fractionation should not be more than 500 μg per sample.
8. While loading 150 μl of protein sample into individual loading chambers, avoid introducing bubbles. The loading chambers are small, so extra care has to be taken. Pipette up and down at least three times during collection of each fraction and wash collection chamber at least three times with HEPES buffer provided with the kit. Make sure there is no "0" reading showing on the machine screen while it runs. If there is a "0", open the lid of the machine and try to remove either any bubbles present and check for empty chambers (without any buffer) since they can hinder current flow.
9. Cover IPG strip during rehydration of strip with mineral oil to avoid any evaporation of sample and drying of the strip. However, wait at least 30 min after adding IPG strip over streaked sample to add mineral oil such that the sample can be evenly adsorbed by the IPG strip.

10. Avoid introducing bubbles between gel and PVDF membrane. Also, do not allow the membrane to dry. While removing the PVDF membrane from the gel, the gel may adhere to the membrane. Separate gel from the membrane by adding buffer using a pipette.
11. Incubate the membrane briefly with Super Signal West Dura Extended Duration Substrate. Be careful not to incubate for too long as it can lead to a dark background on the film and turn the membrane brown.
12. Use sterile scalpel or 18-gauze needle to cut the desired protein spots. Place excised gel samples into labeled eppendorff tubes containing nano-pure water. Wear gloves and head cover to prevent keratin contamination of sample.

References

1. Mitchell TG, Perfect JR (1995) Cryptococcosis in the era of AIDS--100 years after the discovery of *Cryptococcus neoformans*. Clin Microbiol Rev 8(4):515–548
2. Vibhagool A, Sungkanuparph S, Mootsikapun P, Chetchotisakd P, Tansuphaswaswadikul S, Bowonwatanuwong C et al (2003) Discontinuation of secondary prophylaxis for cryptococcal meningitis in human immunodeficiency virus-infected patients treated with highly active antiretroviral therapy: a prospective, multicenter, randomized study. Clin Infect Dis 36(10):1329–1331
3. Park BJ, Wannemuehler KA, Marston BJ, Govender N, Pappas PG, Chiller TM (2009) Estimation of the current global burden of cryptococcal meningitis among persons living with HIV/AIDS. AIDS 23(4):525–530
4. Bozzette SA, Larsen RA, Chiu J, Leal MA, Jacobsen J, Rothman P et al (1991) A placebo-controlled trial of maintenance therapy with fluconazole after treatment of cryptococcal meningitis in the acquired immunodeficiency syndrome. California Collaborative Treatment Group. N Engl J Med 324(9):580–584
5. Galanis E, Macdougall L, Kidd S, Morshed M (2010) Epidemiology of *Cryptococcus gattii*, British Columbia, Canada, 1999-2007. Emerg Infect Dis 16:251–257
6. Datta K, Bartlett KH, Marr KA (2009) *Cryptococcus gattii*: emergence in western North America: exploitation of a novel ecological niche. Interdiscip Perspect Infect Dis 2009:176532.
7. Datta K, Bartlett KH, Baer R, Byrnes E, Galanis E et al (2009) Spread of *Cryptococcus gattii* into Pacific northwest region of the United States. Emerg Infect Dis 15:1185–1191
8. Emergence of *Cryptococcus gattii* (2010) Pacific Northwest, 2004-2010. MMWR Morb Mortal Wkly Rep 59(28):865–868
9. Hagen F, Colom MF, Swinne D, Tintelnot K, Iatta R et al (2012) Autochthonous and dormant *Cryptococcus gattii* infections in Europe. Emerg Infect Dis 18:1618–1624
10. Kwon-Chung KJ, Bennett JE (1984) Epidemiologic differences between the two varieties of *Cryptococcus neoformans*. Am J Epidemiol 120:123–130
11. RJ MC, Phillips R, Perfect JR, Byrnes EJ 3rd, Heitman J et al (2011) *Cryptococcus gattii* genotype VGI infection in New England. Pediatr Infect Dis J 30:1111–1114
12. Byrnes EJ 3rd, Li W, Lewit Y, Perfect JR, Carter DA et al (2009) First reported case of *Cryptococcus gattii* in the Southeastern USA: implications for travel-associated acquisition of an emerging pathogen. PLoS One 4:e5851
13. Biondo C, Messina L, Bombaci M, Mancuso G, Midiri A, Beninati C et al (2005) Characterization of two novel cryptococcal mannoproteins recognized by immune sera. Infect Immun 73(11):7348–7355
14. Kakeya H, Udono H, Maesaki S, Sasaki E, Kawamura S, Hossain MA et al (1999) Heat shock protein 70 (hsp70) as a major target of the antibody response in patients with pulmonary cryptococcosis. Clin Exp Immunol 115(3):485–490
15. Kakeya H, Udono H, Ikuno N, Yamamoto Y, Mitsutake K, Miyazaki T et al (1997) A 77-kilodalton protein of *Cryptococcus neofor-*

mans, a member of the heat shock protein 70 family, is a major antigen detected in the sera of mice with pulmonary cryptococcosis. Infect Immun 65(5):1653–1658

16. Young M, Macias S, Thomas D, Wormley FL Jr (2009) A proteomic-based approach for the identification of immunodominant *Cryptococcus neoformans* proteins. Proteomics 9(9):2578–2588
17. Chaturvedi AK, Weintraub ST, Lopez-Ribot JL, Wormley FL Jr (2013) Identification and characterization of *Cryptococcus neoformans* protein fractions that induce protective immune responses. Proteomics 13:3429–3441
18. Chaturvedi AK, Hameed RS, Wozniak KL, Hole CR, Leopold Wager CM, Weintraub ST, Lopez-Ribot JL, Wormley FL Jr (2014) Vaccine mediated immune responses to experimental pulmonary *Cryptococcus gattii* infection in mice. PLoS One 9:e104316
19. Wormley FL Jr, Perfect JR, Steele C, Cox GM (2007) Protection against cryptococcosis by using a murine gamma interferon-producing *Cryptococcus neoformans* strain. Infect Immun 75:1453–1462

Part II

Design and Delivery

Chapter 11

Beta-Glucan Particles as Vaccine Adjuvant Carriers

Zeynep Mirza, Ernesto R. Soto, Fusun Dikengil, Stuart M. Levitz, and Gary R. Ostroff

Abstract

Glucan particles (GPs) are spherical hollow particles derived from *Saccharomyces cerevisiae* cell walls and mainly consist of β-1, 3-D-glucans. The inner hollow cavity of glucan particles can be loaded with different compounds, including protein antigens, and delivered to macrophages and dendritic cells. Moreover, the GP delivery system possesses β-glucan's intrinsic immunostimulatory properties. Therefore, GPs serve as both an antigen-presenting cell-targeted delivery system and an adjuvant.

Here, we describe the production of GPs from *S. cerevisiae* using hot alkaline and solvent extraction and characterization of these particles for morphology, particle density, and hydrodynamic volume. A detailed protocol for loading and entrapping a model antigen, ovalbumin (OVA), into these particles using yeast RNA is presented. Similar methods are used to load pathogen-specific antigens (peptides, proteins, soluble extracts) which then can be tested in in vivo vaccination models.

Key words Glucan particles, Vaccine production, Cryptococcus, Dectin-1

1 Introduction

While vaccination provides remarkable protection against many diseases, vaccines have remained elusive for many infectious killers. Effective vaccines require antigen(s) delivered in a manner that stimulates protective immune responses. Approved subunit vaccines contain adjuvants such as alum that help stimulate protective antibody responses. However, for many infectious diseases for which a vaccine is not yet available, protection may require adaptive T cell immunity in addition to (or in lieu of) antibody. Thus, there is an urgent need for safe and effective vaccination systems that elicit strong and long-lasting protective immunity to delivered antigens [1].

Glucan particles (GPs) are spherical empty empty and highly purified cell walls of *Saccharomyces cerevisiae* and mainly consist of β-1, 3-D-glucans [2]. GPs are obtained from baker's yeast, using a series of hot alkaline extractions, followed by ethanol and acetone

Markus Kalkum and Margarita Semis (eds.), *Vaccines for Invasive Fungal Infections: Methods and Protocols*, Methods in Molecular Biology, vol. 1625, DOI 10.1007/978-1-4939-7104-6_11, © Springer Science+Business Media LLC 2017

extraction. GPs can be loaded with many classes of drugs due to the porous structure of the shell's hydrocolloid polysaccharide matrix and hollow cavity inside the GPs. Previous studies have shown that proteins (including antigens), DNA, siRNA, and small molecule drugs can be loaded into GPs [3–7].

β-1, 3-D-glucans are the major pathogen-associated molecular patterns (PAMPs) of fungi and are recognized via Dectin-1 (D1), complement receptor 3 (CR3) and scavenger receptors by macrophages, neutrophils, and dendritic cells [8, 9]. Recognition of GPs via these receptors alerts the host phagocytic immune cells and starts a series of events including particle uptake, oxidative burst, and release of pro-inflammatory chemokines/cytokines. After maturation and migration of these antigen-presenting cells, T and B cell responses are also initiated [9–11]. Therefore, GPs can be utilized as a vaccine delivery system with adjuvant properties.

GPs and free antigen co-administration stimulate IgG1 antibody production in vaccinated mice; however, delivering the antigen inside the GPs causes stronger immune response including increased IgG2c and $CD4^{+}$ T cell responses. GPs induce strong $CD4^{+}$ T cell responses and antibody production even at sub-microgram antigen doses [12, 13]. GP-based vaccines containing antigen extracts prepared from *Cryptococcus neoformans* protected mice against lethal *C. neoformans* challenge [14].

This chapter outlines the methods in detail for encapsulating a model antigen (ovalbumin) inside the GPs. The chapter is organized as follows: It begins by presenting the materials to be used, followed by the methods of GP production, particle characterization, and fluorescently labeled ovalbumin loading inside the GPs. Notes are presented at the end of the chapter.

2 Materials

2.1 Production of Glucan Particles

1. *S. cerevisiae* (Fleischmann's baker's yeast) 100 g.
2. Sodium hydroxide.
3. Ethanol—100%.
4. Acetone.
5. Distilled water.
6. Erlenmeyer flask (2 L volume-borosilicate).
7. Magnetic stirring bar.
8. Hot plate with magnetic stirrer.
9. Thermometer.
10. Centrifuge.
11. Spatula.
12. 50 mL conical centrifuge tubes.

13. Fume hood.
14. Polytron homogenizer or equivalent.
15. Centrifuge bottles (0.5 L).

2.2 Particle Density (Number of Particles/mg GP) and Hydrodynamic Volume

1. Dry glucan particles.
2. Microcentrifuge tubes.
3. Analytical balance.
4. Vortex mixer.
5. Pipettor and pipette tips (10, 100, 1000 μL).
6. Hemocytometer.
7. Distilled water.
8. Sonicator.
9. Microscope—200× magnification.

2.3 Fluorescent Labeling of Ovalbumin

1. Ovalbumin solution: Measure and dissolve 100 mg of ovalbumin in 10 mL of 100 mM carbonate buffer, pH 9 in a 15 mL conical centrifuge tube.
2. Fluorescein isothiocyanate (FITC) in DMSO solution: Dissolve 10 mg of FITC in 2 mL of DMSO (5 mg/mL final concentration).
3. 1 M Tris pH 8: Dissolve 121.1 g of Tris base in ~700 mL of distilled water. Adjust pH to 8 using concentrated HCl (~80 mL). Bring final volume to 1 L.
4. 100 mM sodium carbonate-sodium bicarbonate buffer, pH 9.2: Mix 10 mL of 0.1 M sodium carbonate with 90 mL of 0.1 M sodium bicarbonate [15].
5. Fluorescent microplate reader or spectrofluorimeter.

2.4 Fluorescent Ovalbumin Loading

1. Empty GPs 10 mg.
2. FITC-labeled ovalbumin.
3. Torula yeast RNA, type IV (yRNA).
4. 0.9% saline.
5. Microcentrifuge tubes.
6. Heat block.
7. Pipette and pipette tips.
8. Microscope slides and slide covers.
9. Centrifuge.
10. Plate reader and 96-well plate.
11. Fluorescence microscope—200× magnification.
12. Fluorescent microplate reader or spectrofluorimeter.
13. Lyophilizer.

2.5 Sample Preparation for SDS-PAGE

1. FITC-labeled ovalbumin.
2. GP-ovalbumin formulations (experimental and control samples) and also the saved supernatants from the wash steps.
3. 6× SDS-PAGE loading buffer: Mix 3.75 mL of 1 M Tris pH 6.8, 1 g SDS, 5 mL glycerol, 1 mL beta-mercaptoethanol, 30 mg bromophenol blue.
4. 6 M urea: Dissolve 360 mg of urea in 1 mL distilled water.
5. Heat block.
6. Pipette and pipette tips.
7. Cup-sonicator.
8. Centrifuge.

3 Method

3.1 Production of Glucan Particles

1. Add 500 mL water in a 2 L flask and add 100 g of yeast cells (Fig. 1). Use a homogenizer to break up clumps. Insert a magnetic stir bar, and add 20 g of solid sodium hydroxide (*see* **Note 1**). Add distilled water to get 1 L total volume.
2. Place the flask on a stirring hot plate, put a glass thermometer in the flask, and heat to 80 °C for 1 h while mixing. Start timing when the temperature reaches 80 °C. Cover the mouth of

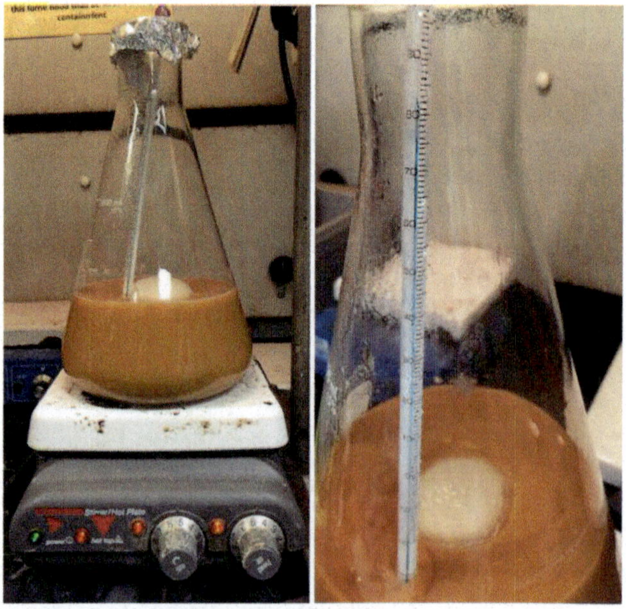

Fig. 1 Alkaline hydrolysis setup for the production of glucan particles

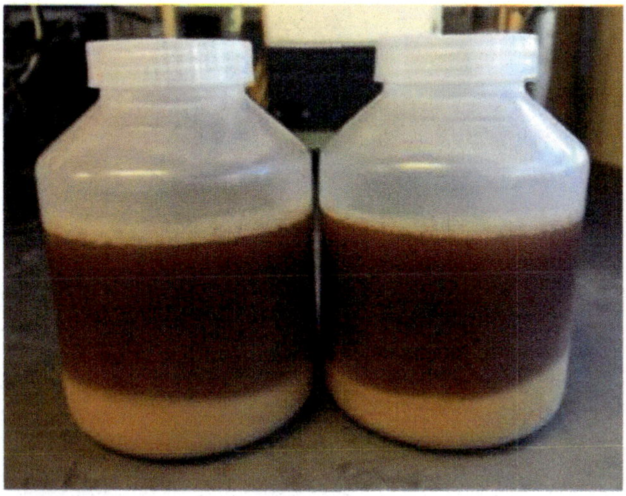

Fig. 2 Centrifuge bottles after first spinning (pH > 10). *Dark brown* supernatant and *white* floating partially saponified lipids must be discarded. Pellet must be washed until the supernatant is clear and pH < 10 (it usually requires four to five washes)

the flask with aluminum foil to prevent evaporation. Maintain temperature between 80 and 85 °C. Caution: hot caustic.

3. Cool down the mixture to room temperature and then transfer the contents to two 500 mL centrifuge bottles.
4. Centrifuge at 2000 × *g* for 30 min, discard supernatant (Fig. 2). Caution: caustic. The supernatant will have a dark brown color and may contain white floating partially saponified lipids, which should also be discarded. Suspend the pellet in 500 mL of distilled water using a Polytron homogenizer (0.5–0.75× full speed until pellet is uniformly suspended) and spin down again. Repeat this wash step until the supernatant is clear and the pH is <10. It usually takes four to five wash steps to achieve a clear supernatant.
5. Adjust the pH of the suspension to pH 6–8 using hydrochloric acid (*see* **Note 2**).
6. Repeat the wash step one more time to remove formed salt.
7. Suspend the pellets in 250 mL of water using the Polytron homogenizer.
8. Divide the suspended pellet into 5–50 mL conical tubes.
9. Collect the insoluble fraction by centrifugation (2000 × *g* for 30 min) and discard supernatant. Packed pellet volume should be <15 mL.
10. Add 30 mL of ethanol per tube. Suspend the pellets using a Polytron homogenizer to achieve a uniform suspension.

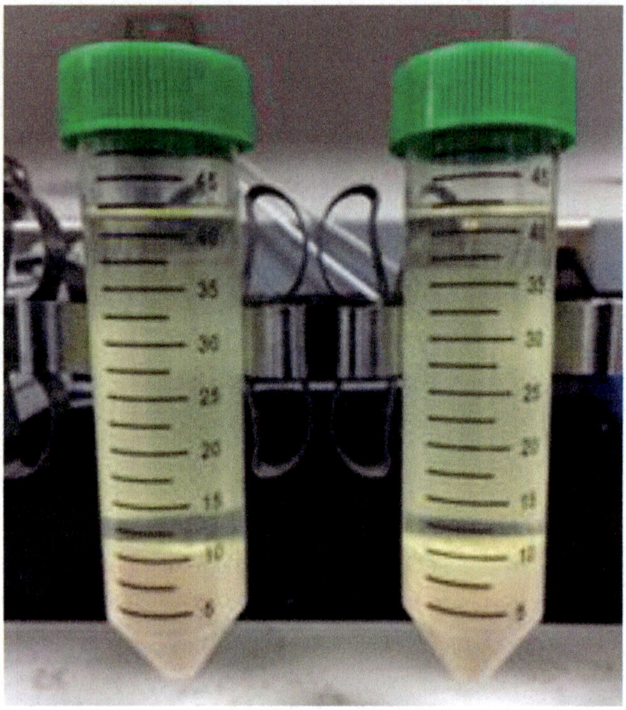

Fig. 3 Centrifuge tubes after first ethanol wash. The supernatant appears slightly *yellow* due to extracted lipids. It typically takes three to four ethanol extractions to obtain a clear supernatant

11. Collect the insoluble fraction by centrifugation (2000 × *g* for 30 min) and discard supernatant. The supernatant appears slightly yellowish at first; repeat until it is clear. It typically takes three to four ethanol extractions (Fig. 3).
12. Suspend the pellet in 20 mL of acetone using a Polytron homogenizer in a fume hood to a uniform suspension. Note: acetone is flammable.
13. Centrifuge and discard acetone as in the previous wash steps. Repeat acetone washes two times.
14. After the last acetone wash, dry the pellet in a fume hood. Use a spatula to break up clumps every 15 min for the first hour, dry at room temperature for 48 h or until constant weight.
15. The final product should be around 8–12 g of an off-white fine powder (Fig. 4). Weigh and characterize the GPs for morphology, number of particles per mg and hydrodynamic volume (water absorption capacity).

3.2 Number of Particles per mg GP

1. Add ~1 mg of GPs to a microcentrifuge tube. Note absolute GP weight. Add 0.5 mL of distilled water and sonicate the tube to obtain single particles.

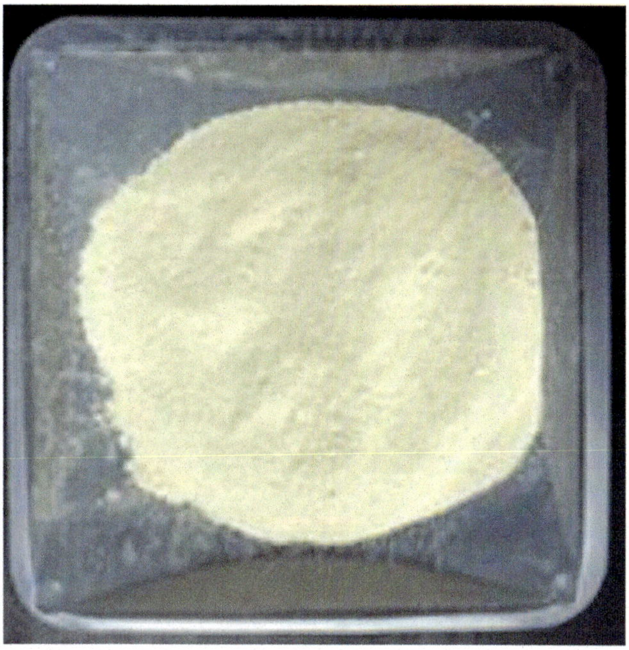

Fig. 4 Final dry GP product

2. Adjust concentration to 1 mg GP/mL with distilled water.
3. Vortex/cup sonicate to uniform suspension.
4. Make 1:100 dilution in water and count particles with a hemocytometer using a microscope with a magnification of ≥200×. The particles will appear as ~4–5 μm slightly ellipsoidal spheres resembling the morphology of the starting yeast material (Fig. 5). If the particles appear as smaller fragments, then the yeast cell source used is unacceptable and the particles are not useful for the encapsulation of antigens.
5. Calculate the number of particles in a 1 mg of GPs (*see* **Note 3**).

3.3 Hydrodynamic Volume of the Particles (Water-Binding Capacity, Fig. 6)

1. Weigh two empty microcentrifuge tubes and record weights (W1). Add ~50 mg of GPs to these tubes. Weigh again and note the measurements (W2).
2. Add 1 mL water to tubes, vortex and cup sonicate to obtain suspension. Incubate the tubes 1 h at room temperature (*see* **Note 4**).
3. Centrifuge at 10,000 × *g* for 10 min.
4. Discard water with fine pipette tip, paying attention to not disturb the pellet.
5. Spin again to remove all water. Weigh tubes and record weights (W3).

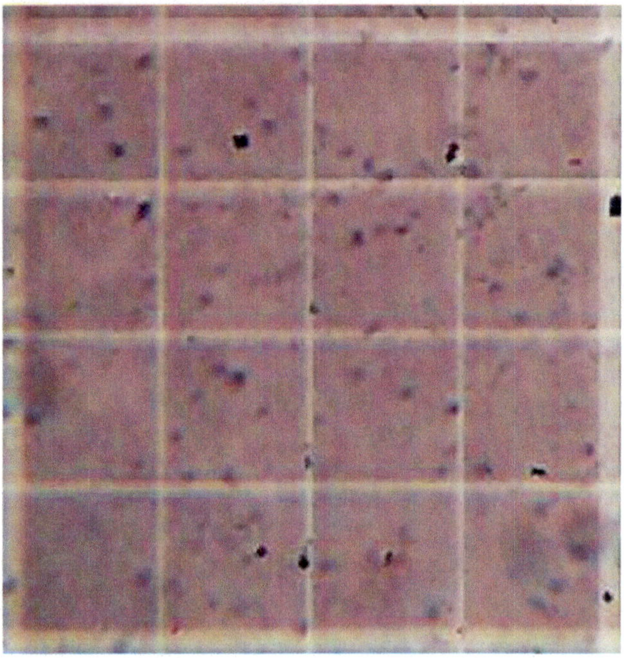

Fig. 5 Image (20×) of glucan particle counting using a hemocytometer

6. Calculate hydrodynamic volume (HV) = $\frac{(W3-W2)}{(W2-W1)}$ mg water/mg GP (*see* **Note 4**).

3.4 Fluorescently Labeling Ovalbumin

1. Mix and add FITC in DMSO solution to ovalbumin solution.
2. Wrap the tube with aluminum foil to prevent photobleaching of fluorescent dye. Place the tube on a rotator and incubate at room temperature overnight.
3. Add 1 mL of 1 M Tris pH 8 to quench unreacted FITC. Incubate for 15 min at room temperature.
4. Purify protein by dialysis against 5 L distilled water until fluorescence of dialysate is equivalent to water. Carry out this step at 4 °C in the dark.
5. Lyophilize the protein to concentrate. Store dry powder at −20 °C.
6. Dissolve the FL-ovalbumin in distilled water at 25 mg/mL for loading experiments, store in aliquots at −20 °C.

3.5 Fluorescent Ovalbumin Loading and Trapping into GPs

1. Weigh 5 mg GPs into two microcentrifuge tubes.
2. Prepare two mixing sticks by sealing the tip of small pipette tips (1–20 μL) and place into tubes (*see* **Note 5** and Fig. 7).
3. Dissolve the fluorescent ovalbumin at 25 mg/mL in sterile water and add 20 μL to each tube. Mix the protein and dry

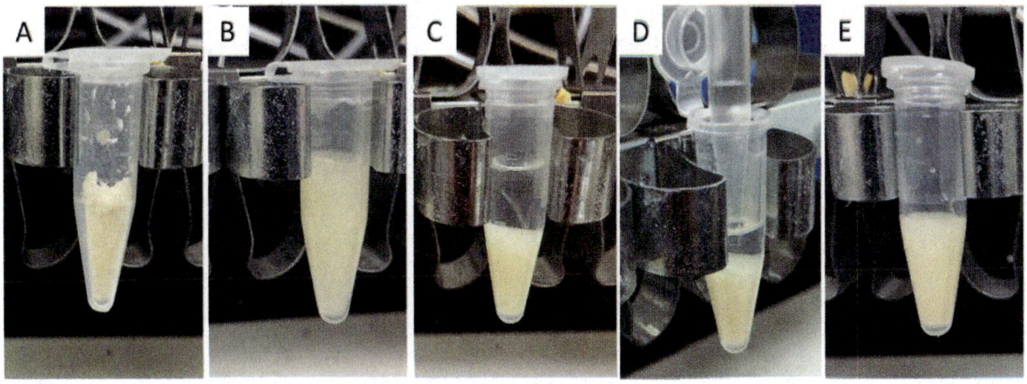

Fig. 6 Hydrodynamic volume, pictures from left to right showing from *left* to *right* (**a**) dry 50 mg GPs sample, (**b**) particles suspended in 1 mL water, (**c**) sample after centrifugation, (**d**) careful removal of excess water, and (**e**) wet pellet

particles into a thick paste using the sealed pipette tip, making sure all of the particles are uniformly wetted. Briefly centrifuge tubes containing the mixing stick (~5 s) to bring the mixture down to the bottom of the tube. Repeat the mixing and centrifugation a total of three times to obtain a homogenous paste. Capillary action draws the soluble protein into the dry particles. A volume of 20 μL of protein is ~1/2 hydrodynamic volume (Subheading 3.3) ensuring most of the protein is absorbed into the GPs.

4. Freeze-dry the tubes in order to remove the water.
5. To push any residual protein either remaining outside the particles, or within the matrix of the particle wall into the hollow cavity of the GPs, add 10 μL of sterile water to each tube (*see* **Note 6**). Mix three times as described above. A volume of 10 μL of protein is ~1/4 hydrodynamic volume (Subheading 3.3) resulting in >95% of the protein inside the GPs.
6. Freeze dry to remove the water as above.
7. Set a heat block to 50 °C. Pre-warm the tubes containing the dry GPs loaded with fluorescent Ova to 50 °C. For labile proteins a temperature of 37 °C can be used.
8. Prepare a supersaturated yRNA solution in 0.9% saline at 25 mg/mL by heating the material in a boiling water bath or microwave until boiling to dissolve the yRNA. Not all the RNA will dissolve. For microwaving, use a 15 mL tube with large headspace and heat the tube 5 s at a time. Mix and immediately transfer the supersaturated yRNA solution into a microcentrifuge tube on a 50 °C heat block. It is important to keep tubes warm; if the mixture cools down, then the yRNA starts to precipitate. Briefly centrifuge at 10,000 × *g* for 5 s to remove

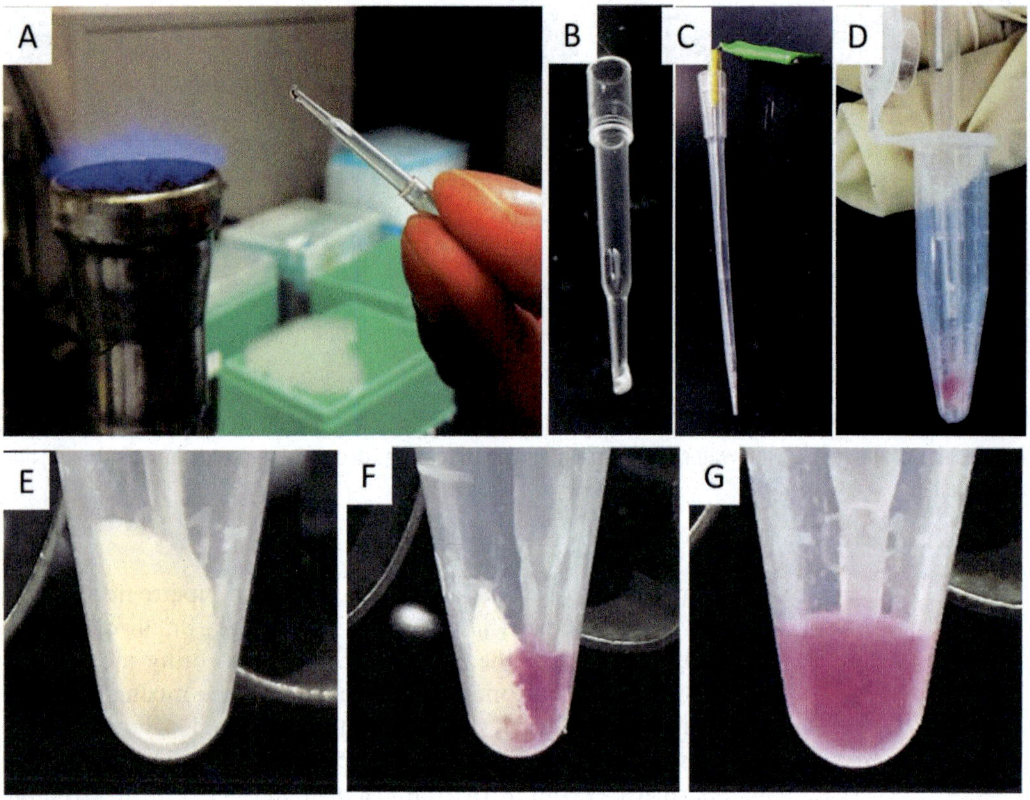

Fig. 7 *Top*: (**a**) sealing of a small pipette tip (1–20 μL) with a Bunsen burner, (**b**) sealed pipette tip for mixing of GP samples, (**c**) image of a mixing stick device, and (**d**) mixing of GP samples and solution into a thick paste using the mixing device inserted into the sealed pipette tip. *Bottom*: Closeup of 5 mg GP pellets (**e**) before addition of loading solution (dry pellet), (**f**) at beginning of mixing the GP sample and solution containing Nile red dye showing dry and wet portions of the pellet, and (**g**) homogenous paste after mixing

insoluble yRNA. Incubate at 50 °C until the yRNA supernatant is clear.

9. Add 25 μL of soluble, clear 50 °C yRNA (25 mg/mL) to the first tube and 0.9% saline at 50 °C to the second tube. Using the mixing stick, mix the yRNA and dry tubes containing GPs loaded with fluorescent OVA while keeping them warm on the heat block. Centrifuge the microcentrifuge tube for 5 s at full speed. Allow the tube to temperature equilibrate to 50 °C and repeat the mixing and centrifugation three times until a uniform paste is obtained. Incubate tubes for an additional 10 min at 50 °C after particles absorb the yRNA. The yRNA complexes with the ovalbumin trapping the protein inside the GPs.
10. Add another 25 μL of yRNA (25 mg/mL) to the first tube and 0.9% saline to the second tube. Mix as above. Incubate for 10 more minutes to continue the trapping reaction.

11. Prepare another yRNA solution at 5 mg/mL in 0.9% saline. Equilibrate to 50 °C to solubilize the yeast RNA. Add 450 μL of soluble 5 mg/mL yRNA to the first tube and 450 μL of 0.9% saline to the second tube. Cup-sonicate tubes and remove the stirring sticks. Microtip sonicate the suspension at setting 7 for 5–10 s or until the particles are suspended into a uniform suspension. Incubate the tubes for 20 more minutes on the heat block to complete the trapping reaction.
12. Centrifuge the tubes at 10,000 × *g* for 5 min. Collect and save the supernatants in two fresh microcentrifuge tubes. Wash the pellets with 250 μL of 0.9% saline three times. Save and combine the supernatants with corresponding supernatants from previous washes. The total volume of supernatant should be ~1 mL for both tubes. These pooled supernatants will be used for loading efficiency assessment (**step 1**).
13. Suspend the pellet in 500 μL of 0.9% saline. Sonicate using a tip sonicator as described above to a uniform suspension and flash freeze the samples using dry ice or liquid nitrogen and store at −80 °C.

3.6 Assessment of Ovalbumin Loading Efficiency

3.6.1 Fluorescence Measurements

1. Prepare free FL-ovalbumin solution for calculations: Put 20 μL of FL-ovalbumin (25 mg/mL) in a microcentrifuge tube. Add 980 μL of 0.9% saline. Transfer 100 μL of this solution into 3 wells of a 96-well microplate plate.
2. Also, transfer 100 μL of pooled supernatants of control and experimental samples to three wells of a 96-well plate.
3. Measure fluorescence using a fluorescent microplate reader (excitation wavelength 494 nm and emission wavelength: 518 nm). Alternatively, a spectrofluorimeter can be used by adjusting standard and sample volumes as necessary. Calculate the encapsulation efficiency using the formula below:

$$\%\ \text{Encapsulation efficiency} = \left(1 - \frac{\text{fluorescence value of the sample's supernatant}}{\text{fluorescence value of the free } FL - ovalbumin}\right) \times 100.$$

Over 90% encapsulation efficiency is expected with this method in tube 1.

3.6.2 Microscopy

1. Prepare microscopic slides from both control saline and yRNA trapped samples. Observe the particles with a fluorescent microscope using a fluorescein filter and 100× objective. Observation of fluorescence inside the GPs indicates a good loading, while fluorescence outside of particles indicates unencapsulated protein (*see* **Note 5**, Fig. 8).

3.6.3 Sample Preparation for SDS-PAGE

Protein loading into GPs can be further confirmed by SDS-PAGE. A standard SDS-PAGE protocol can be used with a minor modification of sample preparation.

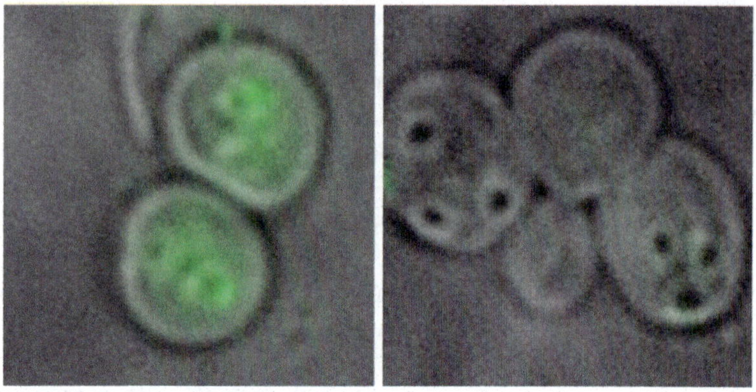

Fig. 8 Fluorescence microscopy image showing a GP-fluorescent ovalbumin core

1. Aliquot 10 μL of GP-ovalbumin formulations (control and experimental samples) into two microcentrifuge tubes.
2. Centrifuge the tubes at 10,000 × *g* for 5 min.
3. Remove the supernatant without disturbing the pellet. Add 15 μL of 6 M urea solution (*see* **Note 6**).
4. Add 3 μL of 6× SDS-page loading buffer to the GP-ovalbumin samples and mix.
5. Cup sonicate the tubes.
6. Aliquot 15 μL of collected supernatants from loading experiments into two microcentrifuge tubes. Add 3 μL of 6× SDS-page loading buffer.
7. Pipette 2 μL of FL-ovalbumin (25 mg/mL), in a tube and mix with 10 μL of distilled water and 3 μL of 6× loading buffer.
8. Place all the tubes on a heat block at 100 °C, boil for 5 min.
9. Supernatants and free ovalbumin control samples are ready to run after this step. However, GP-ovalbumin formulations require additional processing to extract the encapsulated protein. Briefly centrifuge the tubes to bring the condensation down. Cup sonicate the tubes for ~30 s and place on the heat block again for 5 min. Repeat this cup-sonication, heating, and centrifugation steps three times in total in order to extract the protein from GPs.
10. Samples can be stored at −20 °C until the gel is run.
11. Observing ovalbumin identity bands in the experimental GP-ovalbumin sample and not in the corresponding supernatant indicates a good encapsulation. Observing an ovalbumin identity band in the supernatant fraction of experimental sample indicates a poor loading reaction (Fig. 9).

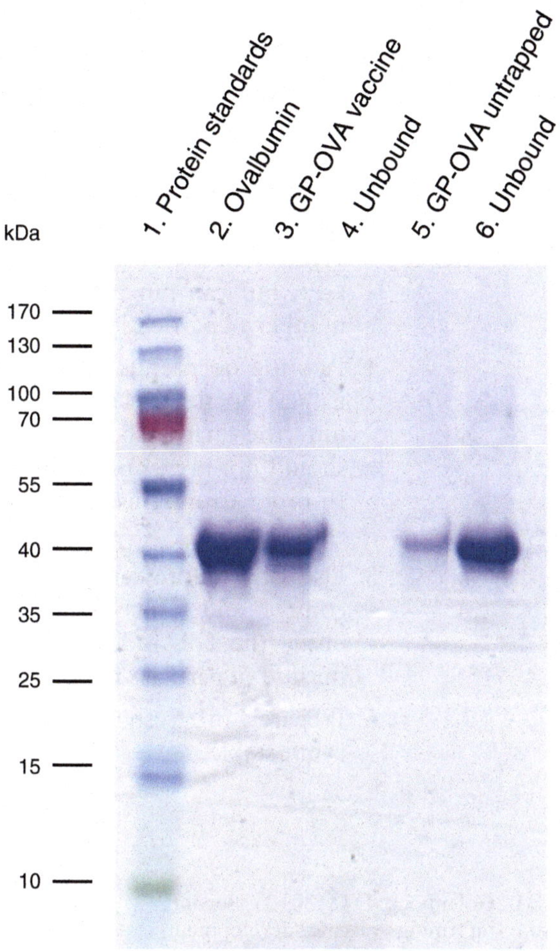

Fig. 9 SDS PAGE analysis of encapsulated (pellet) and unencapsulated (soluble) fractions to assess antigen loading

4 Notes

1. It is important to first add water to the flask and then weigh and add sodium hydroxide to flask for safety reasons. Wear protective goggles, gloves, and lab coat and place the stirring hot plate in a fume hood. Start with concentrated HCl (12.1 N). Add it dropwise in the fume hood, while mixing and measuring the pH. When the pH is close to 8, use a diluted HCl (1 N) solution to prevent sudden pH drop.
2. We usually get ~5 × 10^8 particles/mg GP. The size, lipid and protein content of the yeast and the purification process affect the particles per mg and the hydrodynamic volume. For example, diploid yeast strains yield larger particles than their haploid counterparts; the particles per mg are usually lower with diploid strains. Less pure particles, or particles with a thicker cell wall

also have lower particles per mg. Particles/mg is directly correlated with the hydrodynamic volume.

3. Hydrodynamic volume is the amount of liquid 1 mg of particles can absorb fully. Using a volume less than hydrodynamic volume during loading steps ensures that the "payload" gets fully absorbed into GPs. Soluble payload in the solvent moves into particles along with the solvent by capillary action. Hydrodynamic volume is typically ~10 mg of water per mg GPs, but can range from 8 to 12 mg depending upon the number of particles per mg.
4. Pass the open ends of pipette tips through a Bunsen burner flame. Pipette tips should stay in the microcentrifuge tubes until the final wash step. Therefore, length of the pipette tip should not prevent closing the caps of microcentrifuge tubes. In order to mix, use a secondary pipette tip as shown below (Fig. 7).
5. Use same fluorescence intensity and exposure time for both control and experimental sample. Observing fluorescence inside the GPs indicates a good loading, while fluorescence outside of particles indicates unencapsulated protein.
6. Prepare 1 mL fresh urea solution each time as the urea solution is not stable.

References

1. Levitz SM, Golenbock DT (2012) Beyond empiricism: informing vaccine development through innate immunity research. Cell 148:1284–1292
2. Soto E, Ostroff GR (2012) In: Vetvicka V, Novak M (eds) Biology and chemistry of beta glucan. Bentham science publishers, Oak Park, IL, pp 48–67. doi:10.2174/9781608052103 1110101
3. Tesz GJ et al (2011) Glucan particles for selective delivery of siRNA to phagocytic cells in mice. Biochem J 436:351–362
4. Soto ER, Caras AC, Kut LC, Castle MK, Ostroff GR (2012) Glucan particles for macrophage targeted delivery of nanoparticles. J Drug Deliv 2012:1–13
5. Soto E, Kim YS, Lee J, Kornfeld H, Ostroff G (2010) Glucan particle encapsulated rifampicin for targeted delivery to macrophages. Polymers (Basel) 2:681–689
6. Soto ER, Ostroff GR (2008) Characterization of multilayered nanoparticles encapsulated in yeast cell wall particles for DNA delivery. Bioconjug Chem 19:840–848
7. Aouadi M et al (2009) Orally delivered siRNA targeting macrophage Map4k4 suppresses systemic inflammation. Nature 458:1180–1184
8. Goodridge HS, Wolf AJ, Underhill DM (2009) Beta-glucan recognition by the innate immune system. Immunol Rev 230:38–50
9. Huang H et al (2012) Relative contributions of dectin-1 and complement to immune responses to particulate β-glucans. J Immunol 189:312–317
10. Levitz SM, Huang H, Ostroff GR, Specht CA (2015) Exploiting fungal cell wall components in vaccines. Semin Immunopathol 37: 199–207
11. Huang H et al (2009) Distinct patterns of dendritic cell cytokine release stimulated by fungal beta-glucans and toll-like receptor agonists. Infect Immun 77:1774–1781
12. Huang H, Ostroff GR, Lee CK, Specht CA, Levitz SM (2010) Robust stimulation of

humoral and cellular immune responses following vaccination with antigen-loaded beta-glucan particles. MBio 1:e00164–e00110
13. Huang H, Ostroff GR, Lee CK, Specht CA, Levitz SM (2013) Characterization and optimization of the glucan particle-based vaccine platform. Clin Vaccine Immunol 20: 1585–1591. doi:10.1128/CVI.00463-13
14. Specht CA et al (2015) Protection against experimental cryptococcosis following vaccination with glucan particles containing cryptococcus alkaline extracts. MBio 6:1–11
15. Buffer Reference Center|Sigma-Aldrich. at <http://www.sigmaaldrich.com/life-science/core-bioreagents/biological-buffers/learning-center/buffer-reference-center.html#sodium carbonate>

Chapter 12

Th1-Inducing Agents in Prophylaxis and Therapy for Paracoccidioidomycosis

Thiago Aparecido da Silva, Fabrício Freitas Fernandes, Taise Natali Landgraf, Ademílson Panunto-Castelo, and Maria Cristina Roque-Barreira

Abstract

Adjuvants and immunomodulatory molecules could be included in the treatment of *P. brasiliensis* infection. In this context, we reported that the therapeutic and/or prophylactic administration of Th1-inducing agents, such as immunomodulatory lectins and adjuvants, was able to provide protection against experimental paracoccidioidomycosis. Then, we described the protocols to investigate the effect of immunomodulatory agents on the course of *P. brasiliensis* infection. In this sense, we detailed the measurement of fungal burden and cytokine production, and the histopathological analysis used to evaluate the most effective administration regime.

Key words Adjuvants, Lectins, Immunomodulation, Therapy, *P. brasiliensis*, Paracoccidioidomycoses

1 Introduction

Infections caused by fungi—mycoses—result in manifestations that are dependent on the type and the degree of tissue inflammation and on the host immune response to the pathogen, producing superficial, cutaneous, subcutaneous, or systemic infections. In humans, the fungi can cause a wide spectrum of diseases ranging from mild acute manifestations in mucosa or skin in immunocompetent individuals to life-threatening diseases in immunocompromised patients. The routes of infection can be endogenous, which involve reactivation of previous infections or penetration of mucosal breaches by commensal organisms like *Candida albicans* [1], or exogenous, which include cutaneous, percutaneous, or airborne routes. The latter is a common route of systemic infection by pathogenic dimorphic fungi, such as *Histoplasma capsulatum* and *Paracoccidioides brasiliensis* [2]. The host immune response does not discern between commensal or

Markus Kalkum and Margarita Semis (eds.), *Vaccines for Invasive Fungal Infections: Methods and Protocols*, Methods in Molecular Biology, vol. 1625, DOI 10.1007/978-1-4939-7104-6_12,

ubiquitous fungi, and the balance between pro- and anti-inflammatory mediators is essential for the maintenance of the host-fungus relationship [2]. Although the innate immunity is efficient and stimulates an adaptive immune response against fungi in most people [3], for yet unclear reasons some do not develop this protective immune response. So far, it is known that the differentiation of naive $CD4^+$ T lymphocytes is decisive for the resulting infection. In general, the differentiation in type 1 T helper cells (Th1), which produce interferon (IFN-) γ and activate macrophages, as well as in Th17, which produce interleukin (IL-) 17 and induce neutrophil migration and promote inflammation, favors a protective response against several pathogenic fungi [4]. In contrast, the differentiation into Th2 or regulatory T cells induces an anti-inflammatory environment, via cytokines such as IL-10 and TGF-β, with inhibition of macrophage activation, decrease in inflammatory mediators, and consequent progression of fungal infection. Thus, the candidate targets for vaccines and therapies against invasive fungal infections must trigger cell activation and differentiation mechanisms that account for the development of Th1- or Th17-mediated responses and production of proinflammatory mediators, to improve fungal killing [5, 6].

New strategies, including adjuvants and immunomodulatory molecules, to create efficient fungal vaccines have been investigated. In this context, a modified peptide, P10, derived from a *P. brasiliensis* 43-kDa glycoprotein (gp43) antigen induces a Th1 response and protects mice against fungal infections [7]. Moreover, immunization with a recombinant protein, Pb27, from *P. brasiliensis* [8, 9], along with to fluconazole chemotherapy, showed an additive protective effect [10, 11]. Additionally, the treatment of *P. brasiliensis*-infected mice with complete Freund's adjuvant (CFA) [12] or monophosphoryl lipid A from *Salmonella minnesota* (MPLA-SM) [13], known as Th1 inducers, promoted the reduction of granulomas and yeast cells in the lungs. More recently, it was demonstrated that the therapeutic and prophylactic administration of the immunomodulatory lectins ArtinM and Paracoccin, which recognize glycans N-linked to Toll-like receptors (TLR), induced Th1 response and led to protection against *P. brasiliensis* infection [14–17]. The most effective administration regimen of CFA, MPLA, ArtinM, and Paracoccin was experimentally established [12, 14–17]. Herein, we describe the protocols for lectins and adjuvant administration that were most effective at inducing a protective Th1 response against experimental paracoccidioidomycosis. We also provide protocols for the treatment efficiency analyses.

2 Materials

2.1 Fungal Inoculum

1. YPD medium: solubilize yeast extract (10 g), peptone (20 g), and dextrose (20 g) in 900 mL of distilled water in a glass beaker. Adjust the pH to 6.5 with HCl q.s. and add distilled water q.s. for a final volume of 1 L. Sterilize the medium in an autoclave. Before use, supplement the medium with 4% fetal bovine serum (FBS) (*see* **Note 1**).
2. Ham's F-12 nutrient mixture: Ham's F-12 nutrient mix powder (Gibco®, Thermo Fischer Scientific) and 1.176 g sodium carbonate were solubilized in 1 L of distilled water. The pH of the mixture was adjusted to 7.0 with HCl q.s. before sterilizing it by filtration through a 0.22 μm filter (*see* **Note 1**).
3. Phosphate-buffered saline (PBS): solubilize NaCl (8 g), KCl (0.2 g), Na_2HPO_4 (1.44 g), and KH_2PO_4 (0.24 g) in 900 mL of ultrapure water. Adjust the pH of the mixture to 7.2 with HCl q.s. and add ultrapure water q.s. for a final volume of 1 L. Sterilize the solution in an autoclave.
4. Erlenmeyer flasks (250 mL), glass beaker (1 L), and incubator shaker.
5. 50 mL centrifuge tube/polypropylene and centrifuge.
6. Fluorescein diacetate: 5 mg/mL stock solution (*see* **Note 2**).
7. Ethidium bromide: 1 mg/mL stock solution.
8. Neubauer cell-counting chamber and optical microscope.
9. Trypan blue: 0.4% solution in water.

2.2 Infection and Treatment

1. Anesthetic: ketamine hydrochloride (100 mg/kg) and xylazine hydrochloride (7.5 mg/kg).
2. Sterile PBS (endotoxin-free) (*see* **Notes 3** and **4**).
3. Complete Freund's adjuvant (CFA) containing 1 mg/mL of *Mycobacterium tuberculosis* (Sigma-Aldrich, St. Louis, EUA).
4. 1 mg/mL MPLA-SM (Invitrogen, San Diego, EUA) in dimethyl sulfoxide.
5. Insulin syringe with needle size 12.7 mm × 0.33 mm (22G).
6. Male BALB/c mice at 6–8 weeks of age (*see* **Note 5**).
7. Round-bottom polystyrene Falcon tubes.

2.3 Colony-Forming Unit (CFU)

1. Sterile, round-bottom polystyrene Falcon tubes (*see* **Note 6**).
2. Tissue homogenizer.
3. Brain heart infusion agar (BHI): solubilize BHI (37 g, Difco) and agar (20 g) in 1 L of distilled water, and sterilize the solution in an autoclave. Once the temperature of the BHI is

stabilized at 55 °C, add 4% FBS and 100 μg/mL ampicillin or 96 μg/mL gentamicin.

4. Sterile PBS.
5. Sterile petri dishes (90 mm × 15 mm).
6. Microbiological culture incubator (37 °C).

2.4 Cytokine Measurement

1. Supernatant of tissue homogenization.
2. Kits to measure the levels of cytokines by enzyme-linked immunosorbent assay (ELISA) or cytometric bead array (CBA, Becton, Dickinson Co.) (*see* **Note 7**).
3. 96-well plates with high binding surface and a microplate absorbance reader (for quantification by ELISA).
4. Flow cytometer capable of detecting and distinguishing fluorescence emissions at 576 and 670 nm (for quantification by CBA).

2.5 Histopathology

1. Neutral buffered formalin (3.7%) diluted in PBS (pH 7.2).
2. Ethanol (70% and 95%, v/v) and absolute ethanol (*see* **Note 8**).
3. Mixture of xylene isomers (*see* **Note 8**).
4. Paraffin (melting point range 55–60 °C) and cassettes for tissue processing (*see* **Note 8**) and embedding.
5. Microtome, blade, and cover slips.
6. Hematoxylin-eosin stain.
7. Optical microscope equipped with a digital camera.

3 Methods

3.1 Fungal Inoculum Preparation

1. Use 50 mL of Ham's F-12 nutrient mixture for the fungal inoculum. Incubate at 37 °C with 150 rpm agitation (*see* **Note 9**).
2. After 5 days on the incubator shaker, collect 40 mL of culture supernatant, and centrifuge for 10 min (3000 × *g*, at 25 °C) (*see* **Note 10**).
3. Wash the yeast cell pellet in 40 mL PBS. Repeat the centrifugation under the same conditions as described above.
4. Discard the supernatant and resuspend the yeast cells in 5 mL PBS, followed by cell viability analysis and cell counting.
5. Perform cell viability test with fluorescein diacetate and ethidium bromide [18]. Dilute stock solutions of fluorescein diacetate (5 mg/mL) and ethidium bromide (1 mg/mL) 1/2500 and 1/20, respectively. Add 100 μL of each solution to 100 μL of yeast cells and incubate at 37 °C for 15 min. Transfer the yeast suspension (20 μL) to a glass slide, place cover slip over

the suspension on the slide, and analyze the yeast cells under a fluorescence microscope (*see* **Notes 2** and **11**).

6. Dilute the yeast suspension 1:100 and 1:1000 in 0.4% Trypan blue and determine cell concentration in a Neubauer chamber (*see* **Note 12**).
7. Adjust the cell concentration to 1×10^7 and 5×10^7 yeast cells/mL for intravenous and intranasal infections, respectively (*see* **Note 13**).

3.2 Infection of Mice

1. Anesthetize the BALB/c mice using an insulin syringe with a 100 μL intraperitoneal injection of a mixture of ketamine hydrochloride (10 mg/kg) and xylazine hydrochloride (7.5 mg/kg) diluted in sterile PBS.
2. For the intranasal infection, gently inoculate 40 μL of the fungal suspension into the nostril with a tip. For the intravenous infection, administer 100 μL of the fungal suspension in the ophthalmic plexus using an insulin syringe. Add sterile PBS or vaseline in the eyes of the mice to avoid blindness.
3. Following infection, keep the mice warm until they recovered from the anesthesia.

3.3 Prophylactic and Therapeutic Treatment with Immunomodulatory Agents

1. Adjust the final volume of the agents to 100 μL with PBS to inoculate each mouse (*see* **Note 4**). The optimal concentration of the agents to inoculate should be assessed, and previous studies with immunomodulator lectins used 0.5 μg [14–17].
2. Administer the agents via subcutaneous injections, using an insulin syringe, in the inguinal region. Inoculate slowly to avoid an incision in the mesentery.
3. Prophylactic administration: inoculate the agents 3, 10, and/or 17 days before infection. To evaluate the treatment regimens, consider the following groups (G): control group (PBS administration on 17th, 10th, and 3rd days), G1 (on 17th, 10th, and 3rd days), G2 (on 17th day), G3 (on 10th day), G4 (on 3rd day), G5 (on 10th and 3rd days), G6 (on 17th and 10th days) and G7 (on 17th and 3rd days) (*see* Fig. 1).
4. Therapeutic administration: Inoculate the agents 3, 10, and/or 17 days post-infection. To evaluate the treatment regimens, consider the following groups: control group (PBS administration on 3rd, 10th, and 17th days), G1 (on 3rd, 10th, and 17th days), G2 (on 3rd days), G3 (on 10th day), G4 (on 17th day), G5 (on 3rd and 10th days), G6 (on 10th and 17th days) and G7 (on 3rd and 10th days) (*see* Fig. 1).
5. Remove the lungs 30 days post-infection to verify the fungal burden (Subheading 3.5.1), the levels of cytokines (Subheading 3.5.2), and histopathology (Subheading 3.5.3).

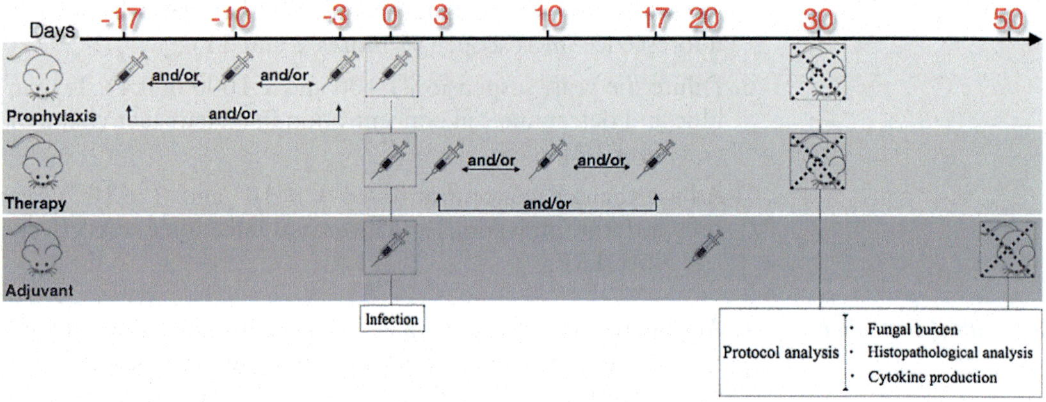

Fig. 1 Protocol to evaluate the effect of immunomodulatory agents on the course of *P. brasiliensis* infection. The scheme indicates the days to investigate the administration regime before (prophylaxis) and after (therapy) infection with *P. brasiliensis*. Moreover, the scheme also demonstrates the most effective administration regimen with adjuvants after infection with *P. brasiliensis*. The effect of the prophylactic and therapeutic administration must be evaluated 30 days post-infection, and the adjuvant therapy must be evaluated 50 days post-infection. The measurements of fungal burden and cytokine production, along with the histopathological analyses, are used to define the most effective administration regimen

6. Collect a portion of the lung for homogenization (*see* **Note 14**) in sterile, round-bottom polystyrene Falcon tubes, which were previously weighed with 1 mL of sterile PBS, and homogenize the tissue. Afterward, weigh the tubes to determine the lung mass that should be considered for CFU measurement (Subheading 3.5.1).
7. Compared to the control group, the most effective administration regimen showed a lower fungal burden, high levels of proinflammatory cytokines, and preserved the organ architecture.

3.4 Adjuvant Treatment

1. Administrate a single dose of 50 μg of CFA [12] or 20 μg of MPLA-SM [13] emulsified with PBS to a final volume of 100 μL, 20 days post-infection via a subcutaneous injection with an insulin syringe into the dorsum (*see* **Note 4**).
2. After 4 weeks of treatments, proceed with the method described in Subheading 3.3 (**steps 5** and **6**) for the analysis of fungal burden (Subheading 3.5.1), cytokine levels (Subheading 3.5.2), and histopathology (Subheading 3.5.3).
3. Both adjuvants have a therapeutic effect on experimental paracoccidioiodomycosis with decreased fungal burden and preservation of lung tissue. It is worth mentioning that the CFA and MPLA induced a Th1 response and reversed the immunosuppression observed in the untreated control group.

3.5 Protocol Analysis

3.5.1 Colony-Forming Unit (CFU)

1. Seed 100 μL of homogenized tissue from each mouse on plate dishes containing BHI agar. Dilute the homogenized tissue from each mouse 1:20 and 1:50 in sterile PBS and seed 100 μL on BHI agar (*see* **Notes** 14 and **15**).
2. Incubate the plates at 37 °C for 7 days and then inspect daily up to 14 days to quantify the colony-forming units.
3. Express the results in terms of CFU/g of organ.

3.5.2 Cytokine Measurement

1. After centrifugation (4000 × *g*, 10 min, 4 °C) of the homogenized tissue, collect the supernatant and store at −20 °C or use immediately to measure the cytokines (*see* **Note 16**).
2. Follow the manufacturer's instructions to measure the cytokine levels by ELISA or CBA (*see* **Note** 7).

3.5.3 Histopathology

1. Remove the lungs, wash with PBS, and transfer to the cassettes (*see* **Note 14**).
2. Place the samples in a bottle containing neutral buffered formalin (*see* **Note** 17) for fixation and incubate for 48 h at 25 °C.
3. Perform the tissue dehydration process with ethanol (70%, 95%, and absolute ethanol) in incubations of 1 h each at 25 °C, additionally two incubations in absolute ethanol for 1 h each as described in **Note 8**.
4. Transfer the tissue to a mixture of xylene isomers (clearing agent) for 1 h at 25 °C (*see* **Note 8**).
5. Place the samples in paraffin at 58 °C for 1 h (*see* **Note 8**). After the incubation period, embed the tissues in paraffin blocks.
6. Cut the tissues into sections of 5 μm thickness using the microtome and place on a glass slide to proceed with rehydration and staining by hematoxylin-eosin.
7. Acquire images with an optical microscope equipped with a digital camera for histopathological analysis.

4 Notes

1. The addition of 4% FBS in the culture medium maintained the fungal virulence [19]. FBS inactivated by incubation at 56 °C for 30 min was used.
2. Fluorescein diacetate was diluted in acetone to obtain the stock solution [5 mg/mL] and stored at −20 °C. The stock solution was diluted in PBS to 1:2.500 at the moment of use [18].
3. The anesthetic was used during intravenous or intranasal infections.

4. Endotoxin-free PBS was used to measure the levels of endotoxin in samples for the treatment. The innate immune system can be activated by high levels of endotoxin, hindering the demonstration of the immunomodulatory activity of the treatment.
5. BALB/c mice are susceptible to *P. brasiliensis* infection; therefore, the treatment of infected BALB/c mice allows evaluating the most effective administration method.
6. Round-bottom polystyrene Falcon tubes allowed for better homogenization, than conical-bottom tubes.
7. Measure the cytokines related to Th1, Th2, and Th17 responses. The homogenized tissue was used to quantify IL-12, IFN-γ, TNF-α, IL-6, IL-10, IL-17, and IL-23 by ELISA or CBA.
8. During the dehydration process, when the sample was incubated in absolute ethanol, it was important to use three different containers of absolute ethanol to avoid decreasing the dehydration efficiency. This procedure was also used during the agent clearing and embedding tissue steps, in which the sample was incubated twice in xylene and paraffin, using different containers.
9. The inoculum was made with a small amount of yeast. Four to five colonies (approximately 2 mm diameter), which were recovered from infected mice and grown on BHI agar plates, were collected. Thus, dead cells in the colony constituted an insignificant part of the total culture. The infection process had to be performed only with inocula of cells with viability above 90%. Excess dead cells alter the results that would be obtained by the treatment.
10. The culture was removed from the incubation shaker and left for 5 min without shaking at 25 °C. Thereafter, 40 mL of the culture supernatant was collected carefully to recover less agglomerated yeast cells. This process made the inoculum more homogenous by separating the cell agglomerates, and aided the passage of cells through the syringe; thus, the cell viability is maintained.
11. The cell viability was determined as the mean of percentages of viable cells (green) in three random fields.
12. Trypan blue was used for the analysis of cell viability. Cells with damaged membranes were stained in blue, and this facilitated the cell counting.
13. The amounts of inoculated yeast cells in each animal during intravenous and intranasal infection were 1×10^6 (100 μL) and 2×10^6 (40 μL) yeast cells, respectively.

14. In all mice, the lung or one lobe of the lung was removed from the same side.
15. Each dilution was performed in duplicate, and two dilutions were chosen for seeding on BHI agar.
16. The supernatant was centrifuged (10,000 × *g*, 4 °C, 10 min), stored at −20 °C to precipitate the aggregates, and only the upper layer was used.
17. Neutral buffered formalin volume was 20 times that of tissue weight (For 1 g of tissue 20 mL of neutral buffered formalin).

References

1. Nobile CJ, Johnson AD (2015) *Candida albicans* Biofilms and human disease. Annu Rev Microbiol 69:71–92
2. Romani L (2011) Immunity to fungal infections. Nat Rev Immunol 11(4):275–288
3. Santamaria R, Rizzetto L, Bromley M, Zelante T, Lee W, Cavalieri D et al (2011) Systems biology of infectious diseases: a focus on fungal infections. Immunobiology 216(11):1212–1227
4. LeibundGut-Landmann S, Wuthrich M, Hohl TM (2012) Immunity to fungi. Curr Opin Immunol 24(4):449–458
5. Spellberg B (2011) Vaccines for invasive fungal infections. F1000 Med Rep 3:13
6. Cassone A, Casadevall A (2012) Recent progress in vaccines against fungal diseases. Curr Opin Microbiol 15(4):427–433
7. de Amorim J, Magalhaes A, Munoz JE, Rittner GM, Nosanchuk JD, Travassos LR et al (2013) DNA vaccine encoding peptide P10 against experimental paracoccidioidomycosis induces long-term protection in presence of regulatory T cells. Microbes Infect 15(3):181–191
8. Reis BS, Fernandes VC, Martins EM, Serakides R, Goes AM (2008) Protective immunity induced by rPb27 of Paracoccidioides brasiliensis. Vaccine 26(43):5461–5469
9. Morais EA, Martins EM, Boelone JN, Gomes DA, Goes AM (2015) Immunization with recombinant Pb27 protein reduces the levels of pulmonary fibrosis caused by the inflammatory response against Paracoccidioides brasiliensis. Mycopathologia 179(1–2):31–43
10. Fernandes VC, Martins EM, Boeloni JN, Coitinho JB, Serakides R, Goes AM (2011) Additive effect of rPb27 immunization and chemotherapy in experimental paracoccidioidomycosis. PLoS One 6(3):e17885
11. Fernandes VC, Martins EM, Boeloni JN, Coitinho JB, Serakides R, Goes AM (2011) The combined use of Paracoccidioides brasiliensis Pb40 and Pb27 recombinant proteins enhances chemotherapy effects in experimental paracoccidioidomycosis. Microbes Infect 13(12–13):1062–1072
12. de Oliveira LL, Coltri KC, Cardoso CR, Roque-Barreira MC, Panunto-Castelo A (2008) T helper 1-inducing adjuvant protects against experimental paracoccidioidomycosis. PLoS Negl Trop Dis 2(3):e183
13. Landgraf TN, Fernandes FF, Peron G, Panunto-Castelo A (2016). Therapeutic effect of monophosphoryl lipid a administration on Paracoccidioides brasiliensis-infected mice. Med Mycol. doi: 10.1093/mmy/myw074
14. Alegre AC, Oliveira AF, Dos Reis Almeida FB, Roque-Barreira MC, Hanna ES (2014) Recombinant paracoccin reproduces the biological properties of the native protein and induces protective Th1 immunity against Paracoccidioides brasiliensis infection. PLoS Negl Trop Dis 8(4):e2788
15. Alegre-Maller AC, Mendonca FC, da Silva TA, Oliveira AF, Freitas MS, Hanna ES et al (2014) Therapeutic administration of recombinant Paracoccin confers protection against paracoccidioides brasiliensis infection: involvement of TLRs. PLoS Negl Trop Dis 8(12):e3317
16. Coltri KC, Oliveira LL, Pinzan CF, Vendruscolo PE, Martinez R, Goldman MH et al (2008) Therapeutic administration of KM+ lectin protects mice against Paracoccidioides brasiliensis infection via interleukin-12 production in a toll-like receptor 2-dependent mechanism. Am J Pathol 173(2):423–432
17. Coltri KC, Oliveira LL, Ruas LP, Vendruscolo PE, Goldman MH, Panunto-Castelo A et al (2010) Protection against Paracoccidioides brasiliensis infection conferred by the prophylactic administration of native and recombinant ArtinM. Med Mycol 48(6):792–799
18. Calich VL, Purchio A, Paula CR (1979) A new fluorescent viability test for fungi cells. Mycopathologia 66(3):175–177
19. Lacaz CS, Porto E et al (2002) Paracoccidioidomicose. In: Tratado de Micologia Médica, 9th edn, pp 639–729

Chapter 13

Nanoparticle-Based Mycosis Vaccine

Swaleha Zubair, Asim Azhar, Nazoora Khan, Ejaj Ahmad, Mohd Ajmal, and Mohammad Owais

Abstract

Many diseases that were considered major affliction of mankind in the past have been successfully eradicated with introduction of appropriate vaccine strategies. In order to expedite new challenges coming up to deal with various infectious diseases, nano-particulate-based subunit vaccines seem to be the demand of ordeal. The nano-vaccines can find better scope for the diseases that were not rampant in the semi-advanced world few years back. For example in present-day circumstances that corroborate with advancement in the field of medical sciences in terms of cancer chemotherapy, organ transplantation, therapy of autoimmune diseases, etc.; along with prevalence of altogether unheard diseases such as HIV infection, people are at risk of infliction with many more pathogens. In this regard, development of an effective prophylactic strategy against many opportunistic infections primarily caused by fungal pathogens needs better understanding of host pathogen relation and role of active immunity against pathogenic fungi. In the present study, we have tried to decipher effectiveness of a nano-sized vaccine delivery system in imparting protection against fungal pathogens.

Key words Antifungal vaccines, Cryptococcosis, Escheriosome, Fibrin, Fungal infections, Liposome, Lipid vesicles, Nanoparticles

1 Introduction

Recent efforts exploiting technologies to uplift quality of the life have benefited mankind in several ways. For example, advancements in the field of medical sciences like the introduction of antibiotics as well as newer chemotherapeutic option in the treatment of cancer and organ transplantation made tremendous impact on general public health. Paradoxically, some of these offer opportunity to infections, mainly those of fungal origin to establish themselves in the host. In fact, human subjects have become more susceptible to a range of opportunistic infections for the last two or three decades. Patients receiving broad-spectrum antibacterial therapy or those subjected to invasive procedures are highly prone to fungal infections [1]. Besides HIV infection, individuals who have undergone organ transplantation or remain on treatment

Markus Kalkum and Margarita Semis (eds.), *Vaccines for Invasive Fungal Infections: Methods and Protocols*, Methods in Molecular Biology, vol. 1625, DOI 10.1007/978-1-4939-7104-6_13, © Springer Science+Business Media LLC 2017

with anticancer drugs are prime targets of such infections [2]. The association of the most of the opportunistic infections in patients with AIDS background significantly exacerbated the situation both in developing and in developed countries. For example, candidiasis occurs in as many as 90% of AIDS patients [3]. The incidences of invasive candidiasis in such patients have increased several folds to become among the first five most common blood culture isolates including it. The recent upsurge in the incidence of candidiasis certainly needs serious attention, since India is poised to register the highest number of HIV infection cases in the world [4].

1.1 Why Nanosized Antigen Delivery Systems

Nanotechnology is the science involving design, synthesis, characterization, and application of materials and devices whose one dimension is at least of nanometer size [5]. Structures, fabricated employing nanotechnology, are categorized as "nanoparticles." One of the most promising applications of nanotechnology is in the realm of medicine and involves the development of nano-sized tools and machines that can act as biosensor, or as a vehicle to deliver drugs to cure diseases and repair damaged tissues, at the molecular level in cells and organelles. The National Institutes of Health, USA, has coined the term "nanomedicine" to refer to the mushrooming innovations in nanotechnology. In other words, nanomedicine is the medical application of nanotechnology. Initially, nanotechnology was used in the form of passive structures (such as in cosmetics); however, later these have been exploited as an active structure that can be developed in the form of new, more effective drug delivery systems. Nanomedicines are now within the realm of reality starting with nano-diagnostics, drug delivery and also as a vehicle to administer subunit vaccine for immunization purposes. The discoveries have been highly instrumental in revolutionizing the temporal and spatial site-specific delivery of biologically active compounds [6]. During nanofabrication, the molecular synthesis and assemblage can be regulated in a controlled fashion so that designed nano-engineered materials exhibit specific and controlled bulk chemical and physical properties.

In order to be successful, therapeutic and preventive strategies not only depend on the appropriate choice of the active principle (drug or antigen) but to a large extent on the use of an appropriate delivery system. This holds true for difficult-to-deliver compounds; in particular drugs having poor solubility (hydrophobic) and undesirable membrane permeability attributes. In fact, the quest to find the ideal therapeutic strategy will continue till a drug with maximum efficacy and no side effects is found. Many of the present-day drugs are plagued by narrow therapeutic window, and their effective use is limited by problems of dose limiting toxic effect. Nevertheless, the bottlenecks need to be circumvented so that the therapeutic effectiveness of existing drugs can be improved through the use of an appropriately designed delivery system that can modify the distribution of the drug in the body by targeting it to desired site and by controlled release of the encapsulated material over the time.

Beside drug delivery, nano-particles offer a formidable platform for antigen delivery as well. Antigen-loaded nano-particles have altogether different types of shortcomings, for example, one of the major challenges is to maintain native structure of the antigen of interest in the formed nano-formulation. In the present scenario, exploitation of nanotechnology to develop nano-particulate delivery systems for drug and antigen delivery has altogether a different purview. Nanotechnology has been increasingly used by the pharmaceutical and biotechnology industries that are likely to make a significant impact on global pharmaceutical planning and marketing (market intelligence and lifecycle management).

The age of nano-structural delivery systems began with the development of liposomes by Bangham [7]. Since then a large number of nanoparticulate systems have been developed and as of this day, the sheer number and types of nano-particulate structures that have been already developed or being researched upon are tremendous. The concept of the "magic bullet" proposed a century ago by Nobel laureate Paul Ehrlich came to reality with the recent appearance of several approved forms of drug-targeting systems for the treatment of certain cancer and serious infectious diseases. An interesting example is the launch of the FDA-approved breast-cancer drug Abraxane (American Pharmaceuticals, U.S.A). Furthermore, many other nano-medicinal formulations for treatment of skin disorders and infections are in the pipeline.

The earliest delivery systems investigated were polymer carriers for accomplishing spatiotemporal release of therapeutics involving both pulsatile dose delivery products and implanted reservoir systems. Various polymers including cellulose derivatives, polyethylene glycol (PEG), and poly (N-vinyl pyrrolidone) are in use for over five decades and their early applications include usage in drug sprays, coating, encapsulation, etc. [8]. A large number of other natural and synthetic drug delivery systems have also been investigated with varying success.

From the drug or antigen delivery perspective, polymer devices can be classified into:

(1) diffusion controlled (monolithic devices), (2) solvent activated (swelling or osmotically controlled devices), (3) chemically controlled (biodegradable), and (4) triggered system [8].

In a manner similar to drug delivery, the use of nanotechnology approaches to antigen delivery focuses on developing nanoscale particles to maximize bioavailability of an antigen at a specific place in the body over an extended period of time. Nanoparticulate systems can be designed to favorably interact with cells and tissues at the molecular level. The small size of these particles and the plausibility to engineer their surface with synthetic polymers or appropriate ligands allow nanoparticulate carriers to be targeted to specific cells, tissues, and extracellular elements in the body. These approaches are aimed at enhancing detection sensitivity in medical imaging, improving therapeutic effectiveness, and minimizing antigen dose for nano-vaccines. Nano-scale engineering may also enable specialized structures that can be activated by change in the environmental pH, chemical stimuli, by the application of a rapidly oscillating magnetic field, or by the application of an external heat source [9, 10]. Such modifications offer control over particle integrity, delivery rates, and the location of load (drug/antigen) release, for example within specific organelles. The nano-carriers can be made to target cell receptors and simultaneously deliver encapsulated material along with biological sensors [11]. The strategies can be applied to deliver drugs, antigens, genetic materials, and diagnostic agents (encapsulated, covalently attached, or adsorbed to such nanocarriers) etc., selectively to specific sites via intravenous and interstitial routes of administration [12–14]. During vaccine development programs, one may deal with both water soluble and hydrophobic membrane proteins as well as other chemical classes of antigens. Nanoparticulate carriers can be useful to stabilize immunogens and protein drugs, such as various cytokines, agents effective against enzymatic and chemical degradations and to increase their bioavailability. Such auxiliary systems can also be employed in the targeting of nucleic acids in gene therapy and antigen for vaccine development. It has been proved that nano-particulate systems provide a useful tool in the trans-dermal and pulmonary antigen administration. Moreover, many immunomodulators and immunosuppressive agents, which require long-term, even lifelong administration, benefit much from being packaged in nano-particles.

1.2 A Brief Overview to Nano-Particle-Based Delivery Systems

A vast array of diverse types of nanoparticles of different shapes, sizes; composition of the assortment materials and with various chemical and surface properties have already been constructed. The nanoparticulate systems comprise a variety of constructs viz. nanospheres, nanocapsules, lipid nanoparticles, microemulsions, macromolecular complexes, ceramic nanoparticles, and vesicular carriers like liposomes, niosomes, etc. Progress in nanotechnology is very dynamic and new systems continue to be developed. Some more common general classes of nanoparticulate delivery systems and their functions are listed as follows:

Bucky balls and carbon tubes are carbon-based lattice like potentially porous structures and are grouped as a fullerene class of systems. Bucky balls are spherical while carbon tubes are cylindrical. In nanomedicine, carbon tubes have been used as carriers for vaccines, drugs, and other molecules.

Nanoshells also called core-shells are few nanometers thick spherical cores composed of a particular compound surrounded by a shell or outer coating of another compound. Their ability to absorb at biologically useful wavelengths, depending on the shell thickness, justifies their use in nanomedicine. For example, silica is used to form the core and some sticky compound to adhere gold particles as the outer shell. Such nanoshells can be injected into a tumor, followed by application of radiation whereby nanoshells heat up enough to kill the tumor cells.

Dendrimers are highly branched structures having hook-like structures on their surfaces that can be used to attach cell-identification tags, fluorescent dyes, enzymes, and other molecules. Dendrimers are of two basic structural types: (a) globular with branches radiating from a central core, (b) a series of highly branched polymers with no central core. Nanomedical applications for dendrimers are many and include nanoscale catalysts and reaction vessels, micelle mimics, imaging agents, chemical sensors, and agents for delivery of drugs, antigens, or genes into cells.

Quantum dots are also known as nanocrystals. Quantum dots behave as semiconductors emitting light in the entire visible light spectrum. These nanostructures confine conduction band electrons, valence band holes, or excitons in all three spatial directions. Examples of quantum dots are semiconductor nanocrystals and core-shell nanocrystals, where there is an interface between different semiconductor materials. They are used for cell labeling and imaging, particularly in cancer imaging studies.

Cross-linked Micelles are self-forming particles that are prepared from individual surfactant molecules that have a water-loving and a water-hating component. The surfactant molecules orientate themselves to form spheres where the water-loving component is on the outside and in contact with the water. The water-hating component remains inside the sphere, preferring to interact with itself rather than with the water. This hydrophobic core makes them ideal carrier systems for water-hating small molecules. Cross-linked micelles are similar. However, they are held in their configuration much more tightly and are therefore more robust. Typically prepared in the size range 5–50 nm, they offer more protection than conventional micelle systems do. Size and physico-chemical properties can be manipulated by varying the composition or molecular weight of the surfactant.

Lipid vesicles are basically highly ordered assemblies of one or several concentric bilayers that are formed when certain amphiphilic building blocks are dispersed in water. The commonly used vesicular systems include liposomes, niosomes, transferosomes, pharmacosomes, ISCOMS, etc. These vesicles can be formed from a diverse range of amphiphilic building blocks. Vesicular carriers are used extensively in the pharmaceutical and cosmetic industries because of their capacity for entering into and breaking down inside cells. Liposomes have the distinction of being the first engineered nanoparticles used for drug delivery. However, their affinity to fuse together in aqueous environments and release entrapped material has led to devising of measures to stabilize them or replacing them with alternative nanoparticles made from more stable materials.

A wide variety of lipids and surfactants can be used to prepare vesicular carriers [15]. The composition of the vesicles influences their physico-chemical characteristics such as size, charge, thermodynamic phase, lamellarity, and bilayer elasticity. The physicochemical characteristics have a significant effect on the behavior of the vesicles and hence on their effectiveness as a drug delivery system. Vesicular systems have been able to address the problems of drug insolubility, instability, and rapid degradation. Encapsulation of an antigen in vesicular structures can be predicted to prolong the existence of the antigen in systemic circulation, and reduce the toxicity if selective uptake can be achieved [16]. Vesicular antigen delivery vehicles reduce the cost of immunization by improved bioavailability of antigens. The antigen comprising of subunit vaccine can be entrapped into the internal aqueous compartment.

When vesicles such as liposomes and niosomes are administered into host they either disintegrate in the bloodstream or may wander in the systemic circulation until picked up, mostly by macrophages. The endothelial lining of healthy blood vessels usually prevents escape of these vesicles from the circulation. During inflammation, the endothelium becomes more permeable thus allowing extravasations of small vesicles. This leads to their rapid clearance from the blood circulation and their capture by the components of the reticulo-endothelial system [17], corresponding to the tissue distribution pattern of some pathogenic microorganisms responsible for intracellular infections. Passive site-specific antigen targeting with vesicles, as it is called, may facilitate lowering of the antigen dosage relative to the amount of the free antigen used, thereby reducing the undesirable features produced by higher doses of the antigen (cf. Anergy or Tolerance Effect). To this end, antibodies or other ligands may be covalently attached to the surface of vesicles allowing uptake of the vesicles by macrophages or dendritic cells. In this regard, grafting anti-DEC antibody on the surface of antigen-bearing vehicles can facilitate specific targeting to dendritic cells. The applications of vesicles in antigen delivery are based on physicochemical and colloidal characterization such as composition, size and loading efficiency and the stability of the carrier, as well as their biological interactions with the cells. A major interaction is lipid exchange, whereby liposomal lipids are exchanged with the lipids of various cell membranes. This depends on the mechanical stability of the bilayer and can be reduced by the addition of cholesterol (which gives rise to improving mechanical properties, such as increased stretching elastic modulus, resulting in stronger membranes and reduced permeability). The second major interaction is adsorption onto cells, which occurs when the attractive forces (electrostatic, electrodynamic, Van der Waals, hydrophobic interaction, hydrogen bonding, etc.) supersede repulsive forces (electrostatic, steric, hydration, undulation, protrusion, etc.). Adsorption onto phagocytic cells is normally followed by endocytosis, or rarely by fusion as well. Fusogenic vesicles mimic the way by which several viruses (HIV, Sendai virus) bind and merge with cell membranes at neutral pH and subsequently release their content into the cytoplasm. In the perspective of treating intracellular infections (where the pathogen resides inside host cells, mainly the macrophages), once the drug-carrying vesicle is endocytosed by the macrophage, the acidic environment of the phagolysosome ruptures the membrane and releases the drug therein. The released drug can access to the cytosol as well. The cytosolic delivery inside the pathogen-harboring macrophage significantly increases the chance of the drug interacting directly with the pathogen leading to efficient killing. Escheriosome-based vesicular carriers, the vesicles composed of *E. coli* membrane lipid are regularly used to deliver drugs, immunogens, genetic materials, and diagnostics agents to specific desired locations [18–20]. Several studies have shown that escheriosomes have been able to overcome the major problem; that is low membrane permeation of drugs to access cytosol of the cells in treating intracellular infections. Phagocytic uptake of drug-loaded vesicular delivery system from the systemic circulation provides an efficient method for cytosolic delivery of encapsulated material. In a manner similar to drug molecules, escheriosome can deliver protein-based antigens to cytosol of target cells. Once in the cytosol, the antigen is likely to be processed by proteasome machinery for the induction of cell-mediated immune response in the host.

Escheriosomes emulate biological membranes that form the ubiquitous delimiting structures that surround and compartmentalize prokaryotic cells and mitochondria or chloroplast of eukaryotic cells. Over the years, lipid vesicles have evolved successfully as vehicles for controlled delivery of encapsulated materials. *E. coli* membrane comprises a great majority of anionic phospholipids that play a pivotal role in membrane-membrane fusion [21]. In vivo administration of escheriosomes encapsulated model antigen-induced antigen-specific strong Cytotoxic T lymphocyte (CTL) responses in the immunized mice. In contrast, the antigen encapsulated in egg phosphatidyl choline- (egg PC) liposomes, in a manner similar to the antigen-Incomplete Freund's adjuvant emulsion, had limited access to the cytosolic pathway of MHC-I-dependent antigen presentation and failed to generate antigen-specific cell-mediated immune response.

Fibrin is a critical blood component responsible for hemostasis and has been used extensively as a biopolymer scaffold in tissue engineering. Fibrin can be prepared from autologous plasma, and is available as glue or as engineered microbeads. Fibrin alone or in combination with other materials has been used as a biological scaffold for stem or primary cells to regenerate adipose tissue, bone, cardiac tissue, cartilage, liver, nervous tissue, ocular tissue, skin, tendons, and ligaments. It is a versatile biopolymer, which shows a great potential in tissue regeneration and wound healing [22].

Fibrin is a biopolymer of the monomer fibrinogen. The fibrinogen molecule is composed of two sets of three polypeptide chains named Aa, Bb, and g, which are joined together by six disulfide bridges [23]. Fibrin is formed after thrombin-mediated cleavage of fibrinopeptide A from the Aa chains and fibrinopeptide B from the Bb chains [24], with subsequent conformational changes and exposure of polymerization sites. This generates the fibrin monomer that has a great tendency to self-associate and form insoluble fibrin. Further, the blood coagulation factor XIIIa is a transglutaminase that rapidly cross-links g chains in the fibrin polymer [25] by introducing intermolecular x-(g-glutamyl) lysine covalent bonds between the lysine of one g-chain and glutamine of the other [26]. This covalent cross-linking produces a stable fibrin network that is resistant to protease degradation [27]. This effect can be reinforced by introducing chemical cross-linkers such as genipin. Fibrin microbeads (FMBs) are small spherical dense beads with a diameter ranging from 50 to 250 microns. FMBs are basically consisting of highly condensed and cross-linked fibrin and produced from plasma fibrinogen obtained by fractionation [28]. The fibrinogen is mixed with thrombin, and the activated fibrin is immediately and quickly stirred in a heated oil emulsion (corn oil: isooctane, 1:1:75 °C) to yield spherical droplets that are further cross-linked into solid beads [29]. Fibrinogen denatures above 50 °C due to the instability of the D-domain, whereas factor XIIIa is much more stable and can cross-link proteins at higher temperatures. Denatured fibrinogen in the FMB is greatly haptotactic to mesenchymal-type cells, such as endothelial cells, smooth muscle cells, and fibroblasts [29]. FMBs have been used widely to isolate and grow mesenchymal stem cells from both bone marrow and blood [28, 30]. Kidney gene and cell therapy have been tested in vitro using FMBs as a three-dimensional platform, since a variety of transduced renal cells grow and differentiate in this material [30]. Further, FMBs in combination with the appropriate cell source can be used in bone regeneration and wound healing [31].

The use of fibrin for tissue engineering has been a popular field of research over the past several years. The ability of fibrin to achieve homeostasis during healing and to naturally act as a scaffold for tissue repair has resulted in a vast field of research aimed at investigating fibrin as a delivery system for cells and biomolecules in tissue engineering. Fibrin has been used as a delivery system for sustained release of embedded antibiotic [32, 33]. Senderoff et al. have investigated different forms of fibrin for sustained drug delivery [34]. Fibrin microparticles, fibrin-coated drug particulates, and fibrin sheets with entrapped drug molecules were assessed for drug release behavior. It was seen that fibrin microparticles prepared by oil emulsion, with entrapped dexamethasone sustained the release of the drug, but only for 4 h. Release kinetics of the drug from fibrin films were evaluated and showed a diffusion coefficient corresponding to near-zero-order release kinetics. Yoshida et al. evaluated the release of different anti-cancer drugs, and it was noted that sustained release can be correlated with the hydrophobicity of the drug [35]. Similarly, Woolverton et al. investigated tetracycline release, as an example of a poorly soluble drug [36]. Tetracycline was delivered within an implanted fibrin scaffold to the peritoneal wall of a mouse model. The animals were subsequently infected with 10^8colony-forming units (CFU) of *S. aureus*. A single treatment of fibrin containing 500 mg/ml tetracycline provided 100% protection against infection in mice for 7 days compared to control mice treated with fibrin only. However, it has been noted that addition of the drug to the fibrin during polymerization results in fragile scaffolds and poor retention of the drug. Therefore, researchers have used freeze-dried fibrin as a possible fabrication method for preventing spontaneous release of the drug [37]. Results exhibited sustained release of tetracycline for 12 days with no initial burst release [37], and release of total drug for 18 days [38]. Fibrin has also been used to deliver chemotherapeutic agents such as carboplatin to the retina [39, 40], sustaining delivery for up to 2 weeks. In the treatment of brain tumors, fibrin has been investigated as a delivery system for emitting radioisotopes in microspheres [41]. Results showed that fibrin adhered to the brain tissue, showing superior adherence than all other tested mucoadhesive materials, thereby preventing migration of microparticles to nearby tissues. Survival data proved the efficacy of this treatment. Recently, a tissue engineering strategy to treat bone fractures suffering infection involved the codelivery of an antibiotic system in addition to bone marrow mesenchymal stem cells via a fibrin scaffold [42]. Vancomycin alginate beads were embedded in a fibrin scaffold, to localize antibiotic exposure at the site of the defect and combat infection. Additionally, bone marrow mesenchymal stem cells were delivered in the scaffold to encourage bone regeneration. In vitro results showed that cell morphology did not change with exposure to antibiotic beads, and cells showed a tendency to proliferate more in fibrin scaffolds containing antibiotic beads. A possible reason for this enhanced proliferation was suggested to be due to the more porous fibrin scaffold resulting from inclusion of the beads, thereby facilitating cellular proliferation.

Biodegradable polymers have emerged as one of the most important polymeric systems with remarkable drug delivery potential. Although molecules that undergo bio-erosion are also classified interchangeably with biodegradation, the two differ; erosion occurs by the dissolution of chain fragments in non-cross-linked systems without chemical alterations to the molecular structure, while biodegradation occurs through the covalent bond cleavage by a chemical reaction. Both biodegradation and erosion can occur as surface or bulk process. In surface degradation the polymeric matrix is progressively removed from the surface but the polymer volume fraction remains almost unaltered. In contrast, during bulk degradation no significant changes occur in the physical size of the polymer until it is nearly completely degraded or eroded. To be biodegradable, a polymer undergoes hydrolysis, usually enzymatic, of a susceptible bond either in the backbone or in the cross-linker. Most of the biodegradable carriers rely on the cleavage of ester bond, ester derivatives like poly (lactic/glycolic acid) and poly (ε-caprolactone) or peptide bond. Other hydrolysable bonds include those of poly(anhydrides), poly(orthoesters), poly(phophoesters). Biodegradable polymers include polymers of diverse origin such as polysaccharide, protein, and synthetic polymers. Among the polysaccharide polymers alginate, dextran, hyaluronic acid, chitosan, and cellulose have been studied extensively. Gelatin, collagen, albumin, and silk fibroin are proteinacious studied in detail. Synthetic polymers investigated for drug delivery include polyphosphazene, polyurethane, polycaprolactone, polyorthoester.

Commercial alginates are extracted from brown algal species that include *Laminaria hyperborean*, *Ascophyllum nodosum*, and *Macrocystis pyrifera*. It is a linear polysaccharide containing varying amounts of 1, 4-linked β-D-mannuronic acid and α-L-gulucronic acid. The exact composition and residue sequence of alginates vary depending on the source. Due to its biocompatibility, low toxicity, non-immunogenic nature, relatively low cost, and ready gelation with divalent cations such as Ca^{2+}, it has been widely used in drug delivery and tissue engineering applications [43]. Cross-linking with various types of molecules has been carried out to control the mechanical and/or swelling properties of alginate gel. The high porosity of alginates makes it more suitable for the entrapments of cells and large molecular weight pharmaceuticals [44]. Alginate has also been studied as an injectable delivery vehicle of cells [45], proteins [46], hormones [47], and various growth factors [48].

Dextrans are a complex, high molecular weight, branched polymer of D-glucose, available in a wide range of molecular dimensions and types. Dextrans have been investigated for numerous applications, including as plasma expanders and blood substitutes in addition to their use as delivery vesicles of drugs. Dextran-based microparticles have been used for the delivery of recombinant human bone morphogenetic protein-2 (rhBMP2) [49]. Acetylated dextran microparticles are potent in vitro delivery platforms for vaccine adjuvants [50, 51], prepared composite BSA-dextran nanoparticles for the delivery of an anticancer drug doxorubicin for the treatment of murine ascites hepatoma H22 tumor-bearing mice. Collagens are a group of naturally occurring proteins found exclusively in animals, especially in the muscle and connective tissues of mammals [52].

Collagens are the main components of connective tissue, and the most abundant proteins in mammals, making up to about 25–35% of the whole body protein content [53]. Collagen gels are visco-elastic thereby semisolid, which facilitates their administration by parenteral route and development of biocompatible drug delivery matrices. They can even be induced to flow under stress (e.g., extrusion from a syringe) [54–57]. In addition, they exhibit good cell and tissue compatibility [54, 58, 59] and thus do not interfere with normal body functions. When injected into the site of interest, collagen matrices release the entrapped pharmaceuticals in their surroundings in a controlled manner [60]. The available forms of injectable collagen gels include suspensions of collagen fibers [54, 56] and non-fibrillar, viscous aqueous solutions [57]. Small molecular weight drugs and therapeutic proteins have also been used with the fibrillar suspensions or viscous collagen solutions [60]. The collagen networks readily retain various cells by physical entrapment [60] and have also been employed as scaffolds in tissue engineering, delivery matrices for cells, and gene therapy [60].

Albumin is the most abundant protein in blood plasma of higher animals and constitutes up to 50% of total mass of plasma. Albumin plays an important role in binding and transport of both endogenous and exogenous substances, including those that are toxic in unbound state. Albumin has the ability to bind to a variety of molecules including fatty acids and a variety of drugs [61] and serves as a circulating depot of several compounds [62]. Nearly all of human body cells degrade albumin making the protein a highly suitable for biomedical applications [63]. Serum albumin can be easily processed into a variety of forms including microsphere, membranes, nanofibers, nanospheres [64]. Human serum albumin microspheres have potential as a slow release drug delivery system. They offer advantages over other types of polymeric microspheres in being non-antigenic, readily metabolizable with potential to bind a variety of drugs in a relatively nonspecific fashion. Albumin conjugated with heparin was used in the preparation of microsphere for some interesting drug delivery applications. Adriamycin-loaded albumin-heparin conjugate microspheres (AHCMS) show an increased anti-tumor efficacy in L1210 tumor-bearing mouse and the CC531 tumor-bearing rat model and reduce its acute toxicity.

A key factor in the design of injectable protein/drug delivery systems is the choice of an appropriate biodegradable polymer. Poly(lactic co-glycolic acid) (PLGA) is one of the polyesters largely used as a drug delivery system because of availability of toxicological and chemical data, biocompatibility/histocompatibility, predictable biodegradation kinetics, ease of fabrication, versatility in properties, chemical integrity, commercial availability, variety in copolymers ratios and molecular weights, lastly and most important is its regulatory approval. Microsphere, composed of chemicals like biodegradable polymer polyvinyl alcohol (PVA) and PLGA, is one of the primary candidates that can be used as a carrier for sustained release of drugs and antigens administered either by oral or parenteral routes [65, 66]. These polymers have demonstrated excellent tissue compatibility. Moreover, the restorable synthetic polymers are nontoxic and have already been used for other biochemical applications including drug delivery [67]. PVA, obtained from poly (vinyl acetate) by alcoholysis, hydrolysis, or aminolysis [68], is useful to deliver proteins in a controlled manner [69]. The PVA is also used to increase the loading content of water-soluble drug molecules into porous PLGA microcapsules [70], as well as for long-term delivery of proteins [71]. DL-PLGA induces only a minimal inflammatory response and biodegrades through the hydrolysis of its ester linkages to yield biocompatible lactic and glycolic acids. The parameters such as co-polymer ratios, different crystallinities, glass transition temperature, and hydrophilicity affect biodegradation profile of PLGA microspheres. Homogeneous degradation involves bulk erosion that is the case in aliphatic polyesters, erosion occurs throughout the device and rate of water penetration is greater than its conversion to water-soluble fragments. Initially, there is random cleavage of hydrogen bonds due to hydration followed by cleavage of covalent bonds. The molecular weight decreases due to continuous cleavage and solubilization of low molecular weight components and complete absorption. The carrier in such situations retains its original shape and mass until significant degradation has occurred (~90%). At a given time point, it attains critical molecular weight that ultimately results in solubilization and mass loss. The poly-lactic acid (PLA) and PLGA chains are cleaved to monomeric acids, i.e., lactic and glycolic acids that are eliminated from the body through Kreb's cycle as CO_2 and water. Role of enzymatic involvement in biodegradation is not clear. It varies depending upon other properties that include molecular weight of the polymer, sequencing and cross-linking within the polymer backbone, surface area of the device, porosity of the matrix, hydrophobicity of matrix and reactive groups present. A ratio of 50/50 poly(DL-lactide-co-glycolide) degrades in approximately 1–2 months, 75/25 in 4–5 months, and 85/15 in 5–6 months [72]. To formulate microspheres from the biodegradable polymer matrix, it is essential to select an encapsulation process, which fulfills the requirements of an ideal controlled release system. The attributes of the encapsulating material are optimal drug loading, high yield of microspheres, stability of the encapsulated drug, batch uniformity, inter-batch reproducibility, adjustable release profiles, low burst effect, free-flowing attributes of formed microspheres. The encapsulation efficiency of the drug molecule should be high. The particles should be formulated in such a way that minimum of the encapsulated drug is released during the burst phase. This will help in extending the release of the core drug for a longer period of time. The encapsulation method used should always produce free-flowing microspheres that do not aggregate. As with all parenteral products, microspheres need to be sterile. This can be ensured by a terminal sterilization step or through aseptic processing. Further, in relation to safety requirements, the excipients and various solvents used in the processing should either be nontoxic or removed from the final product.

The release of active components from the microspheres is dependent both on diffusion through the polymer matrix and on polymer degradation. If during the desired release time, polymer degradation is considerable, then the release rate may be unpredictable and erratic due to breakdown of microspheres. However, the release of encapsulated material depends on the fact that whether microspheres are covered by one or several core material so that release of active component is dependent on its diffusivity through the polymer barrier, solubility of core in bulk phase, size of drug/antigen molecule and distribution of core throughout the matrix, etc. In general, chemical nature of polymer plays a major role in release process. Route of administration of injectable microspheres may also alter the duration of release. Release from PLA and PLGA is dependent on both diffusion and polymer degradation [73]. The possible mechanisms of drug release include: (1) initial release from microsphere surface; (2) release through the pores dependent on spheres structure; (3) diffusion through the intact polymer barrier that is dependent on intrinsic polymer properties and core solubility; (4) diffusion through a water-swollen barrier dependent on polymer hydrophilicity, which in turn depends on polymer molecular weight; (5) polymer erosion and bulk degradation, release affected by the rate of erosion and hydrolysis of polymer chains, leading to pore formation in matrix. All the above-specified mechanisms might together play a crucial role in the release process. Nature of core also influences release kinetics either by increasing polymer degradation or by physically binding with the polymer chain. Drug–polymer interaction leads to decreased release. Additives such as plasticizers decrease Tg (glass transition temperature) which leads to decreased diffusion rates.

Microspheres are capable of forming protein depots that can facilitate release of core protein at the injection site. Interestingly, microsphere size is an important design parameter. Small particles, with sizes smaller than 10 μm, can be directly taken up to macrophages by phagocytosis, whereas larger microspheres (greater than 10 μm) need to undergo biodegradation before phagocytosis can occur. In this case, microspheres are covered by one or several layers of macrophages as a consequence of wound-healing response to injected particles. Consequently, degradation, release, location, and presentation of antigen released from microspheres (size larger than 10 μm) are to be different from smaller ones. Upon administration of the microspheres, a foreign-body response occurs, resulting in an acute initial inflammation. This initial inflammation is followed by the infiltration of small foreign-body giant cells and neutrophils [74]. The immune cells can take up the released protein and produce an immune response. However, if protein is recognized as a self-protein (e.g., homologous), the probability of an immune response by these cells is reduced. It is therefore always essential to release the protein in native conformation. The release of denatured protein from the microspheres may result in an unwanted immune response [75].

1.3 Limitations of the Existing Antifungal Treatment Options

Currently available antifungal drugs have limitations such as toxicity, availability, spectrum of adverse activity in the host. Moreover, when used for long periods of time, they also develop a problem of resistance [76]. Considering these limitations, it is tempting to rely more on body's own defense measures and take help of agents just to supplement immune strategies that ensue in elimination of fungal pathogens. It is important to develop new strategies involving antifungal vaccines in order to reduce the mortality. The idea of an efficient fungal vaccine is to generate immune responses that will lead to immunological memory and protection against a recurrent exposure to fungi and their conidia/spores. Immuno-competency is often required for the generation of immunity against an infectious disease. So, current research is converging on development of vaccines that can be used during immunodeficiency or immediately prior to the development of a severe immunodeficiency among the immune-compromised patients.

Polyene resistance has emerged as a challenge in the field because these drugs are the most effective available antifungals till date. It seems that naturally resistant strains produce modified sterols that bind these drugs with lower affinity. The greater the polyene sterol affinity, the greater is the rate of fungal membrane damages. According to a hypothesis resistance arises due to changes, either quantitative or qualitative, in the sterol content of the cells. Thus, resistant cells with altered sterol content should bind smaller amounts of polyenes than do susceptible cells. Unfortunately, occasionally even the liposomal formulation of antibiotics fails to eliminate less susceptible strains of *Candida* pathogens. Since these fungal infections are restricted mainly to the immunodebilitant subjects, one can speculate that a formulation of Amp B with altered pharmacokinetic properties in combination with some immuno-modulator can synergistically subdue drug-resistant fungal infections.

1.4 Immunomodulation to Rejuvenate Fungal Therapy

Already vexatious with the availability of limited number of antifungal agents, the recent emergence of drug-resistant candidiasis infections against the gold standard Amp B leaves little choice but to opt either for its appropriate replacement by some potent substitute. In this regard, relying on altogether different prophylactic strategy by developing vaccines against the deadly disease could be an effective strategy. Successful efforts were made to evaluate the fully biocompatible and biodegradable delivery system made up of fibrin microsphere for sustained delivery of antifungal drugs/

immunomodulators for the efficient elimination of the fungal pathogens from systemic circulation. Candida cytosolic proteins with immunogenic potential when entrapped in the fibrin network directly or after their encapsulation in appropriate liposome (co-entrapment of antigen-bearing liposomes in fibrin beads to give rise to a dual coated delivery system). The function of the immune system becomes more pertinent in case of opportunistic fungal pathogens that target immunodebilitant subjects mainly. The pathogens that inflict such subjects do not respond to conventional chemotherapy presumably because of collapsing physiological conditions as well as fragile immune system of the host. Concomitant delivery of anti-fungal agents and immunomodulators, using delivery systems that facilitate specific targeting to the pathogen harboring immune cells (macrophages and neutrophils), is expected therefore to be beneficial in eliminating the pathogens from the immunocompromised host. Earlier, our group attempted the development of sustained delivery system using a combination of immunomodulators tuftsin/picroliv along with antifungal drugs and incorporating them in fully physiological and biodegradable fibrin microspheres. A parallel study involving incorporation of *C. albicans* immunogenic proteins (cytosolic/membrane proteins) in fibrin microspheres as candidate vaccine was also undertaken. Both free and liposome-encapsulated antigens were incorporated in the fibrin microspheres and evaluated for its potential to impart protection against experimental murine candidiasis.

Macrophages of the reticuloendothelial system (RES) are capable of rapid recognition and uptake of particulate matter. Such interactions provide a rational approach for specific targeting of nanocarriers to macrophage [9]. Intracellular pathogens, such as *Cryptococcus neoformans*, *Candida spp.*, *Toxoplasma gondii*, *Leishmania spp.*, *Mycobacterium tuberculosis*, and *Listeria monocytogenes*, reside in the lysosome and/or cytoplasm of the host macrophages. Nanoparticulate vehicles containing encapsulated antimicrobial agents passively targeted to such infected macrophages is a favorable strategy for combating intracellular microbes [9, 12, 77, 78]. The endocytic pathway of the macrophage directs drug-loaded nanoparticles to lysosome where pathogens reside. Lysosomal enzymes then degrade the carrier, releasing the drug into the phagosome-lysosome compartment itself or into the cytoplasm of the target cells either by diffusion or by specific transporters, depending on the physicochemical nature of the drug molecule. This strategy has been successfully applied in FDA-approved lipid-based amphotericin B formulations (100–200 nm) for human use, and is recommended for the treatment of visceral leishmaniasis or confirmed infections caused by specific fungal species [12, 77]. This mode of targeting has significantly reduced the required clinically effective quantity of Amp-B for treatment, achieving therapeutic drug concentrations in the infected macrophages. Other beneficial effects include significant reduction in nephrotoxicity, a common side effect associated with Amp-B administration, and pro-inflammatory cytokine release [79]. For example, intravenous injection of tuftsin-bearing liposomes to infected animals has not only resulted in the delivery of liposome-encapsulated drugs to the macrophage phagolysosomes, but also in the nonspecific stimulation of liver and spleen macrophage functions against parasitic, fungal, and bacterial infections [78]. The latter effect is due to the binding of tuftsin to its receptor, which further incites macrophage antimicrobial responses. Intracellular abode of these pathogens to avoid antibody onslaughts and to escape neutralizing agents unable to enter cells combined with apparent lack of vaccines capable of obliterating these pathogens by CTL response persuaded us to develop alternative prophylactic strategies.

Among various immunomodulators, which can modulate immune system nonspecifically, **tuftsin** a tetrapeptide from IgG (289–292 residue of the Fc region) has been found to be effective against cancer as well as infectious diseases. Tuftsin is a natural killer activator of macrophages/monocytes that can easily be grafted onto the surface of liposomes [80]. It is released physiologically as the free peptide fragment after enzymatic cleavage and has been used extensively in a liposomized form both for chemotherapy, prophylaxis and also as an immunoadjuvant. Tuftsin provokes monocytes/macrophages for their natural killer activity against microbes. It has been shown that immunization of animals with Tuft-lip-Ag is effective in increasing antigen-specific antibody titer, T cell proliferation and switching of IgG isotyping to lgG2a.

Grafting of immuno-modulator tuftsin on the surface of nystatin liposomes increases the efficacy of the drug against *C. albicans* isolate, less susceptible to polyenes, upon causing infection in the neutropenic mice. The observed anti-candidal activity of the liposomal drug formulations is likely to be mediated via tuftsin receptors, which have been reported to be present on macrophages, monocytes, granulocytes, etc., the key components of host defense mechanisms. It can be speculated that concomitant delivery of liposomized anti-fungal agents along with an immunomodulator to the pathogen harboring immune cells will not only help in specific targeting but also activate these cells for nonspecific elimination of the pathogens from the body. Upon administration into the host, the liposomes are avidly taken up by macrophages, which subsequently act as secondary depot and help in carrying the active drug molecules to the site of infection. The components of the *C. albicans* cell wall, particularly mannoproteins, have been reported to exert immuno-suppression both in vivo and in vitro, presumably by inhibiting NO production by macrophages which in turn results in the depletion of IL-12. Tuftsin stimulates IL-1 production by human mononuclear cells, which play predominant role in the induction of NO secretion by peritoneal macrophages. In addition, it also helps in maturation and clonal expansion of B-cells so that residual primed B cells respond rapidly to *C. albicans* infection under the effect of tuftsin.

The success of tuftsin-bearing liposomes against both drug-sensitive and drug-resistant fungal infections may be explained on the premise that antifungal activity of amphotericin B could be augmented in the presence of an immuno-modulator, which has the ability to stimulate immune system of the host. Besides, tuftsin-bearing liposomes are specifically recognized by macrophages and neutrophils, and may help in targeting of the drug to these cells, which subsequently act as the secondary depot for the drug. These cells can wander to locate the site of infection (chemotaxis) and help in selective targeting of the antifungal agent. Earlier, it has been demonstrated that prophylactic treatment with muramyl dipeptide resulted in the significant enhancement of antifungal activity of the Amp B.

Immunomodulators such as **Protein A** from *Staphylococcus aureus* (SpA) and **lipopolysaccharide** (LPS) from *E. coli* have been used to rejuvenate the suppressed immune response. When these immunomodulators were used with antigen carrier systems, they stimulate both arms of immune system, i.e., humoral as well as cell-mediated responses presumably by improving uptake of antigen by antigen-presenting cells (APCs) such as macrophages.

Immunotherapy offers a formidable approach to treat fungal infections as it involves stimulation of immune function. In immune-compromised patients, the management of fungal infections becomes problematic due to non-effectiveness of antifungal therapy in such subjects. The therapy involves replacement immunotherapy, which is designed to correct the underlying immunological defects that predispose people to fungal diseases. While augmentative therapy enhances immune function against the pathogens, immune therapy can either be specific or nonspecific. Cytokines, growth factors, and leukocytes can enhance host defense against a range of pathogens and thus constitute nonspecific immunotherapy. In contrast, the administration of immunoglobulins is specific immunotherapy that, similar to antimicrobial therapy, is directed specifically toward the pathogen.

Chloroquine is an anti-malarial drug that has been reported to modulate pH of intracellular compartments of macrophage and thus play important role in survival of pathogens that seek intracellular abode inside them. Chloroquine limits the availability of iron inside the macrophages and promotes killing of *Histoplasma capsulatum*. We have shown chloroquine-mediated elimination of fungal pathogens earlier for example, in case of *C. neoformans*, chloroquine inhibits the intracellular growth by raising phagolysosomal pH and thus affects pathogen survival [81].

GM-CSF promotes differentiation and proliferation of mononuclear cells as well as neutrophils. GM-CSF is used to promote bone marrow recovery after immuno-suppression by chemotherapy [82]. GM-CSF may be effective in the prevention of fungal infections in patients with neutropenia due to chemotherapy for neoplastic diseases and organ transplantation.

IFN-γ is a potent activator of macrophage function that can enhance the activity of murine macrophages against a variety of fungal pathogens both in vitro and in vivo. Antifungal agents show synergy with IFN-γ against *Candida* species, *A. fumigatus* and *C. neoformans.* The rationale for the use of IL-12 as therapy for fungal infections can be correlated with Thl-type cellular responses that seem to be essential for protection against fungal pathogens. With the identification of prophylactically and therapeutically important immunomodulators, it is now possible to alter or manipulate the immune system in favor of the host.

The use of immunomodulators in combination of chemotherapy opens new vistas in treatment of various infectious diseases of fungal and bacterial origin. Moreover, such a strategy would be of great importance in immuno-compromised patients who usually succumb to pathogen assault because of impaired physiological activities.

Other than tuftsin, immuno-modulator **SpA** has been demonstrated to impart prophylactic and therapeutic roles against murine candidiasis. The immuno-modulatory role of SpA against fungal infection is also supposed to be mediated through the production of IFN-γ and related type I cytokines that activate macrophages. The treatment of macrophages with SpA also led to an increased production of nitric oxide and IFN-γ. Besides, it has also been shown to enhance the counts of both polymorphonuclear and mononuclear cells, and helps in the generation of superoxide radicals in both resting and activated neutrophils. During infection with HIV and also in cancer, SpA increases the number of both CD4+ and CD34+ cells and may help in the revival of the immune system in these patients, who are the major targets of fungal pathogens.

During the early phase of host response lipopolysaccharide (**LPS**) isolated from the cell wall of *E. coli* induces a Thl-like response with abundant IFN-γ and tumor necrosis factor alpha (TNF-α) primarily by monocytes and macrophages.

1.5 Immunity to Fungal Infections

The relative contribution of humoral and cellular immunity to host defense against fungal infections has remained a controversial issue. It is considered that cell-mediated immunity (CMI) is the main mode of defense, but certain types of antibody response have also been reported to be protective [83]. Several earlier reports suggest that antibody-mediated immune response can protect the host against fungal infection [84].

In general, the primary protective defense mechanism against invasive fungal infection involves a vigorous Th1 response to fungal antigens. The susceptible hosts who are at risk of invasive fungal infection generally possess a compromised immunity due to a number of factors, including corticosteroid therapy, undergoing cancer chemotherapy or inflicted with HIV. Practically, all medically important fungi carry an impressive line-up of macromolecules with immuno-modulatory functions on their cell surfaces that play significant roles in the fungus-host interaction and immunity. However, CMI mediated by T lymphocytes and nonspecific cellular immunity mediated by macrophages, neutrophils, and natural killer cells account to provide the main defenses against fungi [85].

The cytokine milieu produced by the components of the innate immune system results in the differentiation of CD4+ T-cells toward the Th1 or Th17 subtypes. When activated, these T-cell subtypes can produce pro-inflammatory cytokines like interferon gamma (IFN-γ), tumor necrosis factor alpha, interleukin-6 (IL-6), IL-22, etc. [86]. The cytokines may also help in recruitment of neutrophils and help control systemic fungal diseases [87, 88]. On the other hand, the fungal pathogen-specific antibodies may help in the prevention of adherence, toxin neutralization, antibodyopsonization, and antibody-dependent cellular cytotoxicity [84].

It can be concluded that both the components of immune system work in coordination, and that very diverse components can jointly contribute to the defense of the host. Some parts contribute more than others under certain circumstances, but they are all important for the overall protection against infection.

1.6 Vaccine Development Against Opportunistic Fungal Pathogens

Recent times are witnessing rise of dangerous systemic fungal infections, especially related to immunocompromised patients, premature infants, cancer patients, and those with invasive treatments for long periods in hospital settings, which are known as high-risk groups [89]. Treatments for critical diseases like cancer improve patient's survival rates, but can also affect natural barriers of the body or even significantly influence the competence of the immune system of the individual, contributing to a raised vulnerability to infections caused by fungi [90]. With the development of new treatments for diseases such as cancer and the acquired immune deficiency syndrome pandemic, the number of immunosuppressed patients has risen and, as a consequence, also the number of invasive fungal infections has increased [91]. This is posing threat in the form of new challenges such as emergence of newer type of diseases including opportunistic fungal infections.

The frequency of life-threatening fungal infections has increased dramatically, particularly among cancer, diabetic, and immunocompromised patients [92–95]. On one hand, the observed upsurge could be attributed to the advancement in the field of medical sciences that made possible improved recognition and diagnosis of fungal infections. Besides prolonged survival of patients with defects in their defense mechanisms, more invasive surgical procedures, the use of prosthetic devices and indwelling catheters, increased administration of parenteral nutrition, development of resistance fungal strains to currently available antifungal drugs, the increase in the number of patients contracting AIDS, and the use of peritoneal dialysis and hemodialysis are some of the potential opportunities offered to microbes for their establishment leading to full blown disease. In these patients invasive fungal infections accounted for as many as 30% of deaths. Although the occurrence of fungal drug resistance is far below in comparison to antibacterial agents, historical precedence warns that it is only a matter of time before selective pressures will lead to population shifts resulting in more widespread resistance. Moreover, overuse and inappropriate prescription of antifungal agents has contributed significantly to the situation when pathogens do not respond to the chemotherapy. The emergence of fungi as clinically important pathogens has been well documented, although their role in pathogenesis of human infection has only recently been appreciated [96, 97]. Perhaps more worrisome predicament is the increased occurrence of drug-resistant *Candida* spp. than their emergence as a pathogen [98–100]. There is a strong suggestion that invasive fungal infections have become more common in recent years, with a nearly 500% increase in the incidence of bloodstream infection with *Candida* spp. since the 1980s. Most systemic fungal infections are caused by *Candida* spp., followed by *Aspergillus* and *Cryptococcus* spp. Infections due to *Candida* species are the fourth most important cause of nosocomial bloodstream infection. Systemic fungal infections cause ~25% of infection-related deaths in leukemics. Serious fungal infections may cause 5–10% of deaths in those undergoing lung, pancreas, or liver transplantation. Acquired fungal sepsis occurs in up to 13% of very low birth weight infants. Some of the predisposing factors to the establishment of fungal pathogens in host include: neutropenia, T cell dysfunction, immunosuppression, B cell dysfunction, organ transplantation, AIDS, diabetes, cytotoxic chemotherapy, high dose corticosteroids, long-term antibiotic therapy (broad spectrum), prolonged hospitalization, and burn.

In general, host is continually exposed to many species of fungi that survive at body temperature and establish varying interactions—from symbiotic to pathogenic. The pathogens like *Candida* spp. are well known for their commensal interactions. Others, however, are mostly environmental fungi that can become opportunistic pathogens in immuno compromised hosts, like *C. neoformans* [101], *Aspergillus fumigatus* [102], *Blastomyces dermatitidis* [103], and *Histoplasma capsulatum*. It has been observed that some fungal pathogens may act as primary pathogens that can infect immune-competent individuals as well (many of dimorphic fungi, for instance). These microorganisms infect the host whose immune system fails to control invading spores or conidia. From there, infection progresses to cause an invasive mycosis with high mortality rates [104].

1.6.1 *Candida spp.*

In the last two decades *Candida* spp. has emerged as a major human pathogen. *Candida albicans* is an opportunistic pathogen, which causes life-threatening disease in immune-compromised mammalian hosts [105]. *C. albicans* has been found to account for ~52–63% of all nosocomial fungal infections [100]. It has been proposed that this occurrence may result from selective pressure induced by the increased use of antifungal agents. In 1991, Banerjee and colleagues reported rates of candidemia ranging from 0.28 to 0.61 cases in every 1000 discharges in a hospital participating in the National Nosocomial Infection Surveillance (NNIS) system [96]. This represented a fivefold increase in the detection rate of candidemia in NNIS members between 1980 and 1989 [96]. The upward trend has continued into the 1990s [97]. Among NNIS system centers, *Candida* species have been reported to be the sixth most commonly isolated pathogen and the fourth most prevalent bloodstream pathogen [96]. Factors that are responsible for the exponential rise in the isolation of the *Candida* species include the emergence of AIDS, increased patient exposure to broad spectrum antibiotics resulting in alterations in normal host flora, increasing number of patients with neutropenia, in consequence to cancer treatment and transplantation procedures, and expanded use of intravascular catheter devices. As medical technology progresses, it is likely that we will see the increased number of opportunistic infections in critically ill patients. Consequently, the infection by *Candida* species will probably become even more predominant in the future.

Common Types of C. albicans Infections

(a) **Oropharyngeal Candidiasis(Oral thrush):** This is the most common infection of the mouth that involves buccal mucous membranes, most commonly in infants and AIDS patients. It appears in the form of white adherent patches with minimal erosion of the membrane.

(b) **Vaginal candidiasis (Vulvovaginitis):** It resembles with thrush in feature except that irritation, intense itching, and discharge accompany it. The establishment of vaginal candidiasis is facilitated by loss of the normal bacterial flora (because of antibiotic therapy). The bacteria maintain a low (acid) pH in the vagina that does not allow growth of *C. albicans*, and also not allow it to form pseudo-hyphae that facilitates establishment of infection. Skin infection occurs mostly in moist, warm parts of the body, i.e., axilla, inframammary folds, groin, or inframammary folds. Obesity and diabetes are predisposing conditions for topical fungal infections.

(c) **Chronic mucocutaneous candidiasis:** Chronic mucocutaneous candidiasis (CMC) is a primary immunodeficiency disease presenting with debilitating, persistent, and refractory infections with the opportunistic yeast *C. albicans* [106]. Infections vary from mild to lethal, are characteristically localized to the skin, mucous membranes, and/or nails, and as a rule do not usually progress to disseminated disease or sepsis [107]. The underlying immune defect is poorly understood, although it has been appreciated that mucocutaneous infections with candida other than CMC frequently accompany impairment of T-cell-mediated immunity (HIV, Di George syndrome, etc.) [107].

(d) **Secondary infections:** Fungemia (presence of fungal pathogens in blood) is very common in immuno-suppressed individuals. The infection is not localized to a particular site or organ but distributed in whole body including systemic blood circulation.

C. albicans is a ubiquitous fungal organism that often colonizes the skin and the mucosal surfaces of normal individuals, without causing disease. However, when the normal host defense mechanisms are impaired, *C. albicans* can become a pathogen. First, CMI has consistently been shown to mediate protection against many fungi as demonstrated by adoptive lymphocyte transfer studies, enhanced susceptibility for hosts with CMI deficiencies and the funding that granulomatous inflammation in often essential for control of infection in tissue. Second, humoral immunity has been difficult to demonstrate by either transferring immune sera or correlating antibody titers with protection. Although the notion suggesting that antibody might have a role in protection was controversial because of inconsistent results. CMI remains the primary defense mechanism against fungal infections; however, specific antibodies still play crucial role in complete eradication of intracellular fungal pathogens. The innate immune system not only specifically recognizes various classes of microorganisms, it also initiates and modulates the subsequent adaptive responses that are delivered by T cells and B cells through their interactions with APC. Recognition of an invading pathogen and activating the host response are accomplished by pattern recognition receptors (PRRs), which recognize conserved microbial chemical signatures called pathogen-associated molecular patterns (PAMPs). The cells of the innate immune system recognize elements of both the skeletal and matrix components of the *C. albicans* cell wall. Owing to the localization of mannoproteins and mannans in the outermost part of the cell wall, mannan detection would be expected to be one of the first steps in the recognition of *C. albicans* by the host innate immune system. Pattern recognition receptors (PRRs) enable the innate immune system not only to recognize specific PAMPs, but also to specifically modulate the response that follows.

In addition, by inducing specific cytokine profiles, PRRs bring a certain degree of specificity to the innate response. Phagocytosis of *C. albicans* is mediated by the concerted action of several opsonic and non-opsonic receptors. Complement binding and activation is mediated by the alternative pathway, and complement activation is mainly important for the chemotaxis and opsonization of *C. albicans*. TLRs do not mediate fungal uptake, but they might be involved in directing the subsequent maturation of the phagosome and presentation of antigens. Following uptake, killing of *C. albicans* occurs through both oxidative and nonoxidative mechanisms. Dectin 1 receptor induces the respiratory burst in response to fungi, an activity that can be enhanced by TLR signaling. The respiratory burst is an essential antifungal effector mechanism that results in the production of toxic oxidants and in the activation of granule proteases that can kill *C. albicans*. Dectin 1 induces the production of numerous cytokines and chemokines in response to fungi, including TNF-α, macrophage inflammatory protein 2 (MIP2), macrophage inflammatory protein 1α (MIP1α), granulocyte–macrophage colony-stimulating factor (GM-CSF), granulocyte colony-stimulating factor (G-CSF), IL-10, IL-2, IL-1α, IL-1β, IL-23, and IL-6. Upon recognition of microbial structures, TLRs activate either the NF-κB or MAPK pathway, which lead to the stimulation of pro-inflammatory cytokine production. Recent evidence suggests that the various surface components of the fungus engage different TLRs, for instance TLR4 and TLR2, which protects fungus and results in disease enhancement.

The generation of Abs directed against the virulence fungus traits and capable to tip the protective enhancer balance toward the former is likely to be a convincing response by the immune system against *Candida* spp. There is ample evidence that some *Candida*-specific Abs can do this job by neutralizing the virulent factors and thereby suppress fungus-aggressive potential. In their study, Casanova et al. showed that Fab fragments of a MAb specific for a hyphal cell wall moiety inhibited germ tube formation. Researchers have demonstrated the inhibition of *C. albicans* adherence to polystyrene by two MAbs directed against cell wall antigens of *C. albicans* [108]. Ponton's group has demonstrated the capacity of a MAb directed to a stress mannoprotein of *C. albicans* to exert three different activities (inhibition of adhesion, inhibition of germination, and direct killing) against the fungus and induce protection. There is clear experimental proof that some kind of Abs may indeed be therapeutic, and suggests that Abs play a role under natural course of infection; however, their effect may be concealed by the excess of irrelevant if not disease-enhancing Abs. A strong body of evidence has suggested the protective role of some antibodies in experimental animals. Opsonization and complement deposition are most important for effective protection, in both active and passive vaccination models. However, these antibodies require the presence of cellular effectors, to finally exert their activity, which can be a limiting factor especially in case of immunocompromised patients. Some other antibodies have also been generated following vaccination which work by inhibiting some form of toxicity and enzyme activity. Few highly relevant antibodies can counteract their cognate adhesins, which is a virulent trait of several fungi.

The pathogenic dichotomy of disseminated and mucocutaneous form of candidiasis has led to a very simple immunological explanation. For the prevention of mucocutaneous candidiasis, T cell immunity is required, while neutrophil function is necessary for the prevention of disseminated disease. These observations were made on the basis of the studies on patients with CMC [109, 110]. The observation shows that neutrophil functioning is needed for the prevention of disseminated disease and T cell immunity is essential for the protection against mucocutaneous candidiasis. These studies were limited, however, in patients with rare anomaly of thymic aplasia that exhausts and washes out all T cell population but led to the prediction that CMC could be induced in mice with congenital thymic aplasia (e.g., nu/nu mutant mice). The mice, however, not only resisted attempts to induce mucosal disease, but some even exhibited enhanced resistance to disseminated candidiasis [111, 112]. Apparently T cells are responsible for host defense against mucosal candidiasis but bouts of the vaginal candidiasis apparent in women with normal thymic functions suggest the involvement of non-T-cell factors [113]. Unfortunately, mucosal candidiasis models with any level of severity are not very satisfactory and this complicates attempts to sort out immunological defects that are subtler than those of patients with CMC. The story is further complicated by experimental studies in mice that demonstrate that Thl-dependent cell-mediated immunity is critical to host defense against disseminated candidiasis [114–116]. Mice like humans are highly susceptible to life-threatening disease when rendered neutropenic (Martino et al., 1989). The host defense against hematogenously disseminated candidiasis is thus quite intricate and incumbent upon a number of diverse factors [117–121].

Current antifungal treatment for candidiasis comprises a limited armamentarium mainly of a small number of strategies relying on the differences between the eukaryotic fungal and mammalian cells. The last two decades have however witnessed the emergence of several effective strategies in the treatment of fungal infections. These include use of amphotericin B formulations [122], which target membrane ergosterol and create membrane-spanning channels, several azole derivatives with a broad spectrum of diverse activities such as fluconazole, itraconazole, voriconazole, posaconazole, and allylamines (terbinafine) which target enzymatic synthesis of ergosterol [123–125], the cell wall inhibitors echinocandins that include caspofungin, micafungin, which interfere with the synthesis of the cell wall polysaccharide, p-1, 3-glucan and flucytosine, an anti-metabolite of DNA and RNA synthesis [126]. Unfortunately, success rates for many mycoses remain unacceptably low and drug therapy against candidiasis is often limited by issues like high cost, toxicity, and resistance of the fungus to the drugs [127]. Invasive candidiasis is often fatal because of the diagnostic challenges [117], drug resistance [128, 129], and/or a poor immunologic status [130]. Patients with mucocutaneous disease may either not respond to counter antifungals [131] or develop recurrent disease as noted above. Prevention of candidiasis is more manageable, especially with patients undergoing invasive medical procedures that place them at high risk of developing the disease. It is now a common practice to give such patients antifungal treatment to accomplish a reduction of normal *C. albicans* flora [132]. The importance of preventing certain forms of candidiasis was further recognized when weekly fluconazole therapy was successful in reducing the incidence of recurring vulvovaginal candidiasis in women.

The concept of fungal vaccination as discussed above for humans is sound and apparently feasible but has not attracted remarkable attention in the past because of the relatively low incidence of the infections and the limited geographic distribution of several fungi as compared to many viral and bacterial diseases. However, the advent of AIDS and the increasing use of potent immunosuppressive therapies to combat autoimmune diseases, malignancies, and transplantation rejection have reenergized interest in the search for effective vaccines against clinically important fungi. Fungal diseases are no longer merely considered mysterious infections but recognized as important causes of morbidity and mortality. Ideally, a vaccine should induce a long-term adaptive immune response and avert the invasion or multiplication of its target pathogen without causing significant adverse effect to the host [133]. The efficacy of the immuno-protection invoked by a vaccine depends on the nature of the infecting microbe and the host's immuno-competence. The aspect of immuno-protection is a major concern when one considers the range of candidal infections (i.e., mucocutaneous to disseminated) in humans that necessitate both innate and adaptive immunity for effective protection [134]. Unfortunately in case of the immunocompromised patients who are most vulnerable to mucocutaneous and disseminated candidiasis, induction of active immunity is precluded. Passive immunity therefore appears the most beneficial form of immunotherapy in such patients as it provides immediate protection to the individual, albeit temporarily. On the contrary, active immunization benefits mostly those peoples who are immunocompetent but are highly vulnerable to candidiasis. Women are the major at-risk population for candidiasis and they are the best target subjects for vaccination. The cells of immune system involved in providing protection against candidal vaginitis, particularly recurrent vulvovaginitis, have not yet been identified. However, an effective immunoprophylactic vaccine could potentially prevent the occurrence of vulvovaginal candidiasis, as well as the transfer and subsequent colonization of *Candida* species to new-born infants [134]. Others who should benefit from active immunization are diabetics, denture wearers, patients with predisposing iatrogenic factors (indwelling catheters, corticosteroid treatment, broad-spectrum, or multiple narrow-spectrum antimicrobial chemotherapy) and hospital workers (i.e., nosocomial-derived infections) [135]. Irrespective of whether immuno-protection against *Candida* is mediated by active or passive immunity, availability of an effective immuno-protective agent is the need of the hour in view of the proliferation of the "at-risk" population. Vaccine development against any infectious disease is highly challenging and necessitates both scientific and practical considerations prior to taking up the endeavor [136–138]. Therefore, following is the rationale for initial considerations.

Strong arguments exist in favor of vaccine development against *Candida* spp. These include: (1) the disease causes sufficient morbidity and/or mortality to be considered a significant public health problem, (2) currently available disease treatment and prevention measures are inadequate, (3) the normal history of the disease indicates that specific acquired immunity can either prevent or significantly reduce the disease severity, (4) the etiology of the disease is limited to one or a small number of closely related agents, all or most of which can be affected by an appropriate vaccine formulation.

Understanding of the mechanisms of protection against hematogenously disseminated candidiasis continues to be limited, but new and useful information is surfacing. From clinical observations, it is clear that neutropenia is a significant risk factor [125, 139, 140] and experimental studies on animal models of disseminated candidiasis support this conclusion [125, 130, 131]. Whereas T cell deficiency or dysfunction is not an obvious risk factor in humans [141], animal models of disseminated disease suggest that T-cell-dependent cell-mediated immunity contributes remarkably toward host defense against this form of candidiasis [142]. Although the results obtained from mouse models may help in the understanding of the protective mechanism that is critical to *C. albicans* defense in this species, extrapolating the conclusions to humans may be misleading or overstated. To date, no correlation has been established between the development of disseminated candidiasis in humans and moderate or severe T cell deficiency in HIV/AIDS and CMC, respectively [118, 143]. Whether cell-mediated immunity against disseminated disease is an important factor in humans is, therefore, not known; clearly, humans have other mechanisms of handling this form of disease. Innate and acquired specific immunity acting in concert or independently, could well include phagocytic cells, cell-mediated immune responses, specific antibodies, and a range of associated humoral factors such as complement and cytokines [144]. Furthermore, any host defense element that prevents unrestrained fungal replication should be sufficient to ward off life-threatening invasion of the deep organ systems and morbidity associated with mucosal tissue disease. In order to develop an effective *Candida* vaccine, the complex dichotomy (i.e., commensal and opportunistic pathogen) of *C. albicans* and its interactions with human host needs to be understood thoroughly. There are two divergent postulates that explain fungus-host interaction. The first is based on the idea that *C. albicans* is present in the host as a latent pathogen controlled by the immune system. When the condition of the host becomes devastating this obvious pathogen causes the mucocutaneous and disseminated disease. This idea comes from the transitory occurrence of colonization by *C. albicans* in the healthy individuals [145] and the increased predisposition of the development of candidiasis in the individuals who are colonized prior to immunosuppressive therapy. In contrast, the second postulate states that the *C. albicans*-host interaction is a mutualistic relationship where both microbe and host-derive reciprocal benefit from each other. When the condition of the host becomes debilitated, the interaction shifted from favorable to invasive state. Accordingly, there are two distinctive approaches in the development of a vaccine against candidiasis. One approach involves the complete elimination of the organism from the human system (i.e., immunoprophylaxis) supporting the theory that *Candida* species are pathogens. The other involves inducing and maintaining an immune response against restricted antigens that correlate with an infectious disease state (i.e., immunotherapy), thus permitting the maintenance of the mutualistic *Candida*-host interaction [134].

We tackled disseminated candidiasis in mouse model by rejuvenating the host immune system with liposomized immuno-modulator viz. Tuftsin tetrapeptide as well as liposomes intercalated Amphotericin B-based formulation. The escheriosome-based vaccine that contains cytosolic proteins of *C. albicans* was also found to be effective against disseminated candidiasis in mouse model [146, 147].

1.6.2 *Aspergillus* spp.

Aspergillosis, a systemic fungal disease, becomes life threatening in persons with weak immune system, since these individuals are easy targets of systemic fungal infections. The treatment with antifungal drugs along with some immuno-stimulating agents should offer additional advantage over conventional chemotherapy [78, 80].

1.6.3 *Cryptococcus* spp.

Another important opportunistic fungal pathogen *Cryptococcus neoformans* can live in both plants and animals. Its teleomorph is *Filobasidiella neoformans*, a filamentous fungus belonging to the class Tremellomycetes. It is often found in pigeon excrement. The genome sequence of *C. neoformans* was published in 2005 [148]. Recent studies suggest that colonies of *C. neoformans* and related fungi growing on the ruins of the melted down reactor of the Chernobyl Nuclear Power Plant may be able to use the energy of radiation (primary beta radiation) for "radiotrophic" growth [149]. *C. neoformans* grows as yeast (unicellular) and replicates by budding. *C. neoformans* makes hyphae during mating, and eventually creates basidiospores at the end of the hyphae before producing spores. Under host-relevant conditions, including low glucose, serum, 5% carbon dioxide, and low iron, among others, the cells produce a characteristic polysaccharide capsule [150]. When grown as yeast, *C. neoformans* has a prominent capsule composed mostly of polysaccharides. Microscopically, the India ink stain is used for easy visualization of the capsule. The particles of ink pigment do not enter the capsule that surrounds the spherical yeast cell, resulting in a zone of clearance or "halo" around the cells. This allows for quick and easy identification of *C. neoformans. C. neoformans* grows rapidly on exposure to radiation such as gamma-radiation. Radiation seems to increase the electron-transfer capability of melanin in the fungus, increasing its total metabolic activity.

Infection with *C. neoformans* is termed cryptococcosis. Most infections with *C. neoformans* consist of a lung infection. However, fungal meningitis, especially as a secondary infection for AIDS patients, is often caused by *C. neoformans* making it a particularly dangerous fungus. Infections with this fungus are rare in those with fully functioning immune systems. For this reason, *C. neoformans* is sometimes referred to as an opportunistic fungus. It is a facultative intracellular pathogen [151].

Cryptococcosis that does not affect the central nervous system can be treated with fluconazole alone. Cryptococcal meningitis should be treated for 2 weeks with intravenous amphotericin B 0.7–1.0 mg/kg/day and oral flucytosine 100 mg/kg/day (or intravenous flucytosine 75 mg/kg/day if the patient is unable to swallow). This should then be followed by oral fluconazole 200 mg daily for 10 weeks [152] and then 200 mg daily until the patient's CD4 count was above 100 for 3 months and, if infected, his HIV viral load remained undetectable [153, 154]. Intravenous Ambisome 4 mg/kg/day may be used but is not superior: its main use is in patients who do not tolerate amphotericin B. Flucytosine at dose of 200 mg/kg/day when given orally was not much effective and associated with more side-effects. However, this does not result in cure because it merely suppresses the fungus and does not kill it; viable fungus can continue to be grown from CSF of patients who have taken fluconazole for many months. An increased dose of 400 mg daily does not improve outcomes [155], but preliminary data from Uganda suggested that very high doses at 1200 mg or more per day may be effective. The duration of this treatment and the posttreatment maintenance dose is not known.

C. neoformans is the causative agent of cryptococcosis, a disease typified by an initial pulmonary infection, which can disseminate to produce an ultimately fatal form of meningitis. The diagnosis of the disease relies either on the isolation of the yeast or on the detection of capsular polysaccharide via the latex agglutination test with either cerebrospinal fluid or serum. Thus far, three molecular species have been defined as cryptococcal exo-antigens in culture filtrate: high-molecular-weight glucuronoxylomannan (GXM), galactoxylomannan (GalXM), and mannoprotein. Mannoproteins (MNPs) are major structural and antigenic components of the cell walls of *Saccharomyces* and *Kluyveromyces* spp. as well. The surface location of cell wall MNP of the nonpathogenic yeasts is supported by immunochemical and agglutination data. MNP can be recovered in small amounts from cultural supernatants of the pathogenic yeast *C. neoformans.* MNPs are known to be immunogenic in cryptococcal infections, since antibodies to MNP in the sera of patients with cryptococcosis have been found. Murphy et al. found that *C. neoformans* secreted MNPs elicits a significantly stronger delayed-type-hypersensitivity response in mice than capsular polysaccharide does. Although the function of MNP in the cryptococcal cell and its cellular location are not known, analogy with the above examples suggests that MNP may come from the outer surface of the cell wall.

Cytosolic proteins (Cp) of *C. neoformans* were used in the present study for the development of prophylactic vaccines. The Cp (consisting of primarily T cell antigens) was immunogenic and readily induced formation of specific antibody in the host.

During blood coagulation, the plasma fibrinogen is converted to fibrin that readily undergoes polymerization to form a 3D network, in which various plasma constituents including proteins and blood cells are entrapped. Thrombin catalyzes this process and cleaves fibrinogen to smaller polypeptides that readily aggregate and form the clot [156].

Besides their wide usage in antibiotic delivery system for years, fibrin had been exploited for antigen delivery system as well. The fibrin clots can be readily prepared in vitro in various forms including glues, foams, and beads or can be combined with other polymers to yield more complex preparations [156]. The high antibody titer in the sera of mice immunized with fibrin bead-entrapped Cp vaccine compared to groups of animals receiving the antigen alone suggests the effectiveness of the fibrin cross-linked fibrin beads as effective antigen delivery vehicles. Apparently, the fibrin beads by slow release of entrapped antigen contribute toward the activation of the immune system. The Fib+PLGA-Cp mediated antigen delivery ensued highest up-regulation of Type I cytokines that facilitate induction of CD8+ T lymphocyte response. Thus, immunization with **Fib+PLGA-Cp** formulation induces IFN-γ to levels higher than those by **PLGA-Cp** and **Fib+Cp**. The use of fibrin bead based liposomized antigen leads to the generation of both Th1 and Th2 cells. Since the optimum activation of Th cells requires not only TCR occupancy by the presented MHC-antigens complex, but also a set of specific costimulatory signals provided by APCs. Fibrin beads offer a nearly ideal antigen delivery platform with regard to biocompatibility and biodegradability.

Due to the use of bovine thrombin, the risks of immunological complications arising out of the use of commercial fibrin, thrombin, and factor III preparations as sealants cannot be ignored. Consider that fibrin beads can be prepared rapidly from autologous plasma without the need for added thrombin or other clotting factors. Beaded plasma clots (or fibrin bead) prepared employing autologous plasma; contain cross-linked fibrin, for sustained delivery of pharmaceuticals along with vaccine antigen [156].

2 Materials

1. Tris–HCL buffer (50 mM, pH 7.6) containing 1 mM EDTA, 1 mM DTT, 0.1 mM PMSF.
2. Protease inhibitor cocktail: tosyl-L-lysine chloromethyl ketone, 100 μg/ml; pepstatin A, 50 μg/ml; leupeptin, 50 μg/ml (*see* **Note 1**).
3. PBS stock solution (5 M).
4. Normal saline.
5. Ammonium sulfate, (0.1 g in 1 ml distilled water).
6. Yeast Peptone Dextrose (YPD) broth.
7. SDS-PAGE 12%, β mercapto-ethanol, 0.1% Coosaie Brilliant Blue R-250.
8. Pellet diet ad libitum.
9. PLGA(Poly(lactic co-glycolic acid)), PLA(poly-lactic acid).
10. PBS-Tween 20 buffer.
11. Blocking buffer (3% skimmed milk in PBS-Tween 20).
12. Carbonate-bicarbonate buffer, 0.05 M, pH 9.6.
13. Streptavidin-HRS.
14. Orthophenylene diamine dihydrochloride (OPD.2HCl).
15. 7% H_2SO_4.
16. Biotinylated goat anti-mouse IgG1 and IgG2a.
17. Dichloromethane.
18. Bath-type sonicator.
19. Polyvinyl alcohol (PVA).
20. Silverson L4RT homogenizer.

3 Methods

3.1 Cytosolic ProteinPurification

Preparation of crude extract: All the manipulations to purify the proteins were carried out at 4 °C unless mentioned otherwise.

1. Culture the *C. neoformans* cells in YPD liquid medium for (12–16 h) (*see* **Note 2**).
2. Centrifuge at 6000 × *g* for 20 min., wash three times with normal saline to remove traces of medium.
3. Suspend the cells in 50 mM Tris–HCl buffer pH 7.6 and required amount of the protease inhibitor cocktail.
4. Ground the cells in a chilled mortar followed by sonication for 30 min in a bath-type sonicator (*see* **Note 3**).
5. Centrifuge the resulting homogenate at 10,000 × *g* for 30 min. And the supernatant, which was carefully separated from the fatty layer at the top of the tube by means of a pipette, was referred to as "crude extract."
6. To avoid contamination of lipid components, subject the extract to additional centrifugation at 15,000 × *g* for 30 min and recover the supernatant underlying the fatty layer (*see* **Note 4**).
7. Use Lowry's method to know the concentration of the crude proteins.
8. Add ammonium sulfate to get the desired protein as per the formula:
   $W = \{533 \times (S_2 - S_1) \times 100\}/\{100-(0.3\ S_1)$
   where
   W = Weight of ammonium sulfate to be added per liter of crude protein.
   S_2 = Final amount required.
   S_1 = Initial amount.
9. After ammonium sulfate was dissolved very gently, keep the protein overnight at 4 °C (*see* **Note 5**).
10. Collect the proteins that got precipitated by centrifugation at 15,000 × *g* for 20 min at 4 °C.
11. Suspend the pellet in PBS and dialyze the protein again to remove extra ammonium sulfate.
12. Estimate the protein by Lowery et al. and perform the SDS-PAGE for the characterization of proteins (*see* **Note 6**).

3.2 Ammonium Sulfate Fractionation

1. Ammonium sulfate-mediated fractionations of crude cytosolic protein. Different types of ammonium sulfate cuts were given to the cytosolic crude proteins. The precipitated protein fraction obtained after each cut was dialyzed to remove excess of ammonium sulfate.

2. Determination of the amount of ammonium sulfate needed for the next cut or fraction and dissolve in the rest of crude proteins (157).
3. Bring the crude extract to 20% saturation with solid ammonium sulfate at 4 °C.
4. Allow the preparation to stand for 8 h at 4 °C and collect the precipitate (*see* **Note 7**).
5. Dialyze the suspension overnight against the same buffer with three changes at 4 °C.
6. After dialysis remove the undissolved material by centrifugation at 10,000 × *g* (*see* **Note 8**).

3.3 Gel Electrophoresis

1. Perform SDS-PAGE using 12% polyacrylamide slab gel in the presence of 0.5 ml of β mercapto-ethanol (*see* **Notes 9** and **10**).
2. Detect the proteins by staining the gel with 0.1% Coomassie brilliant blue R-250 (Fig. 1). Apply the ammonium sulfate cuts to the cytosolic crude protein mixture and obtain different fractions of proteins such as 0–20, 20–40, 40–60, 60–80.
3. Calculate the amount of the ammonium sulfate and dissolve very gently into crude cytosolic proteins.
4. Leave overnight at 4 °C.
5. Collect the precipitated proteins by centrifugation at 15,000 × *g* at 4 °C for 10 min.
6. Suspend the proteins in PBS and dialyze to remove the extra ammonium sulfate.
7. Finally, separate the proteins on SDS-PAGE for their characterization.

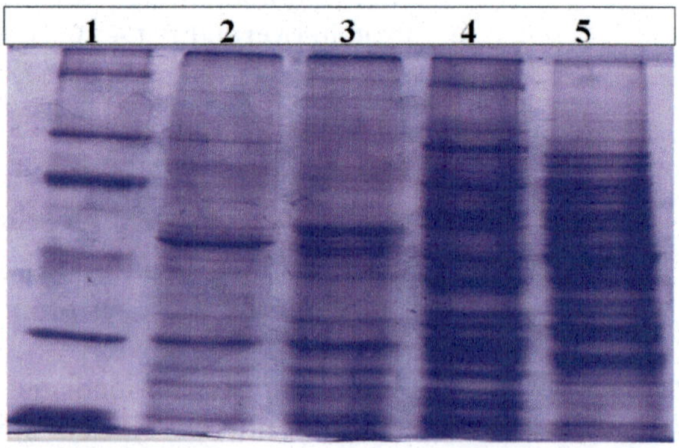

Fig. 1 SDS-PAGE profile of different fractions of C. neoformans cytosolic proteins. Lane1; molecular wt markers, lane 2; 20% amm. Sulfate fraction, lane 3; 40% amm. Sulfate fraction, lane 4; 60% amm. Sulfate fraction lane 5; 80% amm. Sulfate fraction

8. Calculate the amount of ammonium sulfate for the next cut or fraction and add to the rest of crude proteins (supernatant).
9. Follow the above-described procedure to obtain the proteins of this fraction and perform SDS-PAGE again for the study of gel profiles of these proteins.

3.4 Preparation of Cp-Bearing PLGA Nano-Particles

1. Dissolve a known amount (15 mg) of cytosolic protein (Cp) in 0.5 ml PBS.
2. Dissolve 190 mg of PLGA in 1.0 ml of dichloromethane.
3. Mix dissolved protein with PLGA solution in bath-type sonicator (10–15 min) to get an emulsion.
4. Mix the resulting primary emulsion with 100 ml 10% (w/v) PVA.
5. Homogenize using the Silverson L4RT homogenizer.
6. Stir the ensuing (O/W) emulsion at 25 °C for 18 h to allow solvent evaporation.
7. Finally, centrifuge the Cp-bearing microsphere at 10,000 × *g* for 10 min, wash with PBS.
8. Lyophilize the final solution and store at 4 °C until further use.

3.5 Experimental Animals

1. A total of 30 female Balb/c mice of weight 25 ± 2 gm were procured from laboratory animal resources, IVRI, Bareilly, India (*see* **Notes 11** and **12**).
2. Give the animals a standard pellet diet and water ad libitum.
3. Check the animals daily for their mortality and morbidity.
4. Do not include the moribund animals in the study.
5. The techniques used for bleeding, injection etc. are approved by the Institutional Animal Ethics Committee.

3.6 Immunization

Immunize the Balb/c mice with three doses (100 μg antigen/per dose) of control or PLGA-bearing cytosolic protein (Cp), incorporated in fibrin mesh carrier, subcutaneously.

On the 21st day of the first immunization boost the animals with another dose of antigen [158]. Evaluate the immunized animals for the presence of antibodies as well as cell-mediated immune response.

3.7 Protection Studies in Balb/c Mice

1. To perform protection experiments, immunize the Balb/c mice (five animals per group) with free as well as fibrin mesh incorporated cytosolic antigen by subcutaneous route. Ranges of doses regimen schedule were followed for immunization of animals. Other routes of administration were also evaluated to achieve possible better immunological response.

2. Boost the animals with appropriate antigens for three consecutive weeks.
3. On day fifth of the last booster, challenge the Balb/c mice (subcutaneously) with 10^7colony-forming units of *C. neoformans*.
4. Keep the animals under surveillance and assess the efficacy of vaccine on the basis of survival data as well as fungal load in various vital organs.
5. Include various control groups of animals in the study to determine efficacy of the vaccine. The control mice normally die within 10 days of the challenge [159].

3.8 Increased Antibody (IgG) Titer in Mice Immunized with Different Ammonium Sulfate Precipitated Fraction of C. neoformans Cell Extract

1. Determine the antibody response against different delivery systems in sera of immunized mice.
2. Our results showed that mice immunized with antigen-bearing PLGA microspheres entrapped in fibrin beads showed maximum antibody titer. PLGA microspheres entrapped antigen gives superior antibody titer over fibrin bead encapsulated antigens but elicited immune response was not as prominent as PLGA microspheres entrapped in fibrin beads. Various nanoparticle-based vaccines imparted better Abs titer than CFA-Ag (Fig. 2).

3.9 IgG Isotypes Profile in Animals Immunized with Various Vaccine Formulations as Determined by ELISA

The IgG isotype responses in various animals immunized with control free Cp, emulsified form with CFA, PLGA entrapped Cp and fibrin mesh encapsulated Cp or in Cp entrapped in both PLGA and fibrin meshes were determined.

1. Analyze the sera (1:300 dilutions) obtained from normal and experimental animals 5 days post immunization for the presence of Cp-specific IgG by ELISA method (*see* **Note 13**).

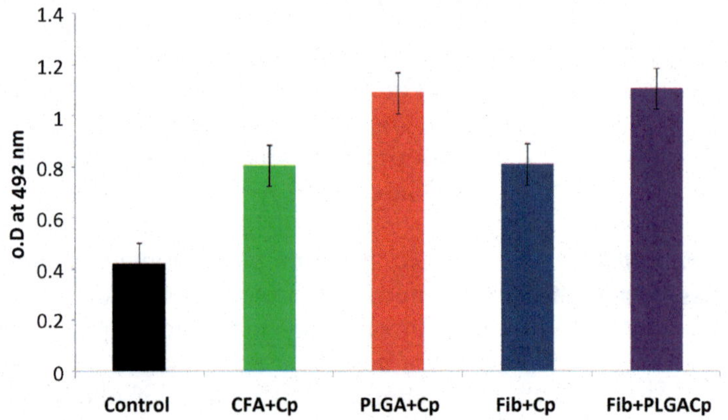

Fig. 2 Immunoglobulin (IgG) titer measured by ELISA in animals immunized with various forms of Cp antigen

2. Coat 96-well microtiter plates overnight with 50 μl of Cp (25 μg/ml) in carbonate-bicarbonate buffer at 4 °C (*see* **Note 14**).
3. After extensive washing with PBS-Tween 20 buffer, apply 300 μl of blocking buffer to the wells followed by incubation at 37 °C for 90 min (*see* **Note 15**).
4. Remove the blocking buffer and add logs 2 dilutions of test and control sera.
5. Allow the reaction to proceed at 37 °C for 2 h.
6. Wash the microtiter plate and add 50 μl of biotinylated goat anti-mouse IgG1 and IgG2a Abs.
7. Incubate the plate at 37 °C for 1 h.
8. After usual steps of washings, add 50 μl of streptavidin-HRP in each well and incubate the plate at 37 °C for 1 h (*see* **Note 16**).
9. Wash the plate once again before the addition of 50 μl of orthophenylene diamine dihydrochloride (OPD.2HCl) and finally incubate at 37 °C for 20 min.
10. Terminate the reaction by the addition of 50 μl of 7% H_2SO_4.
11. Read the absorbance at 492 nm with microtiter plate reader.
12. Express the level of IgG isotypes as absorbance (A 492 nm) of the colored complex developed in the immunosorbant assay (Fig. 3).
13. The data shown in Fig. 3 suggest that IFA-Cp can induce IgG2a isotype antibodies in the host presumably because of its

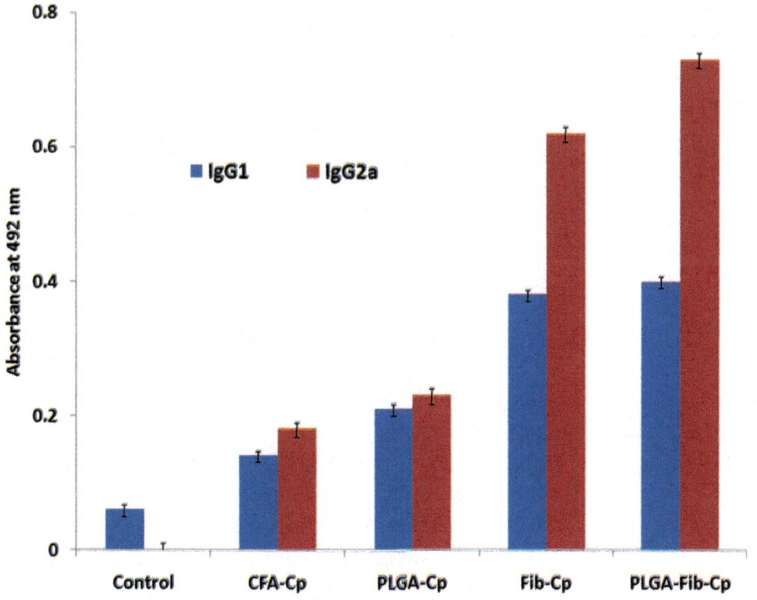

Fig. 3 Effect of various formulations of cytosolic antigen on induction of IgG isotype response in Balb/c mice measured by ELISA

innate T cell antigen properties. Various novel nano-vaccines of Cp antigen described in the study cause further enhancement in the immunogenic potential of Cp antigen. Dual delivery-based antigen carrier system comprising of microsphere/fibrin beads induces maximum antibody production with preponderance of IgG2a class of antibodies in the host. In general, the Th1/Th2 dichotomy plays a crucial role in containment of intracellular pathogens. CD4+ cells with Th1 phenotype activate cell-mediated immune response by upregulating IFN-γ and IL-2 cytokines in the immunized host. IFN-γ can educate B cells for specific production of antibodies with IgG2a isotypes, while cytokines expressed by Th2 helper cells upregulate IgG1 class of antibodies in the host. The ratio of IgG2a versus IgG1 titer thus indirectly reflects Th1/Th2 bias and is widely used as a parameter to define potential of a given vaccine antigen to induce CMI or humoral response in the host. The observed IgG2a/IgG1 ratio (Fig. 3) suggests that the fibrin-based antigen delivery system used in the present study can specifically eradicate fungal pathogens such as *C. albicans* and *C. neoformans* that prefer to reside inside host macrophages during infection in the host.

3.10 Fungal Burden in Vital Organs of Mice Immunized with Ammonium Sulfate Precipitated Fraction of *Cryptococcus neoformans* Cell Extract

Determining fungal load in kidney, spleen, and liver of the infected animals assessed the efficacy of various antigenic formulations.

1. Sacrifice the animals belonging to various treatment groups on day 6, post challenge infection and take out the organs aseptically.
2. Triturate the organs separately with 2 ml of 1.5 M PBS (pH 7.4) and plate an aliquot (100 μl) of this suspension on YPD agar plates after appropriate dilution (*see* **Notes 2** and **17**).
3. Incubate the plates for 48–72 h at 37 °C.
4. Note the development of colonies in each group and calculate the fungal load by multiplying with the respective dilution factor.

Figure 4 clearly shows the high efficacy of novel fibrin based delivery systems in eliminating fungal pathogen from the host. The opportunistic fungal infections as the name suggests are considered to be the disease that establishes in the host with compromised immune system. Recent trend regarding prevalence of opportunistic infections, however, suggests that disease cannot be classified as an opportunistic infection. The pathogen inflicts range of otherwise healthy host especially female human beings. In such circumstances, there is urgent need to evolve a prophylactic strategy that can check establishment and prevalence of fungal infections in the host. In this regard, nano-vaccines hold center stage among other types of existing vaccines.

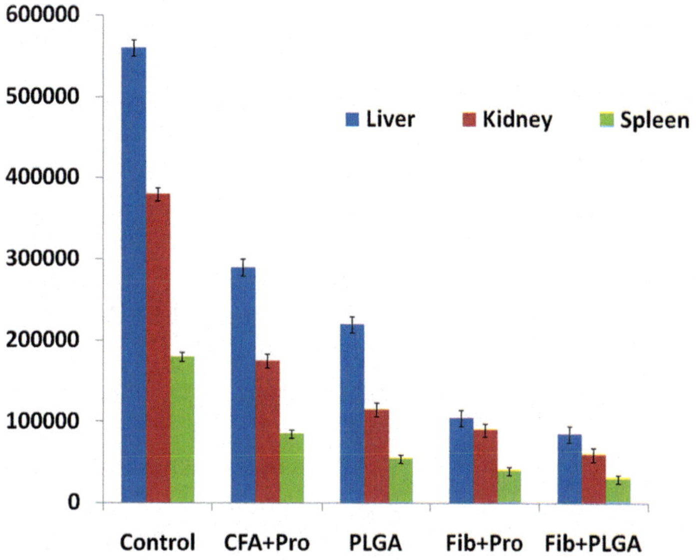

Fig. 4 CFU count on 6th days post infection in the vital organs of animals immunized with various forms of antigen

4 Notes

1. Protease inhibitor cocktail must be used during extraction and purification of protein to prevent degradation caused by proteases.
2. Media (YPD) should be freshly prepared and autoclaved.
3. Avoid heating the sample during sonication.
4. At the time of centrifugation, the centrifuge machine should be handled properly. Lid of high speed centrifuge closed and all the samples in the microcentrifuge tube should be weighed and balanced in a rotor of the machine.
5. While fractionating with ammonium sulfate, add the salt slowly with stirring to avoid temporarily exceeding the desired concentration.
6. Ammonium persulfate should be prepared freshly every time while running SDS-PAGE.
7. Work at 4 °C and keep all protein fractions on ice during purification.
8. At the time of dialysis, be sure the bag is not leaking the protein of interest and is of appropriate mw cut.
9. Always wear gloves and mask while handling and weighing SDS, acylamide, PMSF, etc. and other chemicals as some chemicals are carcinogenic.

10. Keep the apparatus of gel electrophoresis away from sinks or other water sources and turn off power before opening lid or reaching inside chamber.
11. In case of animal handling, one should wear proper cotton gloves to avoid their bite as mice have sharp teeth.
12. Possibility of zoonotic diseases and allergies associated with animals must always be considered. The safest policy is to reduce exposure by wearing protective clothing.
13. While performing ELISA, spillover must be avoided to prevent contamination.
14. All buffers and stock solution should be prepared in deionized water.
15. Use fresh buffers all at the correct pH.
16. Accuracy can be increased by running duplicates for all points in the assay including background, standard, and sample wells.
17. pH of all buffers should be maintained with calibrated pH meter.

Acknowledgment

We thank the coordinator of the department for allowing us to avail required facilities of the department to complete this study. Asim Azhar is thankful to UGC for providing financial assistance in terms of Kothari postdoctoral fellowship.

References

1. Church D, Elsayed S, Reid O et al (2006) Burn wound infections. Clin Microbiol Rev 19:403–434
2. Vivier E, Ugolini S (2011) Natural killer cells: from basic research to treatments. Front Immunol. doi:10.3389/fimmu.2011.00018
3. Buchacz K, Baker K, Palella J Jr et al (2007) AIDS-defining opportunistic illnesses in US patients, 1994-2007: a cohort study. AIDS 24:1549–1559
4. Leena VG, Ravi D, Abhay S (2005) Review of Health care in India. CEHAT, Mumbai. ISBN: 81-89042-40-8
5. Moghimi M, Hunter C, Murray C (2005) Nanomedicine: current status and future prospects. FASEB J 19:311–330
6. Couvreur P, Vauthier C (2006) Nanotechnology: intelligent design to treat complex disease. Pharm Res 23:1417–1450
7. Bangham AD, Standish MM, Miller N (1965) Cation permeability of phospholipid model membranes: effect of narcotics. Nature 208:1295–1297
8. Liechty B, Kryscio R, Slaughter V, Peppas A (2010) Polymers for drug delivery systems. Annu Rev Chem Biomol Eng 1:149–173
9. Moghimi M, Hunter C (2001) Capture of stealth nanoparticles by the body's defences. Crit Rev Ther Drug Carrier Syst 18:527–550
10. Panyam J, Lof J, O'Leary E, Labhasetwar V (2002) Efficiency of dispatch and infiltrator cardiac infusion catheters in arterial localization of nanoparticles in a porcine coronary model of restenosis. J Drug Target 10:515–523
11. Quintana A, Raczka E, Piehler L et al (2002) Design and function of a dendrimer-based therapeutic nanodevice targeted to tumor

cells through the folate receptor. Pharm Res 19:1310–1316
12. Allen TM, Cullis PR (2004) Drug delivery systems: entering the mainstream. Science 303:1818–1822
13. Sahoo SK, Labhasetwar V (2003) Nanotech approaches to drug delivery and imaging. Drug Discov Today 8:1112–1120
14. Sudimack J, Lee J (2000) Targeted drug delivery via the folate receptor. Adv Drug Deliv Rev 41:147–146
15. Sinico C, Fadda M (2009) Vesicular carriers for dermal drug delivery. Expert Opin Drug Deliv 6:813–825
16. Biju S, Sushama T, Mishra R et al (2006) Vesicular systems: an overview. Indian J Pharma Sci 68:141–153
17. Vollmar B, Menger D (2009) The hepatic microcirculation: mechanistic contributions and therapeutic targets in liver injury and repair. Physiol Rev 89:1269–1339
18. Singh S (2011) Membrane permeability in biological systems: a systems biology perspective. J Comput Sci Syst Biol 4:27–32
19. Copland J, Rades T, Davies M et al (2005) Lipid based particulate formulations for the delivery of antigen. Immunol Cell Biol 83:97–105
20. Semple C, Harasym O, Clow A et al (2005) Immunogenicity and rapid blood clearance of liposomes containing polyethylene glycol-lipid conjugates and nucleic acid. J Pharmacol Exp Ther 312:1020–1026
21. Syed M, Khan A, Nasti H et al (2003) Antigen entrapped in the escheriosomes leads to the generation of CD4(+) helper and CD8(+) cytotoxic T cell response. Vaccine 21:2383–2393
22. Ahmed A, Dare V, Hincke M (2008) Fibrin: a versatile scaffold for tissue engineering applications. Tissue Eng Part B Rev 14:199–215
23. Mosesson W (2005) Fibrinogen and fibrin structure and functions. J Thromb Haemost 3:1894–1904
24. Mosesson W, Siebenlist R, Meh A (2001) The structure and biological features of fibrinogen and fibrin. Ann N Y Acad Sci 936:11–30
25. Horan T, Francis W (2001) Fibrin degradation products, fibrin monomer and soluble fibrin in disseminated intravascular coagulation. Semin Thromb Hemost 27:657–666
26. Doolittle F, Chen R, Lau F (1971) Hybrid fibrin: proof of the intermolecular nature of-crosslinking units. Biochem Biophys Res Commun 44:94–100
27. Schense C, Hubbell A (1999) Cross-linking exogenous bifunctional peptides into fibrin gels with factor XIIIa. Bioconjug Chem 10:75–81
28. Gorodetsky R, Clark RA, An J et al (1999) Fibrin microbeads (FMB) as biodegradable carriers for culturing cells and for accelerating wound healing. J Invest Dermatol 112:866–872
29. Marx G, Mou X, Hotovely-Salomon A et al (2008) Heat denaturation of fibrinogen to develop a biomedical matrix. J Biomed Mater Res B Appl Biomater 84(1):49–57
30. Shimony N, Gorodetsky R, Marx G et al (2006) Fibrin microbeads (FMB) as a 3D platform for kidney gene and cell therapy. Kidney Int 69:625–633
31. Gurevich O, Vexler A, Marx G et al (2002) Fibrin microbeads for isolating and growing bone marrow-derived progenitor cells capable of forming bone tissue. Tissue Eng 8:661–672
32. Redl H, Schlag G, Stanek G, Hirschl A et al (1983) In vitro properties of mixtures of fibrin seal and antibiotics. Biomaterials 4:29–32
33. Tsourvakas S, Hatzigrigoris P, Tsibinos A et al (1995) Pharmacokinetic study of fibrin clot ciprofloxacin complex: an in vitro and in vivo experimental investigation. Arch Orthop Trauma Surg 114:295–297
34. Senderoff I, Sheu T, Sokoloski D (1991) Fibrin based drug delivery systems. J Parenter Sci Technol 45:2–6
35. Yoshida H, Yamaoka Y, Shinoyama M et al (2000) Novel drug delivery system using autologous fibrin glue--release properties of anti-cancer drugs. Biol Pharm Bull 23: 371–374
36. Woolverton J, Fulton A, Salstrom J et al (2001) Tetracycline delivery from fibrin controls peritoneal infection without measurable systemic antibiotic. J Antimicrob Chemother 48:861–867
37. Kumar R, Vasantha Bai M, Krishnan K (2004) A freeze-dried fibrin disc as a biodegradable drug release matrix. Biologicals 32:49–55
38. Itokazu M, Yamamoto K, Yang Y et al (1997) The sustained release of antibiotic from freeze-dried fibrin-antibiotic compound and efficacies in a rat model of osteomyelitis. Infection 25:359–363
39. Simpson E, Gilbert A, Rudnick E et al (2002) Transscleral diffusion of carboplatin: an in vitro and in vivo study. Arch Ophthalmol 120:1069–1074
40. Pardue T, Hejny C, Gilbert A et al (2004) Retinal function after subconjunctival injection of carboplatin in fibrin sealant. Retina 24:776–782
41. Häfeli O, Pauer J, Unnithan J et al (2007) Fibrin glue system for adjuvant brachytherapy of brain tumors with 188Re and 186Re-labeled

microspheres. Eur J Pharm Biopharm 65:282–288
42. Hou T, Xu J, Li Q et al (2008) In vitro evaluation of a fibrin gel antibiotic delivery system containing mesenchymal stem cells and vancomycin alginate beads for treating bone infections and facilitating bone formation. Tissue Eng Part A 14:1173–1182
43. Janmey A, McCormick E, Rammensee S et al (2007) Negative normal stress in semiflexible biopolymer gels. Nat Mater 6:48–51
44. Smidsrød O, Skjåk-Braek G (1990) Alginate as immobilization matrix for cells. Trends Biotechnol 8:71–78
45. Atala A, Kim W, Paige T et al (1994) Endoscopic treatment of vesicoureteral reflux with a chondrocyte-alginate suspension. J Urol 152:641–643
46. Wee S, Gombotz R (1998) Protein release from alginate matrices. Adv Drug Deliv Rev 31:267–285
47. Silva A (2006) Nanomedicine: seeing the benefits of ceria. Nat Nanotechnol 1:92–94
48. Kolambkar M, Peister A, Ekaputra K et al (2010) Colonization and osteogenic differentiation of different stem cell sources on electrospun nanofiber meshes. Tissue Eng Part A 16:3219–3230
49. Chen M, Wu F, Wang T et al (2005) Preparation of recombinant human bone morphogenetic protein-2 loaded dextran-based microspheres and their characteristics. Acta Pharmacol Sin 26:1093–1103
50. Bachelder M, Beaudette T, Broaders E et al (2010) In vitro analysis of acetalated dextran microparticles as a potent delivery platform for vaccine adjuvants. Mol Pharm 7:826–835
51. Qi J, Yao P, He F et al (2010) Nanoparticles with dextran/chitosan shell and BSA/chitosan core--doxorubicin loading and delivery. Int J Pharm 393:176–184
52. Müller E (2003) The origin of metazoan complexity: porifera as integrated animals. Integr Comp Biol 43:3–10
53. Di Lullo A, Sweeney M, Korkko J et al (2002) Mapping the ligand-binding sites and disease-associated mutations on the most abundant protein in the human, type I collagen. J Biol Chem 277:4223–4231
54. Wallace D, McPherson J, Ellingsworth L et al (1988) Injectable collagen for tissue augmentation. Collagen, Biotechnology 3:118–144
55. Wallace D, Rhee W, Reihanian H et al (1989) Injectable cross-linked collagen with improved flow properties. J Biomed Mater Res 23:931–945
56. Rosenblatt J, Devereux B, Wallace D (1993) Dynamic rheological studies of hydrophobic interactions in injectable collagen biomaterials. J Appl Polym Sci 50:953–963
57. Chow A, Fuller G, Wallace D et al (1985) Rheo-optical response of rod-like chains subject to transient shear flow:2. Two-color birefringence measurements on collagen protein. Macromolecule 18:793–804
58. Kligman M (1988) Histologic responses to collagen implants in human volunteers: comparison of Zyderm collagen with Zyplast implant. J Dermatol Surg Oncol 14:35–38
59. Stegman J, Chu S, Bensch K et al (1987) A light and electron microscopic evaluation of Zyderm collagen and Zyplast implants in aging human facial skin. A pilot study. Arch Dermatol 123:1644–1169
60. Wallace G, Rosenblatt J (2003) Collagen gel systems for sustained delivery and tissue engineering. Adv Drug Deliv Rev 55:1631–1649
61. Koch-Weser J, Sellers M (1976) Drug therapy. Binding of drugs to serum albumin (second of two parts). N Engl J Med 294:526–531
62. Kragh-Hansen U, Minchiotti L, Brennan O et al (1990) Hormone binding to natural mutants of human serum albumin. Eur J Biochem 193:169–174
63. Prinsen H, de Sain-van der Velden G (2004) Albumin turnover: experimental approach and its application in health and renal diseases. Clin Chim Acta 347:1–14
64. Nair S, Laurencin T (2006) Polymers as biomaterials for tissue engineering and controlled drug delivery. Adv Biochem Eng Biotechnol 102:47–90
65. Eldridge H, Staas K, Meulbroek A et al (1991) Biodegradable and biocompatible poly(DL-lactide-co-glycolide) microspheres as an adjuvant for staphylococcal enterotoxin B toxoid which enhances the level of toxin-neutralizing antibodies. Infect Immun 59:2978–2986
66. O'Hagan T, McGee P, Holmgren J et al (1993) Biodegradable microparticles for oral immunization. Vaccine 11:149–154
67. Pistner H, Gutwald R, Ordung R et al (1993) Poly(L-lactide): a long-term degradation study in vivo. I Biological results. Biomaterials 14:671–677
68. Marten L (2002) Encyclopedia of polymer science and technology. John Wiley & Sons, Inc., New York. doi:10.1002/0471440264.pst384
69. Lee Y, Soon Y (2007) Polymeric protein delivery systems. Prog Polym Sci 32:669–697
70. Mandal K, Bostanian A, Graves A et al (2002) Poly(D,L-lactide-co-glycolide) encapsulated poly(vinyl alcohol) hydrogel as a drug delivery system. Pharm Res 19:1713–1719

71. Yeo Y, Namjin B, Kinam P (2001) Microencapsulation methods for delivery of protein drugs. Biotechnol Bioprocess Eng 6:213–230
72. Middleton C, Tipton J (2000) Synthetic biodegradable polymers as orthopedic devices. Biomaterials 21:2335–2346
73. Makadia K, Siegel J (2011) Poly lactic-co-glycolic acid (PLGA) as biodegradable controlled drug delivery carrier. Polymers (Basel) 3:1377–1397
74. Visscher E, Robison A, Argentieri J (1987) Tissue response to biodegradable injectable microcapsules. J Biomater Appl 2:118–131
75. Cleland L, Powell F, Shire J (1993) The development of stable protein formulations: a close look at protein aggregation, deamidation, and oxidation. Crit Rev Ther Drug Carrier Syst 10:307–377
76. Denning W, Bromley J (2015) Infectious disease. How to bolster the antifungal pipeline. Science 347:1414–1416
77. Veerareddy R, Vobalaboina V (2004) Lipid-based formulations of amphotericin B. Drugs Today (Barc) 40:133–145
78. Agrawal K, Gupta M (2000) Tuftsin-bearing liposomes in treatment of macrophage-based infections. Adv Drug Deliv Rev 41:135–146
79. Shadkchan Y, Keisari Y, Segal E (2004) Cytokines in mice treated with amphotericin B-intralipid. Med Mycol 42:123–128
80. Owais M, Ahmed I, Krishnakumar B et al (1993) Tuftsin-bearing liposomes as drug vehicles in the treatment of experimental aspergillosis. FEBS Lett 326:56–58
81. Masood K, Feroz M, Rukhsana J et al (2004) Prophylactic role of liposomised chloroquine against murine cryptococcosis less susceptible to fluconazole. Pharm Res 21:2207–2212
82. Arellano M, Lonial S (2008) Clinical uses of GM-CSF, a critical appraisal and update. Biologics 2:13–27
83. Blanco L, Garcia E (2008) Immune response to fungal infections. Vet Immunol Immunopathol 125:47–70
84. Polonelli L, Casadevall A, Han Y et al (2000) The efficacy of acquired humoral and cellular immunity in the prevention and therapy of experimental fungal infections. Med Mycol 38:281–292
85. Romani L (2011) Immunity to fungal infections. Nat Rev Immunol 11:275–288
86. Wüthrich M, Deepe S Jr, Klein B (2012) Adaptive immunity to fungi. Annu Rev Immunol 30:115–148
87. van de Veerdonk L, Netea G (2010) T-cell subsets and antifungal host defenses. Curr Fungal Infect Rep 4:238–243
88. Gibson F, Johnston A (2015) Immunity to *Cryptococcus neoformans* and *C. gattii* during cryptococcosis. Fungal Genet Biol 78:76–86
89. Spellberg B (2011) Vaccines for invasive fungal infections. F1000 Med Rep 3:13
90. Paramythiotou E, Frantzeskaki F, Flevari A et al (2014) Invasive fungal infections in the ICU: how to approach, how to treat. Molecules 19:1085–1119
91. Medici P, Del Poeta M (2015) New insights on the development of fungal vaccines: from immunity to recent challenges. Mem Inst Oswaldo Cruz 110:966–973
92. Anaissie E (1992) Opportunistic mycoses in the immunocompromised host: experience at a cancer center and review. Clin Infect Dis 14:S43–S53
93. Pfaller M, Wenzel R (1992) Impact of the changing epidemiology of fungal infections in the 1990s. Eur J Clin Microbiol Infect Dis 11:287–1291
94. Richardson D (1991) Opportunistic and pathogenic fungi. J Antimicrob Chemother 28:1–11
95. Walsh J (1992) Emerging targets in antibacterial and antifungal. Chapman & Hall, New York, pp 249–373
96. Banerjee N, Emori G, Culver H et al (1991) Secular trends in nosocomial primary bloodstream infections in the United States, 1980-1989. National Nosocomial Infections Surveillance System. Am J Med 91:86S–89S
97. Emori G, Gaynes P (1993) An overview of nosocomial infections, including the role of the microbiology laboratory. Clin Microbiol Rev 6:428–442
98. Goff A, Koletar L, Buesching J et al (1995) Isolation of flucanozole-resistant *Candida albicans* from HIV negativepatients never treated with azoles. Clin Infect Dis 20:77–83
99. Nolte S, Parkinson T, Falconer J (1997) Isolation and charecterisation of flucanazole and amphoterecin B resistant *Candida albicans* from blood of two patients with leukemia. Antimicrob Agents Chemother 41: 196–199
100. Nguyen H, Peacock E Jr, Morris J et al (1996) The changing face of candidemia: emergence of non-*Candida albicans* species and antifungal resistance. Am J Med 100:617–623
101. Iannitti G, Carvalho A, Romani L (2012) From memory to antifungal vaccine design. Trends Immunol 33:467–474
102. Behnsen J, Hartmann A, Schmaler J et al (2008) The opportunistic human pathogenic fungus Aspergillus fumigatus evades the host complement system. Infect Immun 76: 820–827

103. Nanjappa G, Klein S (2014) Vaccine immunity against fungal infections. Curr Opin Immunol 28:27–33
104. Del Poeta M, Casadevall A (2012) Ten challenges on *Cryptococcus* and cryptococcosis. Mycopathologia 173:303–310
105. Shapiro S, Robbins N, Cowen E (2011) Regulatory circuitry governing fungal development, drug resistance, and disease. Microbiol Mol Biol Rev 75:213–267
106. Kirkpatrick H (1989) Chronic mucocutaneous candidiasis. Eur J Clin Microbiol Infect Dis 8:448–456
107. Bodey GP (1993) Hematogenous and major organ candidiasis. In: Bodey GP (ed) Candidiasis: pathogenesis, diagnosis and treatment. Raven, New York, pp 279–329
108. Casanova M, Martínez P, Chaffin L (1990) Fab fragments from a monoclonal antibody against a germ tube mannoprotein block the yeast-to-mycelium transition in *Candida albicans*. Infect Immun 58:3810–38112
109. Buckley H, Lucas J, Hattler G Jr et al (1968) Defective cellular immunity associated with chronic mucocutaneous moniliasis and recurrent staphylococcal botryomycosis: immunological reconstitution by allogeneic bone marrow. Clin Exp Immunol 3:153–169
110. Hoh C, Lin P, Chan L et al (1996) Successful allogeneic bone marrow transplantation in severe chronic mucocutaneous candidiasis syndrome. Bone Marrow Transplant 18:797–800
111. Cutler E (1976) Acute systemic candidiasis in normal and congenitally thymic-deficient (nude) mice. J Reticuloendothel Soc 19: 121–124
112. Jones-Carson J, Vazquez-Torres A, Warner T et al (2000) Disparate requirement for T cells in resistance to mucosal and acute systemic candidiasis. Infect Immun 68:2363–2365
113. Tabeta H, Mikami Y, Abe F et al (1984) Studies on defense mechanisms against *Candida albicans* infection in congenitally athymic nude (nu/nu) mice. Mycopathologia 84:107–113
114. Romani L, Cenci E, Menacci A et al (1995) T helper cell dichotomy to *Candida albicans*: implications for pathology, therapy, and vaccine design. Immunol Res 14:148–162
115. Bistoni F, Cenci E, Mencacci A et al (1993) Mucosal and systemic T helper cell function after intragastric colonization of adult mice with *Candida albicans*. J Infect Dis 168:1449–1157
116. Ashman B, Fulurija A, Papadimitriou M (1999) Both CD4+ and CD8+ lymphocytes reduce the severity of tissue lesions in murine systemic cadidiasis, and CD4+ cells also demonstrate strain-specific immunopathological effects. Microbiology 145:1631–1640
117. Bodey P (1986) Infection in cancer patients. A continuing association. Am J Med 81:11–26
118. Nasser M, Melgar R, Longworth L et al (1997) Incidence and risk of developing fungal prosthetic valve endocarditis after nosocomial candidemia. Am J Med 103:25–32
119. Bross J, Talbot GH, Maislin G et al (1989) Risk factors for nosocomial candidemia: a case-control study in adults without leukemia. Am J Med 87:614–620
120. Wey B, Mori M, Pfaller A et al (1989) Risk factors for hospital-acquired candidemia. A matched case-control study. Arch Intern Med 149:2349–2353
121. MacDonald L, Baker C, Chenoweth C (1998) Risk factors for candidemia in a children's hospital. Clin Infect Dis 26:642–645
122. Lopez-Berestein G, Bodey GP, Fainstein V et al (1989) Treatment of systemic fungal infections with liposomal amphotericin B. Arch Intern Med 149:2533–2536
123. Ruhnke M, Schmidt-Westhausen A, Trautmann M (1997) In vitro activities of voriconazole (UK-109,496) against fluconazole-susceptible and -resistant *Candida albicans* isolates from oral cavities of patients with human immunodeficiency virus infection. Antimicrob Agents Chemother 41:575–577
124. Sanati H, Belanger P, Fratti R et al (1997) A new triazole, voriconazole (UK-109,496), blocks sterol biosynthesis in *Candida albicans* and *Candida krusei*. Antimicrob Agents Chemother 41:2492–2496
125. Hazen C, Baron J, Colombo L et al (2003) Comparison of the susceptibilities of Candida spp. to fluconazole and voriconazole in a 4-year global evaluation using disk diffusion. J Clin Microbiol 41:5623–5632
126. Anderson B (2005) Evolution of antifungal-drug resistance: mechanisms and pathogen fitness. Nat Rev Microbiol 3:547–556
127. Richardson D (2005) Changing patterns and trends in systemic fungal infections. J Antimicrob Chemother 56:i5–i11
128. Sangeorzan A, Bradley F, He X et al (1994) Epidemiology of oral candidiasis in HIV-infected patients: colonization, infection, treatment, and emergence of fluconazole resistance. Am J Med 97:339–346
129. Johnson M, Warnock W (1995) Azole drug resistance in yeasts. J Antimicrob Chemother 36:751–755
130. Meunier F, Aoun M, Bitar N (1992) Candidemia in immunocompromised patients. Clin Infect Dis 14:S120–S125

131. White J, Habib R, Vanthuyne A et al (2001) Combined topical flucytosine and amphotericin B for refractory vaginal *Candida glabrata* infections. Sex Transm Infect 77:212–213
132. Kojic M, Darouiche O (2004) *Candida* infections of medical devices. Clin Microbiol Rev 17:255–267
133. Ada G (1991) Vaccine development. Real and imagined dangers. Nature 349:369
134. Mochon B, Cutler E (2005) Is a vaccine needed against Candida albicans? Med Mycol 43:97–115
135. Huang C, Lin Y, Leu S et al (1998) Yeast carriage on hands of hospital personnel working in intensive care units. J Hosp Infect 39:47–55
136. Hilleman R (2002) Overview of the needs and realities for developing new and improved vaccines in the 21st century. Intervirology 45:199–211
137. Milstien J, Lambert S (2002) Emergency response vaccines--a challenge for the public sector and the vaccine industry. Vaccine 21:146–154
138. Owais M, Massod K, Agrewala N et al (2001) Use of liposome as an immunopotentiating delivery system: in perspective of vaccine development. Scand J Immunol 54:125–132
139. Naider F, Shenbagamurthi P, Steinfeld S et al (1983) Synthesis and biological activity of tripeptidyl polyoxins as antifungal agents. Antimicrob Agents Chemother 24:787–796
140. Denning W (2003) Echinocandin antifungal drugs. Lancet 362:1142–1151
141. Farah S, Ashman B, Challacombe J (2000) Oral candidosis. Clin Dermatol 18:553–562
142. Fidel L Jr (2004) History and new insights into host defense against vaginal candidiasis. Trends Microbiol 12:220–227
143. Nucci M, Colombo AL, Spector N et al (1997) Breakthrough candidemia in neutropenic patients. Clin Infect Dis 24:275–276
144. Casadevall A (1995) Antibody immunity and invasive fungal infections. Infect Immun 63:4211–4218
145. Hannula J, Saarela M, Jousimies-Somer H et al (1999) Age-related acquisition of oral and nasopharyngeal yeast species and stability of colonization in young children. Oral Microbiol Immunol 14:176–182
146. Chauhan A, Zubair S, Nadeem A et al (2014) Escheriosome-mediated cytosolic delivery of PLK1-specific siRNA: potential in treatment of liver cancer in BALB/c mice. Nanomedicine (Lond) 9:407–420
147. Singha H, Mallick I, Jana C et al (2008) Escheriosomes entrapped DNA vaccine co-expressing Cu-Zn superoxide dismutase and IL-18 confers protection against *Brucella abortus*. Microbes Infect 10:1089–1096
148. Loftus J, Fung E, Roncaglia P et al (2005) The genome of the basidiomycetous yeast and human pathogen *Cryptococcus neoformans*. Science 307:1321–1324
149. Dadachova E, Bryan RA, Huang X et al (2007) Ionizing radiation changes the electronic properties of melanin and enhances the growth of melanized fungi. PLoS One 2:e457
150. Joseph H, Thomas K, Kyung K et al (1998) Book ISBN: 978-1-55581-501-1
151. Alvarez M, Burn T, Luo Y et al (2009) The outcome of *Cryptococcus neoformans* intracellular pathogenesis in human monocytes. BMC Microbiol 9:51. doi:10.1186/1471-2180-9-51
152. Saag MS, Graybill RJ, Larsen RA et al (2000) Practice guidelines for the management of cryptococcal disease. Infectious Diseases Society of America. Clin Infect Dis 30:710–718
153. Martínez P, Gil L, López-Ribot L et al (1998) Serologic response to cell wall mannoproteins and proteins of *Candida albicans*. Clin Microbiol Rev 11:121–141
154. Vibhagool A, Sungkanuparph S, Mootsikapun P et al (2003) Discontinuation of secondary prophylaxis for cryptococcal meningitis in human immunodeficiency virus-infected patients treated with highly active antiretroviral therapy: a prospective, multicenter, randomized study. Clin Infect Dis 36: 1329–1331
155. Schaars F, Meintjes A, Morroni C et al (2006) Outcome of AIDS-associated cryptococcal meningitis initially treated with 200 mg/day or 400 mg/day of fluconazole. BMC Infect Dis 6:118
156. Ahmad E, Fatima T, Owais M et al (2011) Beaded plasma clot: a potent sustained-release, drug-delivery system. Ther Deliv 2:573–583
157. Wingfield T (2001) Protein precipitation using ammonium sulfate. Curr Protoc Protein Sci. doi:10.1002/0471140864.psa03fs13
158. Ahmad N, Masood K, Owais M (2001) Fusogenic potential of prokaryotic membrane lipids. Implication in vaccine development. Eur J Biochem 268:5667–5675
159. Pietrella D, Mazzolla R, Lupo P et al (2002) Mannoprotein from *Cryptococcus neoformans* promotes T-helper type 1 anticandidal responses in mice. Infect Immun 70: 6621–6627

Chapter 14

Yeast Expressing Gp43 Protein as a Vaccine Against *Paracoccidioides brasiliensis* Infection

Aline Ferreira Oliveira and Paulo S.R. Coelho

Abstract

Paracoccidioidomycosis (PCM) represents the most frequent systemic mycosis in Latin American. The disease is caused by the pathogenic thermally dimorphic fungus *Paracoccidioides brasiliensis*, and is initially characterized by pulmonary lesions, which can subsequently disseminate to other organs, resulting in secondary injuries. Although its high incidence, there is no commercially available vaccine against fungal diseases. A novel strategy, using *Saccharomyces cerevisiae* yeast as a vehicle for immunization against PCM, was recently successfully described. Herein, we describe strategies for the construction of the suitable *S. cerevisiae* vaccine, and protocols of administration and evaluation of the efficacy of the vaccine against experimental PCM.

Key words *Saccharomyces cerevisiae*, Paracoccidioidomycosis (PCM), Gp43 recombinant protein, *Paracoccidioides brasiliensis*, Vaccine

1 Introduction

In the past few years, *Saccharomyces cerevisiae* has been tested as a vaccine against many mycoses. Vaccination of mice with heat-killed *S. cerevisiae* provides protection against experimental aspergillosis, coccidioidomycosis, candidiasis, zygomycosis, and paracoccidioidomycosis [1–6]. This yeast has also been tested in clinical trials as immunotherapeutic vaccine for cancers and chronic infections [7]. Some aspects make yeast a promising vaccine vehicle. Yeast delivers antigens to antigen-presenting cells that elicit both CD4 and CD8 T cells. In addition, yeast presents intrinsic adjuvant characteristics, by having β-glucan as a component of its cell wall. Due to its genetic tractability, yeast can be genetically engineered to express pathogen-specific antigens. Here, we describe a method to construct a yeast strain that expresses gp43, the *P. brasiliensis* dominant antigen. We also describe methodologies to evaluate the efficacy of this vaccine against experimental paracoccidioidomycosis.

Markus Kalkum and Margarita Semis (eds.), *Vaccines for Invasive Fungal Infections: Methods and Protocols*, Methods in Molecular Biology, vol. 1625, DOI 10.1007/978-1-4939-7104-6_14, © Springer Science+Business Media LLC 2017

2 Materials

2.1 Gateway Cloning of gp43 into a Yeast Expression Plasmid

2.1.1 Gateway Vectors

1. Entry vector: pDONR201 (Thermo Fisher).
2. Destination vector: BG1805 (Dharmacon—GE healthcare).

2.1.2 Construction of Expression Vector

1. LR Clonase and BP clonase and buffers (Thermo Fisher).
2. Deoxynucleotide 5′-triphosphates (dNTPs).
3. Platinum High Fidelity *Taq* DNA polymerase (Thermo Fisher).
4. Luria Bertani (LB) broth.
5. Electrocompetent *Escherichia coli* DH10B competent cells.
6. Ultrapure agarose.
7. Primers of 1st PCR (Polymerase Chain Reaction):

   Forward: 5′-*CAAAAAAGCAGGCT* TC **ATG** AAT TTT AGT TCT CTT AAC CTG G- 3′.

   Reverse: 5′-*GTACAAGAAAGCTGGGT* C CCT GCA TCC ACC ATA CTT-3′.

   Gp43 translation start codon is in bold, partial *AttB* sequence is in italics.
8. Primers of 2nd PCR:

   Forward: 5′-*GGGGACAAGTTTGTACAAAAAAGCAGG CTT*-3′.

   Reverse: 5′-*GGGGACCACTTTGTACAAGAAAGCTGG GTC*-3′.
9. Deoxyribonucleic acid (DNA) gel purification kit.
10. Thermal cycler.
11. DNA gel electrophoresis equipment.

2.2 Detection of Expressed Recombinant Protein

1. Lysis buffer: 50 mM Tris–HCl at pH 7.5, 150 mM NaCl, 1 mM EGTA, 10% glycerol, 0.1% Triton X-100, 0.5 mM DTT, 1 mM PMSF, 1× Complete protease inhibitors.
2. Complete Mini, EDTA-free protease inhibitor.
3. 0.5 mm Zirconia/Silica Beads (Biospec Products, INC.).
4. Calf Serum.
5. Rabbit anti-HA antibody.
6. Goat anti-rabbit antibody.
7. ECL Plus Western Blotting.
8. SDS-PAGE and Western blotting transfer equipment.
9. Mini BeadBeater 16-cell disrupter (Biospec Products, INC.).
10. Yeast strain: Y258-MAT**a***pep4-3*, *his4-580*, *ura3-53*, *leu2-3, 112*.

2.3 Inducing Protein Expression with Galactose

All buffers should be prepared with high quality, filtered and endotoxin-free water.

1. SC-ura media: Dissolve 1.7 g of yeast nitrogen base without amino acids, 5 g of ammonium sulfate, 2 g of SC-ura dropout mix, and 20 g of dextrose in H_2O to a final volume of 1 L, and autoclave.
2. SC-ura raffinose media: Dissolve 1.7 g of yeast nitrogen base without amino acids, 5 g of ammonium sulfate, 2 g of SC-ura dropout mix, and 20 g of raffinose in H_2O to a final volume of 1 L, and autoclave.
3. 3× YP + 6% galactose (wt/vol): Dissolve 30 g of yeast extract and 60 g of peptone in 700 mL of H_2O and autoclave. Add 300 mL of sterile 20% galactose solution (wt/vol) under sterile conditions (*see* **Notes 1** and **2**). Mix well and store at 4 °C. Galactose should not be autoclaved.

2.4 Vaccine Preparation and Mice Administration

1. Erlenmeyer flasks of 250 mL and incubator shaker (*see* **Note 3**).
2. Sterile 50 mL conical polypropylene centrifuge tube and centrifuge.
3. Standard phosphate-buffered saline (PBS): suspend 8 g NaCl, 0.2 g KCl, 1.44 g Na_2HPO_4, and 0.24 g KH_2PO_4 in 900 mL of ultrapure water, under vigorous agitation for solubilization. Adjust pH to 7.2 with HCl and make up to 1 L with ultrapure water. Autoclave at 121 °C for 20 min.
4. Trypan blue: 0.4% solution in water.
5. Neubauer Chamber Cell Counting and optical microscope (*see* **Note 4**).
6. Heat plate to kill *Sacharomyces cerevisiae* yeast.
7. Male BALB/c mice (4–6 weeks of age).
8. 1-mL insulin syringe fitted with 29-Gauge 0.5 needle.

2.5 Cultivation of *P. brasiliensis* and Experimental Infection

1. *Paracoccidioides brasiliensis* 18 yeast cells (1×10^6/mice).
2. YPD liquid medium: add 10 g Yeast Extract, 20 g Peptone, and 20 g Dextrose in a glass beaker and solubilize in 900 mL of distilled water. Afterward, adjust the pH to 6.5 with 1 M HCl and make up to 1 L with distilled water. Autoclave at 121 °C for 15 min.
3. Erlenmeyer flasks of 250 mL and incubator shaker (*see* **Note 5**).
4. Sterile 50 mL conical polypropylene centrifuge tube and centrifuge.
5. Trypan blue: 0.4% solution in water.
6. Neubauer Chamber Cell Counting and optical microscope (*see* **Note 6**).

7. Sterile PBS buffer.
8. 1 mL insulin syringe fitted with 29-Gauge 0.5 needle.
9. Male BALB/c mice (4–6 weeks of age).
10. Anesthetics for mice: dissolve ketamine hydrochloride (150 mg/kg) and xylazine hydrochloride (7.5 mg/kg) in sterile PBS buffer, endotoxin-free (*see* **Note 1**).

2.6 Histo-pathological Analysis

1. Gloves.
2. Process/embedding cassettes.
3. Stock phosphate buffer 0.2 M: suspend 5.52 g $NaH_2PO_4.H_2O$ and 22.72 g Na_2HPO_4 in 900 mL of ultrapure water, under vigorous agitation for solubilization. Adjust pH to 7.3 and make up to 1 L with ultrapure water. Filter the solution, using number one filter paper, and store at 4 °C for up to 1 month.
4. 4% Paraformaldehyde solution (*see* **Note 7**): add 4 g of paraformaldehyde in 45 mL of distilled water heated at 55 °C and stir continuously on heat/stir plate for 15 min. Do not allow temperature to exceed 60 °C, because at higher temperature, formic acid decomposition can occur. Add a few drops of 1 N NaOH until solution turns clear (*see* **Note 8**). Filter the solution, using number one filter paper. Complete the volume to 100 mL, using stock phosphate buffer 0.2 M, pH 7.3 (*see* **Note 9**).
5. Absolute ethanol, 95%, 90%, 80%, 70%, and 50% ethanol.
6. Xylene.
7. Paraffin in melting point ranges from 56 to 58 °C (*see* **Note 10**).
8. Microtome, blade, and cover slip.
9. Hematoxylin-eosin (H&E) stain.
10. Grocott's methenamine silver stain [8].
11. Optical microscope equipped with a digital camera.
12. KS-100 software (Carl Zeiss, Germany).

2.7 Assay for Organ Colony-Forming Units (CFU)

1. Sterile falcon round-bottom polystyrene tubes.
2. Sterile PBS buffer.
3. Scales.
4. Tissue homogenizer.
5. Brain heart infusion agar (BHI): Add 37 g of BHI and 15 g of agar in a glass beaker and solubilize in 900 mL of distilled water. Afterward, complete to 1 L with distilled water, and proceed with the autoclave sterilization at 121 °C for 15 min. Next, wait the medium temperature to reach 55 °C and add 4% FBS (*see* **Note 11**) and 100 μg/mL ampicillin or 96 μg/mL gentamicin (*see* **Note 1**).

6. Sterile Petri dishes (90 mm × 15 mm)).
7. Microbiological culture incubator at 37 °C.

2.8 Quantification of Cytokines by ELISA

1. 96-well polypropylene ELISA plates.
2. Microplate reader able to measure absorbance at 450 nm.
3. Precision pipettes and Multichannel pipettor, 50–200 μL, and tips that hold at least 100 μL.
4. Distilled or deionized water.
5. Automated washer.
6. 1.5 mL polypropylene tubes for diluting standards.
7. Plate sealers.
8. Coating buffer: 0.1 M Sodium Carbonate, pH 9.5 or 0.2 M Sodium Phosphate, pH 6.5 (*see* **Note 12**).
9. Assay diluent: PBS with 10% FBS, pH 7.0.
10. Wash buffer: PBS with 0.05% Tween-20 (*see* **Note 13**).
11. Substrate solution: 3,3′,5,5′-tetramethylbenzidine dihydrochloride (TMB) (*see* **Note 14**) and Hydrogen peroxide (*see* **Note 15**).
12. Stop solution: 2 N H_2SO_4.
13. Recombinant cytokines, specific antibodies, and horseradish peroxidase enzyme are from BD OptEIA™ Set Mouse IFN-γ or IL-12(p40) kits.

3 Methods

The methods used for the construction of a yeast strain expressing *P. brasiliensis* gp43 and for the evaluation of this strain as a vaccine against PCM are described in the following sections. The steps are (1) cDNA cloning into a yeast expression vector, (2) yeast transformation and detection of recombinant protein, (3) vaccine preparation and mice administration, (4) cultivation of *P. brasiliensis* and experimental infection, (5) histopathological analysis, (6) assay for organ colony-forming Units (CFU), and (7) quantification of cytokines by ELISA.

3.1 gp43 ORF Cloning into a Yeast Expression Vector, Construction of Expression Plasmid

The cloning method described below uses the commercially available Gateway technology [9] and basic recombinant DNA techniques [10]. The Gateway technology is a method for rapid and efficient transfer of DNA sequences into vectors designed for protein expression. A PCR product is obtained, containing gp43 open reading frame (ORF) flanked with *attB* bacteriophage lambda sequences. By in vitro site-specific recombination (BP reaction), the ORF is transferred to an *attP*-containing entry vector (pDONR201). In a final recombination reaction (LR reaction), the ORF is transferred to a destination vector (BG1805). The resulting yeast plasmid carries the gp43 ORF in an in-frame C-terminal fusion with a tandem affinity tag that includes a hemagglutinin (HA) tag, 6× histidine tag, a protease C cleavage site, and the ZZ domain of protein A. Other relevant features of BG1805 are (1) the ORF is under the control of the *GAL1* promoter, (2) the plasmid carries a *URA3* transformation marker. In principle, the method described can be applied to cloning of any heterologous protein.

1. Perform reverse transcription of *P. brasiliensis* mRNA (RT-PCR) and PCR clone gp43 cDNA into a bacterial plasmid vector. This cDNA will be used as a template in the next PCR reaction (*see* **Note 16**).
2. Perform a 2-step amplification of full-length gp43 coding sequence. The advantage of a 2-step PCR is that there is no need to use long and expensive primers that contain template specific and *attB* sequences. Instead, in the first step template-specific primers containing 14–17 nucleotides of the *attB* sites are used in 15 cycles of PCR to amplify the cDNA. In the second step a portion of the reaction mixture is transferred to a second PCR containing universal *attB* adapter primers to amplify the full *attB* PCR product. The C-terminal primer of the first PCR reaction should include one additional nucleotide to maintain the frame with *attB* and the tandem tag in BG1805 expression vector (*see* **Note 16**).
3. Check the presence and correct size of the PCR product (1.3 kb) by agarose gel electrophoresis.
4. Clean the PCR product. A commercial kit supplied by GE can be used.
5. Perform Gateway BP reaction to transfer the purified fragment coding gp43 into entry vector (pDONR201).
6. Use a portion of the BP reaction (2 μL) to transform DH10B competent cells and plate transformants into kanamycin-containing plates.
7. Purify plasmid DNA from individual kanamycin-resistant colonies.
8. Check the presence of the insert by PCR.
9. Perform Gateway LR reaction to transfer the coding gp43 from the entry vector to the destination vector (BG1805).
10. Repeat **steps 6–8**.
11. Check the construct by sequencing.

3.2 Detection of Expressed Recombinant Protein

Before using as a vaccine, the authors should check if galactose-induced yeast cells are expressing the recombinant gp43 by western blotting. Protocols for yeast transformation with the plasmid harboring the expression construct and selection of URA+ transformants are described elsewhere [11].

1. Transfer the yeast harboring the expression construct to a 10-mL Falcon tube and pellet cells for 1 min at room temperature and 6000 × *g*.
2. Discard the supernatant and resuspend cells with 1 mL 1× PBS.
3. Transfer cells to a 2 mL eppendorf tube and centrifuge for 1 min at room temperature and 6000 × *g*.
4. Harvest cells by centrifugation at 6000 × *g* for 1 min at 4 °C.
5. Discard supernatant and add 1 cell volume of zirconia beads (~300 μL; 0.5 mm) and 2 cell volume of lysis buffer.
6. Disrupt the cells in a Mini BeadBeater 16-cell disrupter using 10 cycles of 20 s beat, 1 min rest (for cooling) in a cold room.
7. Samples are centrifuged (10,000 × *g*, 1 min, 4 °C), and transfer the supernatant to an eppendorf tube.
8. Quantify the protein quantity with the Bradford method.
9. Separate total yeast proteins with 10% SDS-PAGE.
10. Electrotransfer proteins to PVDF, and probe membrane with anti-HA antibody (1:2000). You should detect a 61 kDa recombinant protein (including the 19 kDA tandem fusion tag).

3.3 Inducing Protein Expression with Galactose

1. Grow *S. cerevisiae* cells carrying the construct overnight in SD-uracil, then dilute 1 mL overnight culture into 25 mL SC-uracil +2% raffinose and grow for several hours at 30 °C, followed by dilution into 300 mL SC-ura + raffinose and overnight growth to OD600 1.0.
2. Induce recombinant protein expression by the addition of 150 mL 3× YP + 6% galactose, followed by growth for 6 h; harvest the cells by centrifugation at 3000 × *g*, wash with 5 mL cold H_2O, centrifuge again and store in two aliquots at −70 °C.

3.4 Immunization of Mice

1. Kill the cells by heating at 56 °C during 1 h, and adjust the cell concentration to 2×10^7 yeast/0.1 mL (*see* **Note 4**).
2. Inoculate the *S. cerevisiae* suspension in mice weekly (on days 0, 7, and 14), through intraperitoneal route (i.p.), by using 1 mL insulin syringe (*see* **Notes 17** and **18**) (Fig. 1).

3.5 Experimental Infection with *P. brasiliensis*

1. Grow *P. brasiliensis* yeast (Pb 18 strain) in YPD medium, at 37 °C, 150 rpm, for 10 days (*see* **Note 19**).
2. Harvest the yeast cells by centrifugation at 3000 × *g*, 10 min, 4 °C, and wash twice with sterile PBS buffer (*see* **Note 1**).

3. Suspend the cells with 1 mL sterile PBS buffer and adjust the concentration to 1×10^6 yeast/0.1 mL PBS (*see* **Notes 6** and **20**).
4. 1 week after the last immunization (day 21), anesthetize the BALB/c mice intraperitoneally with 100 μL ketamine hydrochloride and xylazine hydrochloride, and inoculate the *P. brasiliensis* yeast suspension intravenously, through ophthalmic plexus, by using 1 mL insulin syringe (*see* **Note 17**) (Fig. 1).
5. Following infection, add sterile PBS in the eyes of mice to avoid blindness. Afterward, keep the animals in a warm condition until they recover from the anesthesia.
6. On days 30 and/or 60 post-infection, sacrifice mice by cervical dislocation.
7. Remove fragments of the lung and spleen from all mice in order to perform the histopathology analysis (Subheading 3.5), and measure the fungal burden (Subheading 3.6), and the levels of cytokines produced (Subheading 3.7) (*see* **Notes 1** and **21**).

3.6 Histopathological Examination of Infected Mice

1. Collect fragments of the right lobe of the lung from all mice on days 30 and 60 post infection and put them inside appropriated cassettes (*see* **Note 22**).
2. Immerse the cassettes in a bottle, containing 4% paraformaldehyde diluted in 0.1 M phosphate buffer, for fixation, at room temperature (*see* **Notes 23** and **24**).
3. After 12–24 h (*see* **Note 25**), dehydrate the tissues through a series of graded ethanol baths to displace the water, and then embed them in paraffin (*see* **Note 26**).

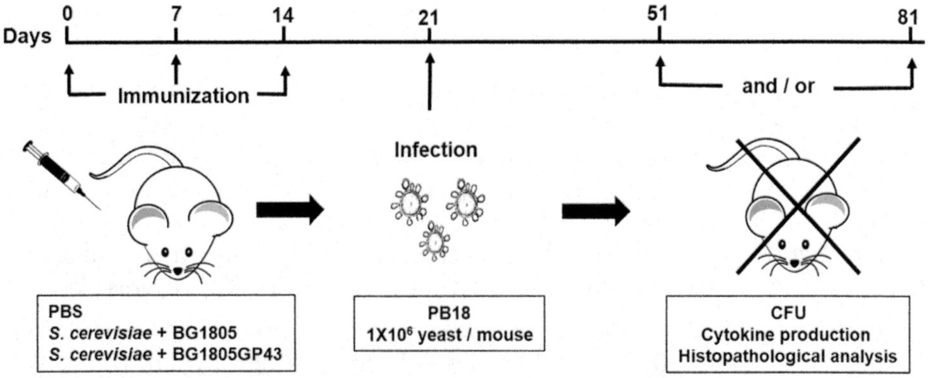

Fig. 1 Protocol of mice immunization and infection with *P. brasiliensis* yeasts. On days 0, 7, and 14, groups of mice were inoculated, through intraperitoneal route, with *S. cerevisiae* yeast carrying the GP43 protein (*S. cerevisiae* BG1805GP43), with *S. cerevisiae* yeast carrying the empty vector (*S. cerevisiae* BG1805), or with buffer alone (PBS). On day 21, all mice were intravenously infected with 1×10^6 *P. brasiliensis* yeast per mouse. Several aspects of the immune response mounted by these mice and the protection conferred by vaccination were evaluated 30 and 60 days post-infection, as summarized in the figure

4. After solidification of the paraffin, cut the tissues into 5-μm-thick-sections, using a microtome (*see* **Note 27**).
5. Pick the tissue sections up with a fine paintbrush and float them on the surface of the 37 °C water bath.
6. Transfer the sections onto the surface of clean glass slides.
7. Place the slides in a 65 °C oven for 20 min (*see* **Note 28**).
8. Afterward, let the slides air-dry at room temperature or dry them up at 56 °C overnight in an oven.
9. Perform the deparaffinization and rehydration of the sections, using xylene, ethanol in decreasing concentrations, and water (*see* **Note 29**).
10. Stain the sections with hematoxylin and eosin (H&E), for the analysis of the inflammatory reactions and granulomas formation.
11. Stain the sections with Grocott's methenamine silver impregnation, to detect polysaccharides in the fungal cell wall, generally localized inside the granulomas.
12. Use an optical microscope equipped with an integrator lens to obtain images of the lung sections and measure the granuloma area (mm^2) by using a KS-100 software.

3.7 Colony-Forming Unit (CFU) Assay

1. Collect aseptically specific fragments of the lung and spleen, and transfer to sterile falcon round-bottom polystyrene tubes, which were previously weighed with 1 mL of sterile PBS buffer.
2. Weigh the tubes again, in order to determine the value of mass of tissue that will be used to calculate the number of colony-forming units (CFU)/mL/g of tissue.
3. Perform the tissue homogenization (*see* **Note 30**) and spread 100 μL into sterile Petri dishes containing BHI agar, supplemented with 4% FBS, plus ampicillin or gentamicin, in duplicate (*see* **Note 31**).
4. Incubate the plates during 7–14 days, at 37 °C (*see* **Notes 32** and **33**).
5. Express the fungal burden as CFU/mL/g of tissue.

3.8 Cytokines Quantification

1. After plating the tissue homogenates for the determination of the CFU, centrifuge the tubes at 2000 × *g*, at 4 °C, for 10 min. Collect the lung and spleen supernatants for cytokines quantification (*see* **Note 34**).
2. Analyze the supernatants by ELISA, according to the manufacturer's instructions (*see* **Note 35**).

4 Notes

1. Perform this procedure only in a clean and confined environment, or ideally, in a sterile laminar flow hood.
2. Sterilize the 20% galactose solution by filtration, using a 0.22-μm filter.
3. Grow *S. cerevisiae* recombinant strains in 100 mL of medium.
4. Dilute *S. cerevisiae* cells in 0.4% Trypan blue solution (1:100) and count, using Neubauer Chamber, for the adjustment of the desired cell concentration.
5. Grow *P. brasiliensis* yeast in 100 mL of medium.
6. Dilute *P. brasiliensis* cells in 0.4% Trypan blue solution (1:100) and count, using Neubauer Chamber, for the adjustment of the desired cell concentration.
7. Paraformaldehyde has to be prepared in fume hood, because of its toxicity.
8. Flocculent material may remain, in a small amount.
9. 4% Paraformaldehyde solution should be freshly prepared.
10. Paraffin can be purchased with melting points at different temperatures, the most common for histological use being about 56 °C–58 °C. At its melting point, it tends to be slightly viscous, but this decreases as the temperature is increased.
11. FBS: Heat inactivated fetal bovine serum.
12. The 0.1 M Sodium Carbonate buffer is used for the quantification of IFN-g, and the 0.2 M Sodium Phosphate is used for IL-12(p40) quantification.
13. PBS-TW buffer: make it fresh or filter-sterilize and store at 4 °C.
14. Dissolve 3,3′,5,5′-tetramethylbenzidine dihydrochloride to 0.75% (w/v) in water and filter to 0.22 μm to remove any undissolved material. Store in 1 mL aliquots at −20 °C.
15. Hydrogen peroxide should be stored at 4 °C, but it has a limited shelf life, and should be replaced every 6 months.
16. The reactions are split into four tubes that are pooled after the PCR to prevent the possible predominance of a mutation that may occur early in one of the PCR reactions.
17. Inoculate 0.1 mL of the cell suspension per mouse.
18. Three groups of mice are used: one group is immunized with recombinant yeast expressing the gp43 protein (yMAgp43; Vaccine group), and the other two groups of mice are used as controls: one group is immunized with yeast cells carrying an empty plasmid (yMA; Vector Group) and the other with vehicle only (PBS Group).

19. The Pb18 isolate is chosen based on its high virulence and ability to induce granulomatous reaction [12].
20. The cells viability is verified using the Trypan blue solution. Only the suspension containing higher than 90% of yeast live should be used for mice inoculation.
21. It is important to collect fragment of the same region of the tissue from all animals for each assay.
22. Cut the tissues to be fixed and processed no thicker than 3 mm.
23. Fixative volume should be adjusted to a ratio of 1/20 (tissue weight per total volume); use 20 mL of 4% paraformaldehyde buffer per 1000 mg of tissue.
24. Place the bottle in a vacuum system, at 25 Hg, during the enough time to make the cassettes, containing floating lung fragments, settle to the bottle bottom. This procedure is extremely important to remove the air from the lungs, allowing its replacement by the fixative.
25. The tissues can become very brittle if the fixation process takes longer than 24 h.
26. The dehydration process is done as follows:

    Solution 1: water—15 s.

    Solution 2: 50% ethanol—1 h.

    Solution 3: 70% ethanol—1 h.

    Solution 4: 80% ethanol—1 h.

    Solution 5: 90% ethanol—1 h.

    Solution 6: absolute ethanol—1 h.

    Solution 7*: absolute ethanol—1 h.

    Solution 8: Clearing reagent (xylene)—1 h.

    Solution 9*: Clearing reagent (xylene)—1 h.

    Solution 10: Paraffin 1–1 h.

    Solution 11*: Paraffin 2–1 h.

    Solution 12*: Paraffin 3–1 h.

    *The repetition of some steps is important occasionally to remove water and/or previous solution.
27. Once the tissue is embedded, it is stable for many years and can be stored at room temperature.
28. During this step, the paraffin starts to melt, and it favors the tissue bonds to the glass.
29. The deparaffinization and rehydration of tissue slides are done as follows:
    (a) Deparaffinize the slides in two changes of xylene for 5 min each.

(b) Transfer the slides to absolute alcohol, make two changes for 3 min each, and transfer once to 95% alcohol for 3 min.

(c) Transfer the slides to 90%, 80%, 70%, and 50% alcohol, respectively.

(d) After rinsing the slides in distilled water they are ready for the staining procedure.

30. Tissue homogenizer speed: 3000 × *g*

31. Dilute 1:10 or 1:100 the homogenized tissue from each mouse in sterile PBS sterile, before plating the 100 μL on BHI agar.

32. Seal the plates with parafilm to avoid medium dryness.

33. Check the plates daily to inspect the growing yeast colonies.

34. Tissues homogenates: use immediately after centrifugation or store at −20 °C.

35. All the assay procedures and buffer preparations were done in accordance with the manufacturer's recommendations of the ELISA (OptEIA set; Pharmingen, San Diego, CA, USA).

References

1. Capilla J, Clemons KV, Liu M, Levine HB, Stevens DA (2009) *Saccharomyces cerevisiae* as a vaccine against coccidioidomycosis. Vaccine 27:3662–3668
2. Liu M, Clemons KV, Johansen ME, Martinez M, Chen V et al (2012) *Saccharomyces* as a vaccine against systemic candidiasis. Immunol Invest 41:847–855
3. Liu M, Capilla J, Johansen ME, Alvarado D, Martinez M et al (2011) *Saccharomyces* as a vaccine against systemic aspergillosis:'the friend of man' a friend again? J Med Microbiol 60:1423–1432
4. Majumder T, Liu M, Chen V, Martinez M, Alvarado D et al (2014) Killed *Saccharomyces cerevisiae* protects against lethal challenge of *Cryptococcus grubii*. Mycopathologia 178: 189–195
5. Luo G, Gebremariam T, Clemons KV, Stevens DA, Ibrahim AS (2014) Heat-killed yeast protects diabetic ketoacidotic-steroid treated mice from pulmonary mucormycosis. Vaccine 32: 3573–3576
6. Assis-Marques MA, Oliveira AF, Ruas LP, dos Reis TF, Roque-Barreira MC et al (2015) *Saccharomyces cerevisiae* expressing Gp43 protects mice against *Paracoccidioides brasiliensis* infection. PLoS One 10:e0120201
7. Ardiani A, Higgins JP, Hodge JW (2010) Vaccines based on whole recombinant *Saccharomyces cerevisiae* cells. FEMS Yeast Res 10:1060–1069
8. Grocott RG (1955) A stain for fungi in tissue sections and smears using Gomori's methenamine-silver nitrate technic. Am J Clin Pathol 25(8):975–979
9. Hartley JL, Temple GF, Brasch MA (2000) DNA cloning using in vitro site-specific recombination. Genome Res 10:1788–1795
10. Green M, Sambrook J (2012) Molecular cloning, a laboratory manual, 4th edn. Cold Spring Harbor Laboratory Press, Cold Spring Harbor, NY
11. Xiao W (ed) (2006) Yeast protocols in molecular biology protocols. Humana Press
12. Kashino SS, Calich VL, Burger E, Singer-Vermes LM (1985) In vivo and in vitro characteristics of six Paracoccidioides brasiliensis strains. Mycopathologia 92(3):173–178

Chapter 15

Vaccination with Phage-Displayed Antigenic Epitope

Yicun Wang and Li Wang

Abstract

Phage-displayed antigenic epitope is able to induce both humoral and cell-mediated immune responses, which could be used as an delivery system to design vaccines without compromising safety and tolerability. Here, we describe the vaccination with phage-displayed antigenic epitope (M13 phage-displayed SLAQVKYTSASSI) against *Candida albicans* infection in BALB/c mice by this method.

Key words Phage display, Vaccine, Epitope

1 Introduction

Phage display technique allows us to insert exogenous DNA into the genes of the coat proteins [1], then the peptides are displayed on the surface of phage coat proteins with natural construction [2, 3]. The filamentous bacteriophages (fl, fd, M13) are commonly used for phage display, which are composed of a single-strand DNA genome and surrounded surface coat proteins [1, 2]. The major coat protein pVIII consists of about 4000 copies on the lateral surface, and five copies of four minor coat proteins (pIII, pVI, pVII, and pIX) located at two filament ends [4, 5]. Since the coat proteins are encoded by the DNA within the phage, the surface of the phage can be genetically modified by fusing a foreign peptide to the N-terminal end of the coat proteins.

The challenge for vaccine development is to design vaccines that induce long-lasting protective immune response without compromising safety and tolerability [6, 7]. Phage particles are naturally immunostimulatory [8], which could be taken up and processed by the MHC class I and II pathways and then activate antigen-specific $CD4^{+}T$ cell, induce the antibody response and prime cytotoxic T lymphocytes (CTL) response [9, 10]. Unlike other virus vectors, phage cannot replicate in a eukaryotic host [11], it has been approved in food safety by FDA. Phage vaccines are cheap, highly stable, and can be produced easily on a large scale.

Markus Kalkum and Margarita Semis (eds.), *Vaccines for Invasive Fungal Infections: Methods and Protocols*, Methods in Molecular Biology, vol. 1625, DOI 10.1007/978-1-4939-7104-6_15, © Springer Science+Business Media LLC 2017

Now, phage is widely used as an antigen delivery system for B and T cell epitopes [12], the immunogenicity of epitopes is enhanced when they are displayed on the phage [13].

Candidaalbicans (*C. albicans*) infection causes high mortality rates within immunocompromised patients [14], it is important to develop an antifungal vaccine. Nevertheless, there are a few experimental vaccines against candidiasis [15]. Only two anti-candida vaccines, NDV-3 and PEV-7, made it to clinical trials, but are not approved for clinical use yet. The secreted aspartyl proteinase 2 (Sap2) plays a protective role in systemically infected BALB/c mice, and peptide SLAQVKYTSASSI was the IgG epitope of Sap2 in *C. albicans*[8]. We displayed the epitope SLAQVKYTSASSI on phage and evaluated whether the phage-displayed epitope represents a potential vaccine candidate without adjuvant [8]. Our result demonstrated that the phage-displayed epitope could be a potential vaccine against *C. albicans* infections, which induced strong immune responses in the animal model (Fig. 1). Here, we introduce the procedure of vaccination with the phage-displayed antigenic epitope.

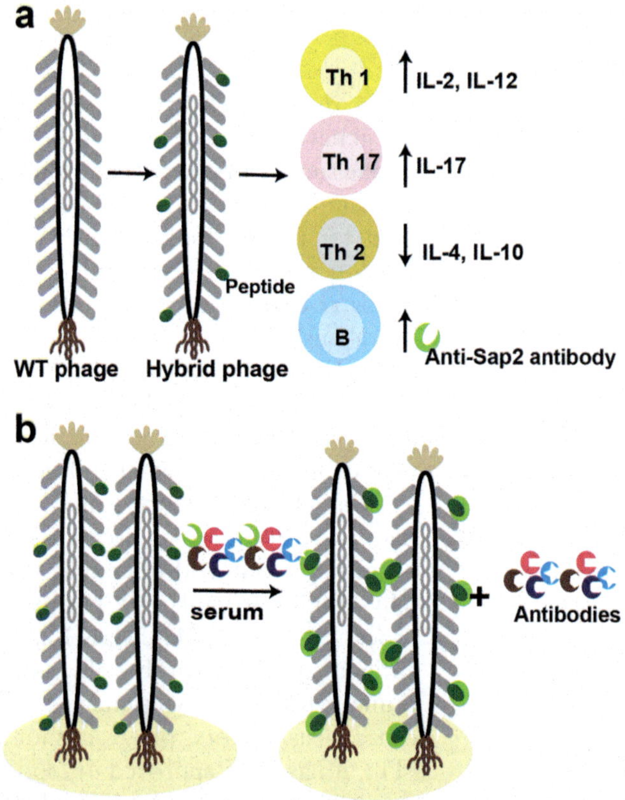

Fig. 1 Schematic of hybrid phage for protection and detection. (**a**) Schematic of WT phage and hybrid phage displayed peptide on the pVIII, and schematic of the host immune response to hybrid phage; (**b**) The peptides on hybrid phage capture anti-Sap2 antibodies

2 Materials

Prepare all the solutions using ultrapure water (prepared by purifying deionized water following Millipore construction) and analytical grade reagents. Prepare and store all the reagents at room temperature (unless otherwise indicated).

2.1 Preparation of Hybrid Phage

1. Phagemid pfd8SHS and wild-type phage.
2. CutSmart® Buffer.
3. Restriction enzymes *SacII* and *Bst*BI (New England Biolabs).
4. T4 DNA ligase kit (New England Biolabs).
5. DNA purification kit (TIANgel Midi Purification Kit).
6. *Escherichia coli* (*E. coli*) strain: TG1.
7. IPTG stock solution (1 M): Dissolve 1.19 g IPTG in 5 ml water, sterilize it through a 0.22 μm filter (*see* **Note 1**), store at −20 °C.
8. Ampicillin stock solution (100 mg/ml): Dissolve 1 g ampicillin in 10 ml water (*see* **Note 2**), sterilize it through a 0.22 μm filter, store at −20 °C.
9. LB medium: Dissolve 10 g yeast extract, 5 g tryptone, and 5 g NaCl in 1 l water, autoclave the medium (*see* **Note 3**), store at 4 °C.
10. PEG6000 (20%)/2.5 M NaCl solution: Dissolve 200 g PEG6000 and 146.1 g NaCl in 1 l water (*see* **Note 4**).
11. TE Buffer: 1.0 mM EDTA, 0.01 M Trisl, adjust pH with HCl to pH 8.0.

2.2 Assessment of Hybrid Phage

1. Blocking solution: Dissolve 5 g non-fat milk powder in 100 ml of TBS buffer (vortex for 1 min). Freshly prepare the solution.
2. SDS-loading buffer: 4% SDS, 20% glycerol, 100 mM Tris–HCl, pH 8.3, 0.2% bromophenol blue.
3. Tris–Tricine buffer: Dissolve 17.9 g Tricine, 12.11 g Tris, 1 g SDS in 1 l water.
4. Antibodies (Sigma): Rabbit anti-mouse antibody, HRP-conjugated Rabbit anti M13 antibody; HRP-conjugated goat anti-human IgG.
5. TBS buffer: 50 mM Tris, 150 mM NaCl, adjust pH with HCl to pH 7.6.
6. TBS-T buffer: 50 mM Tris, 150 mM NaCl, 0.05% Tween 20, adjust pH with HCl to pH 7.6.
7. Silver staining buffer: Dissolve 0.2 g $AgNO_3$ in 200 ml water, and keep in a dark place (*see* **Note 5**).
8. Stationary buffer I: Add 100 ml methyl alcohol and 10 ml acetic acid in water to 200 ml.

9. Stationary buffer II: Add 10 ml methyl alcohol and 10 ml acetic acid in water to 200 ml.
10. Developing solution: Add 8.16 g sodium carbonate anhydrous and 120 μl oxymethylene into 200 ml water (*see* **Note 6**).
11. Nitrocellulose membranes.
12. Tris/glycine buffer: Dissolve 5.8 g Tris, 2.9 g glycine, 0.37 g SDS, and 200 ml methyl alcohol in water to make 1000 ml.
13. 3-amino-9-ethylcarbozole (AEC) reagent: Dissolve AEC 1 mg in 1 ml DMF, add into 2 ml 0.025 mol/l sodium acetate solution, before developing, add 10 ul 30%H_2O_2.

2.3 Immunization

1. PBS buffer (10× stock): Dissolve 2.4 g KH_2PO_4, 14.1 g $Na_2HPO_4{\cdot}H_2O$, 2 g KCl and 80 g NaCl in 1 l water. This buffer gives a pH of 7.4 when diluted to 1× PBS (*see* **Note 7**).
2. PBS-T: Add 100 ml of 10× PBS and 500 μl Tween 20– into 900 ml water.
3. YPD medium: Dissolve 10 g yeast extract, 10 g tryptone, and 20 g glucose in 1000 ml water, autoclave the medium (*see* **Note 8**).
4. Female BALB/c mice: Between 6 and 8 weeks of age, purchased from the Specific-Pathogen-Free Animal Facility.
5. *C. albicans* ATCC10231: Culture *C. albicans* on YPD medium for 16 h at 28 °C. Collect the yeast cells and adjust the concentration (2×10^8cells/ml) for infecting mouse.
6. LB solid media: Dissolve 10 g tryptone, 5 g yeast extract, 10 g NaCl, 15 agar in 1000 ml water, autoclave the medium.

2.4 Assessment of Cell Proliferation

1. Sterile PBS.
2. 100-gauge wire mesh sieve.
3. Centrifuge.
4. Flat-bottom 96-well plates.
5. RPMI 1640 medium supplemented with 10% FBS.
6. CO_2 incubator at 37 °C.
7. MTT (5 mg/ml): Add 5 mg MTT into 1 ml sterile PBS to mix by vortexing or sonication until dissolved (*see* **Note 9**).
8. DMSO.
9. Microplate Reader.

2.5 Challenge

1. *C. albicans* conidial suspension.
2. Glass pestle.
3. Sterile saline.
4. YPD solid medium.

3 Methods

Carry out all procedures at room temperature unless otherwise specified.

3.1 Preparation of Recombinant Phagemid

1. Digest plasmid pfd8SHS in CutSmart® Buffer at 37 °C with SacII, then add *Bst*BI and raise temperature to 65 °C, follow the manufacturer's instruction.
2. Purificiate enzyme-digested plasmid by TIANgel Midi Purification Kit, follow the manufacturer's instruction.
3. Synthesize and anneal complementary oligonucleotides encoding the epitope SLAQVKYTSASSI(5′-GGAGGGTTCTTTGG CTCAAGTCAAATATACTTCTGCTTCCAGTATTCCAT-3′,5′-CGATGGAATACTGGAAGCAGAAGTATATTTG ACTTGAGCCAAAGAACCCTCCGC-3′) (*see* **Note 10**).
4. Mix the digested vector with the synthetic exogenous DNA fragments at a molar concentration of 1: 3 in a total reaction volume of 10 μl at 16 °C in T4 DNA Ligase Reaction Buffer over night, follow the manufacturer's instruction.

3.2 Transfection

1. Add 10 μl recombinant phagemid into 100 μl of competent TG1 cells, place the cell on ice for 30 min.
2. Place the cell in 42 °C water bath for 90 s (*see* **Note 11**), then quickly transfer to the ice bath for 2 min, add 800 μl LB broth, culture at 37 °C for 45 mins, shake at 100 rpm/min.
3. Centrifuge (5000 × *g*) for 5 min, discard the supernatant, culture remaining part on an LB solid media containing 100 μg/ml ampicillin, 37 °C overnight.
4. Select single colony, inoculate to 2 ml LB medium containing 100 μg/ml ampicillin, 37 °C overnight, and sequence DNA.

3.3 Production of Hybrid Phage

Phage was prepared based on a procedure described by P. Malik [16].

1. Take transformed cells with correct insertion recombinant phagemid on LB plates (100 μg/ml ampicillin).
2. Inoculate the colony to 3 ml LB medium containing 100 μg/ml ampicillin, 37 °C overnight.
3. Transfer 0.5 ml of the culture into 100 ml LB medium with ampicillin (100 μg/ml) and wild-type phage (5 ng) for 4 h at 37 °C (*see* **Note 12**), shake at 200 rpm/min.
4. Centrifuge the culture at 2000 × *g* for 10 min, resuspend the bacteria pellet in 100 ml of fresh LB medium (1 mM IPTG), incubate overnight at 37 °C (*see* **Note 13**).
5. Centrifuge at 8000 × *g* for 10 min at 4 °C, recover phage particles in the culture supernatants, and purify it in polyethylene

glycol-6000 (final concentration 5% polyethylene glycol-6000, 0.5 M NaCl) by two consecutive precipitations for 12 h.

6. Centrifuge at 8000 × *g* for 30 min 4 °C, resuspend phage pellet in 20 ml TE buffer.
7. Centrifuge at 12,000 × *g* for 20 min at 4 °C, discard the precipitate, and add 5 ml PEG6000 (20%)/2.5 M NaCl solution into supernatant, 4 °C stand for 5 h.
8. Centrifuge at 12,000 × *g* for 20 min at 4 °C, resuspend phage pellet in 1 ml TE buffer.
9. Estimate the amount of phage by spectrophotometry, which an OD of 1.0 at 270 nm represents a concentration (μg/μl) of 1/3.84.

3.4 Assessment of Hybrid Protein

1. Boil phage samples for 5 min in an equal volume of loading buffer.
2. Subject the 30 μg phage samples to 20% SDS-PAGE using Tris–Tricine buffer, 80 V for 1 h and 120 V for 2.5 h according to the method described previously [17].
3. Incubate the gel in stationary Buffer I for 1 h.
4. Incubate the gel in stationary Buffer II for 1 h.
5. Wash the gel five times by water, and silver stain the gel by incubation in the silver staining buffer for 30 min in a dark place (*see* **Note 14**).
6. Develop the gel by 50 ml developing solution for 30 s, and exchange 150 ml developing solution until band presenting (*see* **Notes 15** and **16**) (Fig. 2).

Fig. 2 SDS-PAGE for hybrid phage and WT phage. Lane 1, WT phage, lane 2, Hybrid phage [8]

7. Perform western blotting with patient sera containing an antibody to *C. albicans* or healthy individual sera to test antigenicity of the phage-displayed epitope SLAQVKYTSASSI, according to the method described by Matthews et al. [18].
8. Transblot the separated proteins onto nitrocellulose membrane in Tris/glycine buffer, 60 V for 4 h.
9. Wash the nitrocellulose membrane by TBS.
10. Block nitrocellulose membrane overnight at 4 °C in blocking solution.
11. After washing four times with TBS-T, incubate the nitrocellulose membrane with diluted serum in TBST-5% nonfat milk at 37 °C for l h.
12. After further washing, incubate the membrane with peroxidase-conjugated IgG at 37 °C for 1 h, stain with AEC reagent as a chromogen until the band presenting.

3.5 Immunization

1. Select no-pregnant female BALB/c mice (18–20 g) (6–8 weeks).
2. Using a 22-G needle, inject mice intraperitoneally four times (*see* **Note 17**) at weekly intervals, with 25 μg hybrid phage particles mixed in 100 μl TE.
3. Collect 100 μl blood, 7 days after every immunization by cutting the tail with sterile sharp scissors (*see* **Note 18**), and get the serum for determining the antibody titer by ELISA (Fig. 3) and western blotting. Coat the ELISA with rSap2. The titer was given as the reciprocal of the highest dilution with an OD450 that was 2.5-fold greater than the OD of TE treated mice sera at the same dilution [8].

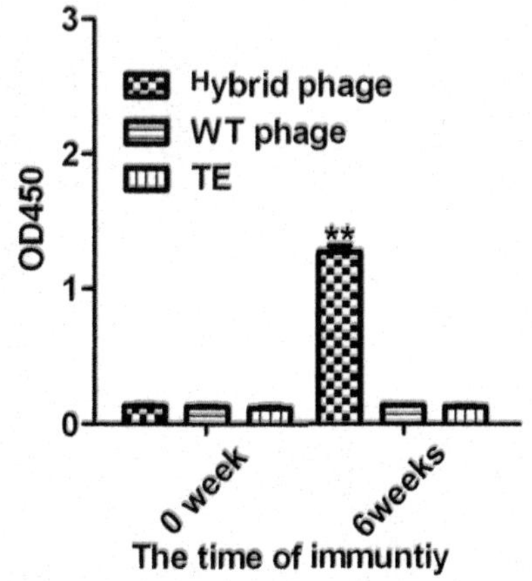

Fig. 3 IgG determination by ELISA. Serum IgG responses in mice vaccinated with hybrid, WT phage on weeks 0 and 6. Sera were collected on 1 day prior to each immunization, and tested by ELISA using rSap2. The titer was given as the reciprocal of the highest dilution with an OD450 that was 2.5-fold greater than the OD of TE treated mice sera at the same dilution [8]

3.6 Cell Proliferation

1. One week after the last immunization, collect spleen tissues from mice, wash with PBS, and tease the spleen gently using a sterile needle and forceps from the tissue under aspetic condition, and prepare single-cell suspension by passage through a 100-gauge wire mesh sieve.
2. Centrifuge at 1000 × *g* for 5 min at 4 °C, discard the supernatant, collect cells, and count cells by using a small aliquot of cell suspension.
3. Culture the cells in triplicate wells of flat-bottom 96-well plates at a concentration of 2.5×10^4 cells/ml in 200 μl RPMI 1640 medium (10% FBS) alone or in medium containing a pool of hybrid phage (25 μg/ml), incubate plates in a humidifier CO_2 incubator at 37 °C for 72 h.
4. Add 20 μl MTT (5 mg/ml) to all wells and incubate for 4 h at 37 °C.
5. Pipette out the spent media along with suspension of cultured cells, add DMSO (150 μl/well), and mix to dissolve the formazan crystals, then measure the absorbance by using a Microplate Reader at 492 nm (Fig. 4).

3.7 Challenge

1. Mice are immunized three times, 2 weeks after the final immunization, inject mice with 10^6 *C. albicans* by tail intravenous injection.
2. Seven days after the infection, sacrifice mice, remove and weigh the kidney and spleen under aspetic condition.

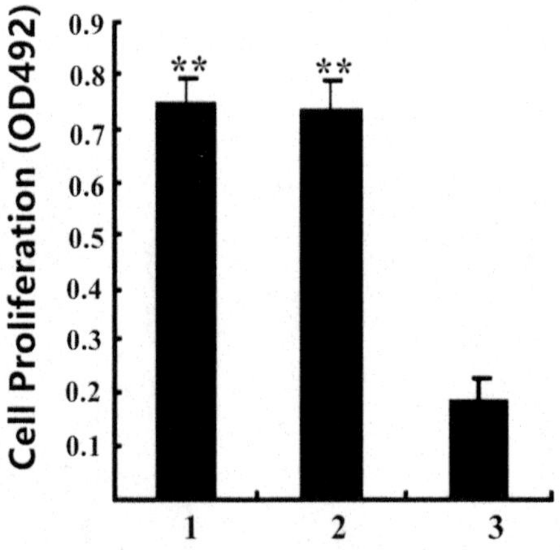

Fig. 4 Splenocytes proliferation measured by MTT. Cells were seeded into a 96-well plate with the density of 5×10^3 cells per well and cultured with stimulus at 37 °C. The MTT assay was performed after 72 h. The data shown are means ± SD of three independent experiments. Group 1, hybrid phage immunized mice; group 2, WT phage immunized mice; group 3, TE injected mice. **Statistically significant ($P < 0.01$) [8]

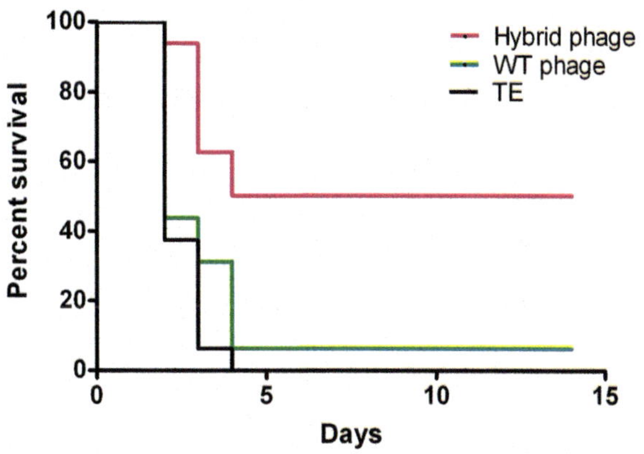

Fig. 5 Hybrid phage was used to induce protection against *C. albicans* infection. Percent survival in mice immunized with different immunogens. Eight mice of each group were inoculated with 10^7 *C. albicans* after the final immunization. The survival rates were evaluated for 15 days after challenge [8]

3. Grind up the samples using glass pestle, dilute the homogenate using normal saline (1:100) and culture 100 μl diluent on YPD solid medium 20 °C for 48 h, count the colony-forming units.
4. Two weeks after the final immunization, inject mice with 10^7 *C. albicans* by tail intravenous injection, observe and calculate survival for 15 days (Fig. 5).

4 Notes

1. IPTG is used to induce the expression of cloned genes, and the aliquots can be stored at −20 °C for at least 1 year.
2. For bacteria use the final working concentration (in media) of ampicillin is 100 μg/ml, aliquots can be stored at −20 °C for at least 1 year.
3. The LB medium can be stored for up to 6 months at 4 °C or for 1 month at RT, when preparing the LB medium with ampicillin, cool down the medium until it is cool enough to be held in the hands (about 40 °C), and then add the ampicillin.
4. Dissolving PEG and NaCl requires stirring for several hours. If using a glass beaker, it can be dissolved faster when the water is warmed to about 37 °C.
5. Prepare and precool silver staining buffer when it will be used; it needs to be fresh each time.
6. Prepare and precool the developing solution when it will be used, it is best to be fresh each time.
7. Autoclave the buffer and store it for months at RT.

8. YPD medium can be stored for up to 6 months at 4 °C or for 1 month at RT.
9. Occasionally, there may be some particulate material that will not dissolve; this can be removed by filtration or centrifugation. Once prepared, the MTT solution can be stored for 4 weeks at 4 °C protected from light.
10. The oligonucleotides should be designed to avoid forming large secondary structures (hairpins), or it will not be annealed to ligate into the vector.
11. The temperature and time are performed strictly, or it will fail to transfect the phagemid to the competent cells.
12. The time cannot be more than 4 h.
13. The time cannot be more than 16 h.
14. Avoid touching gel when sliver staining.
15. If developing solution turns yellow, which often appears within 30 s, discard and replace with fresh 150 ml developing solution.
16. Expression of the epitope by hybrid phage is analyzed by SDS-PAGE, and bands are revealed by silver-staining. If the hybrid protein is successfully expressed, two bands appear on the sheet. Top band is hybrid protein with epitope, and the bottom is the wild-type filamentous phage coat protein band.
17. Mice need to be immunized three or four times, 7 days after every immunization, detect the antibody titer, stop immunizing when antibody titer is more than 10,000.
18. To collect blood plasma, use tubes that contain EDTA as an anticoagulant (5 μl of 0.1 M EDTA for 100 μl of blood) and place on ice. Spin whole blood samples at 2100 × *g* in a refrigerated centrifuge (4 °C) for 10 min within 10 min of collection. Separate the plasma, avoiding disturbing the red and white blood cell layers.

References

1. Smith GP (1985) Filamentous fusion phage: novel expression vectors that display cloned antigens on the virion surface. Science 228(4705):1315–1317
2. Marvin D, Hale R, Nave C, Citterich MH (1994) Molecular models and structural comparisons of native and mutant class I filamentous bacteriophages: Ff (fd, f1, M13), If1 and IKe. J Mol Biol 235(1):260–286
3. Scott JK, Smith GP (1990) Searching for peptide ligands with an epitope library. Science 249(4967):386–390
4. Fuh G, Sidhu SS (2000) Efficient phage display of polypeptides fused to the carboxy-terminus of the M13 gene-3 minor coat protein. FEBS Lett 480(2–3):231–234
5. Weiss GA, Roth TA, Baldi PF, Sidhu SS (2003) Comprehensive mutagenesis of the C-terminal domain of the M13 gene-3 minor coat protein: the requirements for assembly into the bacteriophage particle. J Mol Biol 332(4):777–782
6. Koff WC, Johnson PR, Watkins DI, Burton DR, Lifson JD, Hasenkrug KJ, McDermott AB, Schultz A, Zamb TJ, Boyle R (2006) HIV vaccine design: insights from live attenuated SIV vaccines. Nat Immunol 7(1):19–24
7. Bachmann MF, Jennings GT (2010) Vaccine delivery: a matter of size, geometry, kinetics

and molecular patterns. Nat Rev Immunol 10(11):787–796

8. Wang Y, Su Q, Dong S, Shi H, Gao X, Wang L (2014) Hybrid phage displaying SLAQVKYTSASSI induces protection against *Candida albicans* challenge in BALB/c mice. Hum Vaccin Immunother 10(4):1057–1063
9. Del Pozzo G, Mascolo D, Sartorius R, Citro A, Barba P, D'Apice L, De Berardinis P (2010) Triggering DTH and CTL activity by fd filamentous bacteriophages: role of CD4+ T cells in memory responses. Biomed Res Int 2010:894971
10. Prisco A, De Berardinis P (2012) Filamentous bacteriophage fd as an antigen delivery system in vaccination. Int J Mol Sci 13(4): 5179–5194
11. Jepson CD, March JB (2004) Bacteriophage lambda is a highly stable DNA vaccine delivery vehicle. Vaccine 22(19):2413–2419
12. Fehr T, Skrastina D, Pumpens P, Zinkernagel RM (1998) T cell-independent type I antibody response against B cell epitopes expressed repetitively on recombinant virus particles. Proc Natl Acad Sci 95(16):9477–9481
13. di Marzo VF, Willis AE, Boyer-Thompson C, Appella E, Perham RN (1994) Structural mimicry and enhanced immunogenicity of peptide epitopes displayed on filamentous bacteriophage. The V3 loop of HIV-1 gp120. J Mol Biol 243(2):167–172
14. Vonk AG, Netea MG, van der Meer JW, Kullberg BJ (2006) Host defence against disseminated *Candida albicans* infection and implications for antifungal immunotherapy. Expert Opin Biol Ther 6(9):891–903
15. Cassone A, Casadevall A (2012) Recent progress in vaccines against fungal diseases. Curr Opin Microbiol 15(4):427–433
16. Malik P, Terry TD, Gowda LR, Langara A, Petukhov SA, Symmons MF, Welsh LC, Marvin DA, Perham RN (1996) Role of capsid structure and membrane protein processing in determining the size and copy number of peptides displayed on the major coat protein of filamentous bacteriophage. J Mol Biol 260(1):9–21
17. Schägger H, Von Jagow G (1987) Tricine-sodium dodecyl sulfate-polyacrylamide gel electrophoresis for the separation of proteins in the range from 1 to 100 kDa. Anal Biochem 166(2):368–379
18. Matthews RC, Burnie JP, Tabaqchali S (1987) Isolation of immunodominant antigens from sera of patients with systemic candidiasis and characterization of serological response to *Candida albicans*. J Clin Microbiol 25(2): 230–237

Chapter 16

Preparation of an Oral Vaccine by Proteome Analysis and Molecular Display Technology

Seiji Shibasaki and Mitsuyoshi Ueda

Abstract

In recent years, genetic engineering and protein expression technologies have promoted the development of recombinant protein vaccines. To accelerate the development of efficient vaccines for mycosis, screening candidate antigens, and determining the optimal route of administration are indispensable steps. Two methods for identifying novel antigens and producing antigens specific to *Candida albicans*, as a model causative pathogen of mycosis, are discussed in this chapter. Specifically, the application of liquid chromatography/tandem mass spectrometry using a long monolithic column for proteome analysis to identify virulence factors of *C. albicans*, followed by molecular display technology to produce an oral vaccine using antigens found by the proteomic study, is described.

Key words Oral vaccine, Molecular display, *Saccharomyces cerevisiae*, *Lactobacillus casei*, LC-MS/MS, Proteome analysis, Cell surface, *Candida albicans*

1 Introduction

The use of recombinant proteins is a route for vaccine development that presents an alternative to the use of attenuated virulent organisms. For example, vaccines for hepatitis B virus and human papilloma virus are made using genes from each pathogen to produce antigens, which generate a protective immune response. Each gene is inserted into an expression system capable of producing the protein antigen. The gene for the hepatitis B virus antigen has been inserted into yeast cells, which produce large quantities of the antigen [1]. However, these conventional methods need several complicated steps to recover the antigen from the protein fraction of microbial cells to produce an efficient and high-purity vaccine. On the other hand, the development of mycosis vaccines first requires the identification of efficient antigenic proteins, because no clinically efficient antigen has yet become available. This chapter describes technologies that can be applied to find a novel antigen and conveniently produce the antigen for the development of a mycosis vaccine.

Markus Kalkum and Margarita Semis (eds.), *Vaccines for Invasive Fungal Infections: Methods and Protocols*, Methods in Molecular Biology, vol. 1625, DOI 10.1007/978-1-4939-7104-6_16, © Springer Science+Business Media LLC 2017

1.1 Screening for Antigens Using Proteomics

In recent years, new approaches to the study of vaccine development have involved screening for antigenic proteins. For instance, a proteomic analysis of hyphal induction as an infectious phenotype in *Candida albicans* identified characteristic cell wall protein profiles [2]. In another study, the virulent protein of *C. albicans* cultured in serum was examined by liquid chromatography/tandem mass spectrometry (LC-MS/MS) using a long monolithic capillary column [3]. For this analysis, *C. albicans* was cultured in fetal bovine serum (FBS) for 0–180 min, and the time-dependent variations of protein abundance in the cultured cells were quantified by LC-MS/MS. A clustering analysis of the results identified some FBS-induced proteins that were associated with virulence factors.

1.2 Molecular Display Technology

We can choose a convenient tool for the preparation of antigenic proteins using an engineered microbial cell surface. This approach is called "cell surface engineering" or "molecular display technology" [4–6]. In general, the method involves the genetic fusion of a heterologous protein to a cell wall protein, which results in the hybrid protein being displayed on the microbial cell surface. The use of molecular display technology to produce target proteins has recently been especially well established for use with *Saccharomyces cerevisiae* and *Lactobacillus casei*. *S. cerevisiae* and *Lactobacillus* species are organisms that are "generally recognized as safe" for human consumption, and engineered cells of these strains can be used to prepare oral vaccines without purification, unlike recombinant proteins produced in *Escherichia coli* [7].

Interestingly, the oral delivery of yeast cells that displayed Eno1p on their surfaces (Fig. 1a) protected 60% of mice against candidiasis [8]. A similar study of *L. casei* also suggested that the molecular display of antigenic proteins on microbial cell surfaces (Fig. 1b) has a high potential to generate oral vaccines against infectious diseases [9]. For the application of molecular display technology, the only requirement is the availability of a DNA sequence that encodes the antigenic protein; no purification step is needed to produce oral vaccines (Fig. 2).

2 Materials

2.1 Strains

1. *C. albicans* strain SC5314 (American Type Culture Collection, Manassas, VA, USA).
2. *S. cerevisiae* strain BY4741 (*MATα his3-1 leu2 met15 ura3*) (GE Healthcare, Little Chalfont, UK).
3. *Lactobacillus casei* strain 525 [10].

2.2 Vectors and Primers

1. pULD1 *S. cerevisiae* expression vector [8].
2. pKV-Pald-pgsA380L *L. casei* expression vector [10].

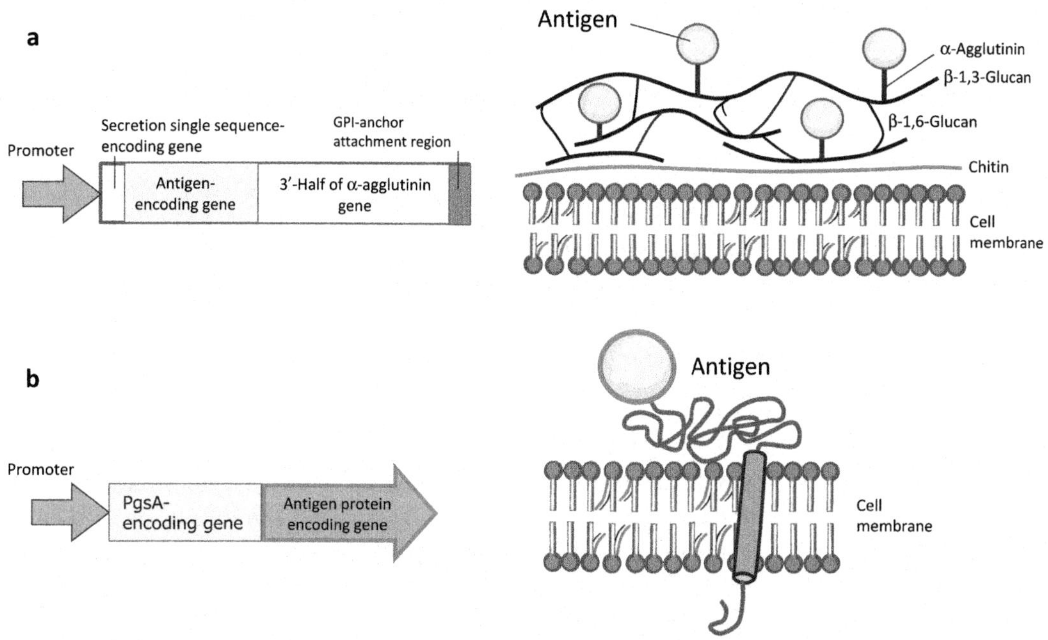

Fig. 1 Strategies for molecular display and cell architectures. (**a**) *S. cerevisiae* cell surface display. (**b**) *L. casei* surface display

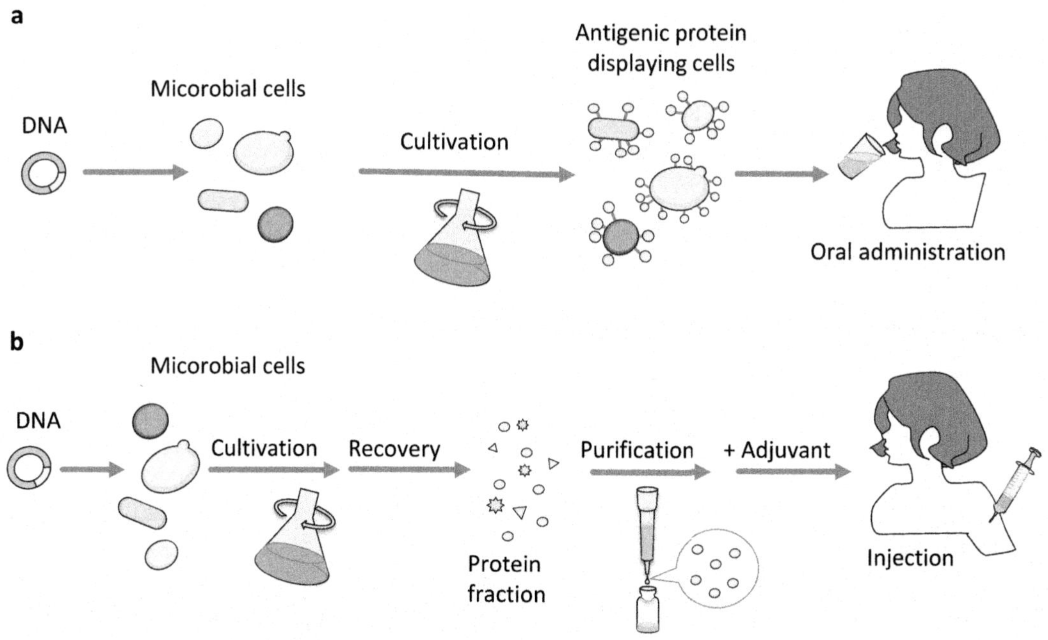

Fig. 2 Oral vaccines by molecular display technology and conventional recombinant vaccines

3. Primers for yeast display; ENO1-ydF (5′-ACGCGGCCGCTCTTACGCCACTAAAATCCACGCC-3′) and ENO1-ydR (5′-TGCTCGAGCAATTGAGAAGCCTTTTGGAAATCTTTACC-3′).
4. Primers for yeast display; ENO1-LDF (5′-CGGGATCCATGTCTTACGCCACTAAAATCCAC-3′) and ENO1-LDR (5′-GCTCTAGATTACAATTGAGAAGCCTTTTGGAAATCTTTACC-3′).

2.3 Media and Buffers

1. Yeast extract–peptone–dextrose (YPD) medium: 1% (w/v) yeast extract, 2% (w/v) glucose, and 2% (w/v) peptone.
2. Fetal bovine serum (FBS).
3. Phosphate-buffered saline.
4. SDC medium: 2% (w/v) glucose, 0.67% (w/v) yeast nitrogen base without amino acids, 1% (w/v) casamino acids, and supplemented with appropriate amino acids.

2.4 Reagents

1. Lysis buffer: 4% (w/v) 3-(3-cholamidepropyl)dimethyl ammonio-1-propanesulfonate, 1% (w/v) dithiothreitol, 1% (v/v) protease inhibitor cocktail, 7 M urea, and 2 M thiourea.
2. 200 mM triethyl ammonium bicarbonate (TEAB).
3. 200 mM Tris-(2-carboxyethyl) phosphine.
4. 375 mM iodoacetamide.
5. TMT (tandem mass tag) 6-plex labeling kit (Thermo Fisher Scientific, Waltham, MA, USA).
6. Sequencing-grade modified trypsin (Promega, Madison, WI, USA).
7. Protein Assay Bicinchoninate Kit (Nacalai Tesque, Kyoto, Japan).

2.5 Equipment

1. BeadSmash 12® cell disruptor.
2. 0.5 mm glass beads.
3. LC-MS/MS: LC (UltiMate® 3000; Thermo Fisher Scientific); MS (LTQ Orbitrap Velos™; Thermo Fisher Scientific).

3 Methods

3.1 Protein Preparation for Proteome Analysis

1. Precultivate *C. albicans* in 300 mL YPD media for 24 h. Collect *C. albicans* cells (5 g wet weight) by centrifugation at 4000 × *g* for 5 min at 25 °C and resuspend in fresh 300 mL YPD media. Incubate the cells for 2 h at 37 °C to maintain the exponential growth phase (Fig. 3a).

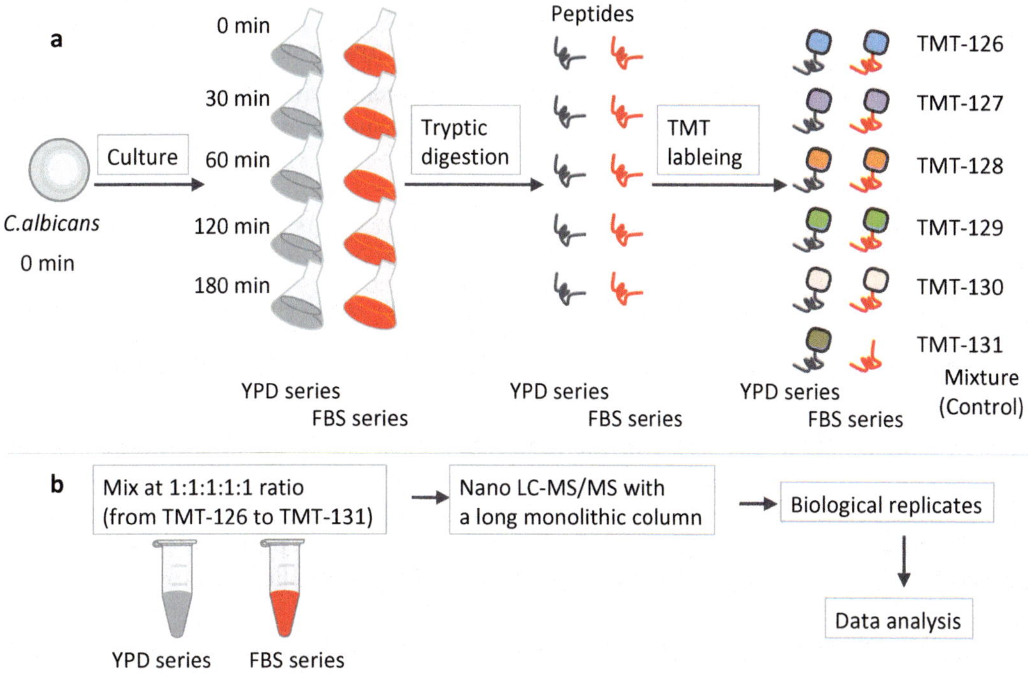

Fig. 3 Workflow of the identification of proteins. (**a**) Steps are shown from cultivation to TMT-labeling of tryptic digests of samples from the 0, 30, 60, 120, and 180 min time points in the YPD and FBS series. (**b**) Steps are shown after TMT-labeling to data analysis

2. Collect *C. albicans* cells and transfer to 50 mL buffered YPD media or FBS (30 mg wet weight of cells/mL). Immediately shake the media for 0, 30, 60, 120, and 180 min at 37 °C (*see* **Note 1**).
3. After incubation, cool each cell sample in ice-cold water and centrifuge at 7000 × *g* for 2 min at 4 °C.
4. Wash the collected cells twice with PBS to eliminate serum proteins (*see* **Note 2**).
5. Resuspend cells in 700 μL lysis buffer. Mix the solution with 200 mg of 0.5-mm glass beads and disrupt mechanically ten times using a BeadSmash 12® cell disruptor at 4 °C with 4000 agitations per minute for 1 min.
6. Centrifuge the solution at 3000 × *g* for 15 min at 4 °C, and collect the supernatant.
7. Mix each supernatant (350 μL) with 135 μL of 200 mM TEAB and 30 μL of 200 mM Tris-(2-carboxyethyl) phosphine. Incubate the solution at 55 °C for 1 h for reduction.
8. Add 60 μL of 375 mM iodoacetamide to the solution and incubate for 30 min.

9. Mix the reactant with 4 mL of ice-cold acetone and incubate at −20 °C for 2 h to precipitate the proteins.
10. Resuspend precipitated proteins with 100 μL of TEAB and mix with 2 μL of 1 μg/μL sequencing grade modified trypsin at 37 °C for 12 h.

3.2 TMT Labeling

1. Dissolve the TMT-labeling reagents in 41 μL of acetonitrile and mix with 30 μL of each tryptic digest.
2. Quench the reactants by the addition of 8 μL of 5% (w/v) hydroxylamine and then lyophilize after mixing the six solutions in either the YPD or FBS series labeled with TMT-126 to TMT-131 together in a 1:1:1:1:1:1 ratio (Fig. 3b).
3. Reconstitute the dried samples in 90 μL of 0.1% (v/v) formic acid.

3.3 LC–MS/MS Analysis

1. Inject tryptic digests and separate peptides by reversed-phase chromatography using a long monolithic silica capillary column (*see* **Note 3**).
2. Produce a solvent gradient by changing the mixing ratio of the two eluents: A, 0.1% (v/v) formic acid; and B, 80% (v/v) acetonitrile containing 0.1% (v/v) formic acid.
3. Start the gradient with 5% B and increase to 45% B over 600 min, then further increase to 95% B to wash the column.
4. Observe the separated analytes by MS with a full-scan range of 350–1500 m/z in the positive mode followed by 10 data-dependent high-energy C-trap dissociation (HCD) MS/MS scans acquired for TMT reporter ions.
5. Apply an ESI voltage of 2.4 kV directly to the LC buffer distal to the chromatography column using a MicroTee. Use a normalized collision energy of 80% for HCD scans with an activation time of 0.1 ms. Set the ion-transfer tube temperature on the LTQ Velos™ ion trap to 300 °C.
6. Proteome Discoverer™ 1.2 (Thermo Fisher Scientific) can be used for protein quantification. Protein identification can be performed using MASCOT (Matrix Science, London, UK) with the assembly database at the *Candida* Genome Database [11].

3.4 Plasmid Construction for Yeast Surface Antigen Display

1. To construct the pULD-eno1 plasmid for the display of Eno1p (*C. albicans* antigen protein) from pULD1, amplify the *Eno1p* coding sequence by polymerase chain reaction (PCR) using the primers ENO1-ydF and ENO1-ydR and the genomic DNA of *C. albicans*.
2. Insert the fragment of the gene encoding *ENO1* into the pULD1 plasmid. The resulting plasmid is referred to as pULD-eno1 in the following sections (Fig. 4a) (*see* **Note 4**).

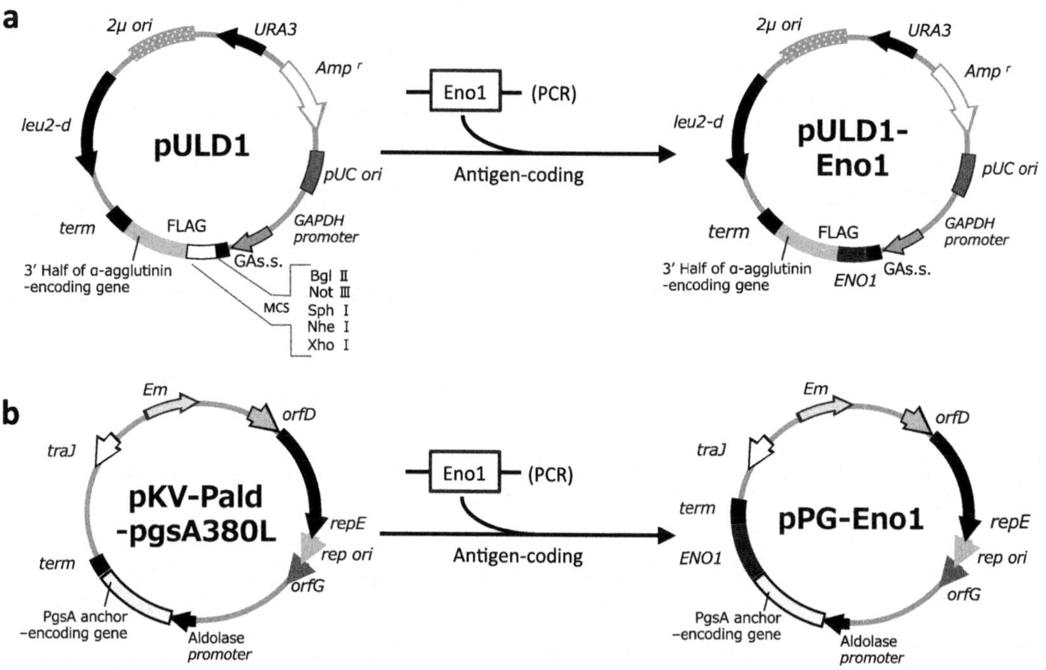

Fig. 4 Construction of plasmids for the microbial surface display of antigens. (**a**) Plasmid for *S. cerevisiae* cell surface display. (**b**) Plasmid for *L. casei* surface display

3. Introduce the pULD1-eno1 plasmid and parent pULD1 plasmid (as a control) into *S. cerevisiae* using the lithium acetate method [12] to achieve the surface display of the antigenic protein Eno1p.
4. Select the cells harboring these plasmids using uracil-deficient SDC (SDC-ura) medium.

3.5 Plasmid Construction for L. casei Surface Antigen Display

1. Amplify the *ENO1* gene by PCR with the primers ENO1-LDF and ENO1-LDR and the genomic DNA of *C. albicans.*
2. Insert the *ENO1* PCR product into pKV-Pald-pgsA380L. The resulting plasmid is referred to as pPG-eno1 in the following sections (Fig. 4b) (*see* **Note 4**).
3. Introduce the constructed plasmid (pPG-eno1) into *L. casei* 525 using the previously described electroporation protocol for microorganisms [9].
4. To assess the transformation of *L. casei* with the recombinant plasmid, select colonies and perform PCR with primers flanking a region on the PgsA-Eno1-FLAG sequence.

3.6 Oral Administration of Cells Displaying C. albicans Antigen

1. Select a colony of cells harboring a plasmid for an antigenic protein on the cell surface and place it in SDC-ura liquid medium.
2. Cultivate cells in SDC-ura liquid medium at 30 °C overnight.

3. Take 1 mL of cultivated liquid medium and pour it into fresh SDC-ura liquid medium. Cultivate cells at 30 °C overnight.
4. Collect yeast cells by centrifugation at 6000 × *g* for 5 min.
5. Wash the cell pellet with PBS and store at 4 °C until administration.
6. Check the display of Eno1p by immunofluorescence staining (Fig. 5) [8].
7. Adjust the concentration of *S. cerevisiae* or *L. casei* cells displaying Eno1p on their surfaces to 1.6×10^9 cells in 400 μL using PBS.
8. Administer solutions to mice at weeks 0, 1, and 3 (priming) and at week 7 (booster) (*see* **Note 5**).

4 Notes

1. In cultures of *C. albicans* grown in FBS, we observed hyphal development, while cells maintained the yeast-type morphology in YPD media.
2. The cells were frozen quickly using liquid nitrogen and preserved at −80 °C until required.
3. The monolithic column is prepared from a mixture of tetramethoxysilane and methyltrimethoxysilane (470 cm long, 0.1 mm internal diameter) as described previously [13].

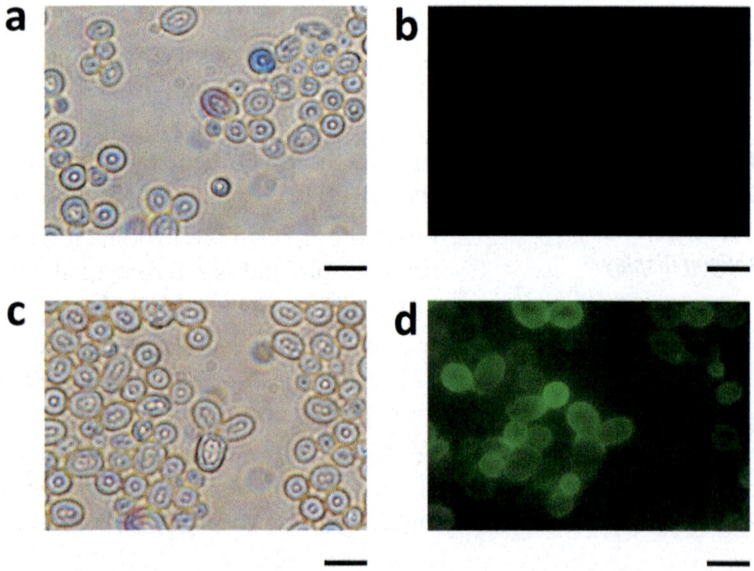

Fig. 5 Immunofluorescence staining of antigens displayed on cell surface. (**a**, **b**) *S. cerevisiae* BY4741 (control cells). (**c**, **d**) *S. cerevisiae* harboring pULD1-eno1. (**a**, **c**) Bright-field images. Scale bars = 10 μm

4. Check the nucleotide sequence of the plasmid using an ABI PRISM® 3130 Genetic Analyzer (Applied Biosystems, Foster City, CA, USA).
5. Suspend all inocula in PBS (400 μL per animal) and administer via an intragastric tube after 2 h of fasting, once per day, 5 days per week.

References

1. WJ MA, Buynak EB, Maigetter RZ, Wampler DE, Miller WJ, Hilleman MR (1984) Human hepatitis B vaccine from recombinant yeast. Nature 307:178–180
2. Heilmann CJ, Sorgo AG, Siliakus AR, Dekker HL, Brul S, de Koster CG et al (2011) Hyphal induction in the human fungal pathogen *Candida albicans* reveals a characteristic wall protein profile. Microbiology 157:2297–2307
3. Aoki W, Tatsukami Y, Kitahara N, Matsui K, Morisaka H et al (2013) Elucidation of potentially virulent factors of *Candida albicans* during serum adaptation by using quantitative time-course proteomics. J Proteome 91:417–429
4. Shibasaki S, Ueda M (2014) Bioadsorption strategies with yeast molecular display technology. Biocontrol Sci 19:157–164
5. Shibasaki S, Maeda H, Ueda M (2009) Molecular display technology using yeast—arming technology. Anal Sci 25:41–49
6. Shibasaki S, Kawabata A, Ishii J, Yagi S, Kadonosono T et al (2007) Construction of a novel synergistic system for production and recovery of secreted recombinant proteins by the cell surface engineering. Appl Microbiol Biotechnol 75:821–828
7. Shibasaki S, Karasaki M, Ueda M (2014) Combining proteomic strategies and molecular display technology for development of vaccines against *Candida albicans*. J Proteomics Bioinform 7:134–138
8. Shibasaki S, Aoki W, Nomura T, Miyoshi A, Tafuku S et al (2013) An oral vaccine against candidiasis generated by a yeast molecular display system. Pathog Dis 69:262–268
9. Shibasaki S, Karasaki M, Tafuku S, Aoki W, Sewaki T, Ueda M (2014) Oral immunization against candidiasis using *Lactobacillus casei* displaying Enolase 1 from *Candida albicans*. Sci Pharm 82:697–708
10. Adachi K, Kawana K, Yokoyama T, Fujii T, Tomio A, Miura S et al (2010) Oral immunization with a *Lactobacillus casei* vaccine expressing human papillomavirus (HPV) type 16 E7 is an effective strategy to induce mucosal cytotoxic lymphocytes against HPV16 E7. Vaccine 28:2810–2817
11. Arnaud MB, Costanzo MC, Skrzypek MS, Binkley G, Lane C, Miyasato SR et al (2005) The Candida genome database (CGD), a community resource for *Candida albicans* gene and protein information. Nucleic Acids Res 33:358–363
12. Ito H, Fukuda Y, Murata K, Kimura A (1983) Transformation of intact yeast cells treated with alkali cations. J Bacteriol 153:163–168
13. Motokawa M, Kobayashi H, Ishizuka N, Minakuchi H, Nakanishi K, Jinnai H et al (2002) Monolithic silica columns with various skeleton sizes and through-pore sizes for capillary liquid chromatography. J Chromatogr A 961:53–63

Part III

Endpoint Assessment

Chapter 17

Precise and Efficient In-Frame Integration of an Exogenous GFP Tag in *Aspergillus fumigatus* by a CRISPR System

Chi Zhang and Ling Lu

Abstract

As one of the most common airborne fungal pathogenic species, *Aspergillus fumigatus* infection is the increasingly fatal threat to immunocompromised patients worldwide. Setting up an efficient live-cell pathogen-labeling system will give insight into the dynamic process of the pathogen invasion in host, which offers us opportunities to explore the pathogenesis of *A. fumigatus*. In this chapter, we have described an efficient CRISPR-Cas9 system, which enables a precise in situ tag-insertion of an exogenous GFP tag at the predicted site with or without marker insertion in *A. fumigatus*. According to the detectable proportional fluorescence intensity, it is possible to in vivo track the *A. fumigatus* infection and to assess the fungal burden in relative organs.

Key words GFP, CRISPR-Cas9, *Aspergillus fumigatus*

1 Introduction

The CRISPR (clustered regularly interspaced short palindromic repeats)-Cas9 system has emerged as a powerful tool for the genome editing technology across varied species [1]. This bicomponent system consists of a Cas9 endonuclease and a single guide RNA (sgRNA) that recruits Cas9 to a site-specific target in the genome [2]. The sgRNA consists of a CRISPR RNA (crRNA) and a transactivating crRNA (tracrRNA) module. The ribonucleoprotein complex composed of Cas9 and sgRNA generates a double-stranded break (DSB) in the target region [3]. The nick generated by the complex is sealed by both endogenous repair mechanisms: nonhomologous-end joining (NHEJ) and homology-directed repair (HDR) [1]. Based on this principle, we have established a high-efficiency CRISPR mutagenesis system with which we can efficiently target the genome and introduce changes via microhomology-mediated end joining (MMEJ) with only very short (approximately 35-bp) homology arms [4]. Through this approach, we can carry out precise and efficient in-frame integration

Markus Kalkum and Margarita Semis (eds.), *Vaccines for Invasive Fungal Infections: Methods and Protocols*, Methods in Molecular Biology, vol. 1625, DOI 10.1007/978-1-4939-7104-6_17, © Springer Science+Business Media LLC 2017

of an exogenous GFP tag at the predicted site without marker insertion (approximately 95–100% accuracy rate). Moreover, we found that this MMEJ-CRISPR mutagenesis occurs via a *ku80*-independent pathway, indicating that this system may serve as a powerful and versatile genome-editing tool in clinical *Aspergillus* isolates.

The CRISPR approach would make for an excellent methodology that could be applied to endpoint assessment in vaccine studies. In order to evaluate antifungal vaccine protection, vaccinated laboratory animals can be infected with a constantly GFP-expressing *Aspergillus* strain. Fungal fluorescence emission allows in vivo monitoring of *A. fumigatus* infection and assessment of fungal burden in organs, which are directly proportional to fluorescence intensity.

2 Materials

2.1 Strains and Reagents for Aspergillus Transformation

1. *A. fumigatus* strain A1160 (*Δku80; pyrG1*) was obtained from FGSC [5].
2. *A. fumigatus* strain ZC03 (*Δku80; pyrG1; AMA1::PgpdA::Cas9::pyr4*) was constructed from A1160 transformed by plasmid FM-6 and this strain could constitutively express Cas9 [4].
3. Glucanex (lysing enzymes from *Trichoderma harzianum*; Sigma-Aldrich, cat. no. L1412-5G) and Yatalase (Takara, cat. no. T017); Hygromycin B 200 mg/mL, 0.2 μm filtered.
4. Yeast extract and agar.
5. 20× salt solution (1 L): 120 g $NaNO_3$,10.4 g KCl, 10.4 g $MgSO_4 \cdot 7H_2O$, 30.4 g KH_2PO_4. Add ddH_2O up to 1 L, autoclave and store at room temperature (RT).
6. Trace elements (100 mL): 2.20 g $ZnSO_4 \cdot 7H_2O$, 1.10 g H_3BO_3, 0.50 g $MnCl_2 \cdot 4H_2O$, 0.16 g $FeSO_4 \cdot 7H_2O$, 0.16 g $CoCl_2 \cdot 5H_2O$, 0.16 g $CuSO_4 \cdot 5H_2O$, 0.11 g $(NH_4)_6Mo_7O_{24} \cdot 4H_2O$, 5.00 g Na_4EDTA, put in 80 mL ddH_2O in the order shown, make sure each component is dissolved, add water up to 100 mL, you may need to add KOH to fully dissolve trace elements solution, store at 4 °C.
7. Minimal media (MM) (100 mL): 1 g glucose, 2 g agar, 0.1 mL trace elements and 5 mL 20× salt solution, store at 4 °C.
8. YAG (100 mL): 0.5 g yeast extract, 2 g agar (BD Difco), 1 g glucose, and 0.1 mL trace elements, store at 4 °C.
9. Liquid Minimal Medium (LMM) (100 mL): 1 g glucose, 5 mL 20× salt solution, 100 μL trace elements, 0.1 g yeast extract (optional), supplements. Adjust pH to 6.5 prior to autoclaving.

10. Stabilized Minimal Medium (SMM) (1 L): 10 g glucose, 50 mL 20× salt solution, 1 mL trace elements, 218.6 g sorbitol (1.2 M), 1 g yeast extract. Adjust pH to 6.5, add 10 g agar prior to autoclaving.
11. Osmotic Medium buffer (OM buffer) (500 mL): 147.9 g $MgSO_4$ (1.2 M), 10 mM NaPhosphate buffer (can be made from a 2 M NaPB stock, which has 90.9 g Na_2HPO_4 and 163.4 g NaH_2PO_4 per liter). Adjust pH to 5.8 with 1 M Na_2HPO_4, filter sterilize and store at 4 °C.
12. Trapping buffer (1 L): 109.3 g Sorbitol (0.6 M), 0.1 M Tris–HCI, pH 7.0 (can be made using 100 mL 1 M Tris), autoclave and store at 4 °C.
13. STC buffer (1 L): 218.6 g sorbitol (1.2 M), 1.11 g $CaCl_2$ (10 mM), 10 mM Tris–HCI, pH 7.5 (can be made using 10 mL 1 M Tris), autoclave and store at 4 °C.
14. PEG solution (1 L): 60% PEG 4000, 5.55 g $CaCl_2$ (50 mM), 50 mM Tris–HCI, pH 7.5 (can be made using 50 mL 1 M Tris), autoclave and store at RT.

2.2 Material Preparation for sgRNA and GFP Repair Template (Donor DNA)

1. Plasmid pX330 (Addgene, plasmid ID: 42230). This plasmid contains a codon-optimized human Cas9 gene and a sgRNA scaffold.
2. Takara DNA polymerase PrimeSTAR® HS and PrimeSTAR® Max DNA Polymerase.
3. MEGAscript T7 Kit (Life Technologies, cat. no. AM1333).
4. Gel Extraction Kit and PCR Purification Kit.
5. Phenol/chloroform/isopropanol (25:24:1, pH > 7.8), Chloroform, Isopropanol, RNase-free Water.

2.3 Materials and Equipment

1. 15 and 50 mL Centrifuge tubes.
2. 1.5 mL MaxyClear Snaplock Microcentrifuge Tube, Polypropylene, Clear, Nonsterile, (AXYGEN, cat. no. MCT-150-C).
3. 50 and 250 mL conical flask.
4. Incubator and Thermal cycler.

3 Methods

3.1 Design Principle and Preparation for sgRNA (See Note 1)

1. Design for the optimal crRNA target sequence (Fig. 1).
   (a) Guanine-cytosine (GC) content for the crRNA sequence must be limited to a range within 40–60% [6, 7].
   (b) The GC content of the six nucleotides adjacent to proto-spacer adjacent motif (PAM) should be more than 40% [8].

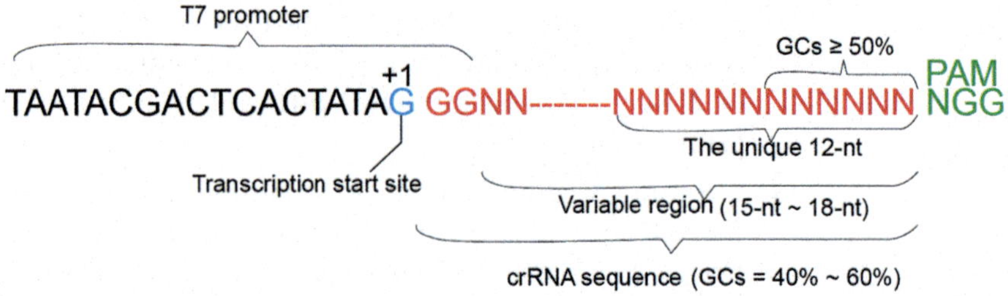

Fig. 1 Schematic illustration of the rules for designing the optimal crRNA target sequence

T7-sgRNA-F

TAATACGACTCACTATAGGGNNNNNNNNNNNNNNNNGTTTTAGAGCTAGAAATAGCAAGTTAAAATAAGGCTA

GTCCGTTATCAACTTGAAAAAGTGGCACCGAGTCGGTGCTTTTTT
CCGTGGCTCAGCCACGAAAAAA

sgRNA-R

Fig. 2 Schematic illustration for design of primers T7-sgRNA-F and sgRNA-R

(c) A short crRNA sequence only with an 18-nt targeting sequence is able to significantly decrease off-target rate while with a similar mutagenesis efficiency to a 20-nt targeting sequence [8, 9].

(d) crRNA target sequence must be included two or three nucleotides Gs in its 5′-sequence for the efficient transcription of T7 promoter.

(e) At least 12-nt unique sequences adjacent to the PAM are required for the design of crRNAs, which can be checked in website http://www.aspergillusgenome.org/cgi-bin/compute/blast_clade.pl (Input the crRNA sequence with PAM—select intended Target Genomes—select complete genome sequence as Target Sequence Dataset—Run blast).

2. Primers containing T7 promoter and crRNA sequences are designed according to the rule shown in Fig. 2. After finishing preparation of PCR, the followed procedure is carried out.
3. Mix PCR components in a PCR tube (Table 1).
4. Place the PCR reaction in a Thermal cycler, and run program as shown in Table 2.
5. Run all the PCR products on a 2% (wt/vol) agarose gel to check the presence of an approximate 120 bp amplicon.
6. Purify the intended amplicon by an appropriate Gel Extraction Kit (*see* **Note 2**).
7. Transcribe the sgRNA via the T7 MEGAscript kit (Life Technologies) according to the manufacturer's instructions (Table 3).
8. Incubate the reaction mixture at 37 °C for 16 h.

Table 1

PCR components for the dsDNA template

Component	Amount per reaction (μL or ng)	Final concentration
5× PrimeSTAR buffer (Mg^{2+} plus)	10 μL	1×
dNTP Mixture (2.5 mM each)	4 μL	200 μM each
10 μM T7-sgRNA-F	2 μL	0.4 μM/μL
10 μM sgRNA-R	2 μL	0.4 μM/μL
pX330	200 ng	4 ng/μL
PrimeSTAR HS DNA polymerase ddH_2O	0.5 μL	1.25 units/50 μL
	Up to 50 μL	

Table 2

PCR program for dsDNA amplification

Cycle number	Denature	Anneal	Extend
1	98 °C, 2 min		
2–34	98 °C, 10 s	48–51 °C, 20 s	72 °C, 15 s
35			72 °C, 5 min

Table 3

The recipe for sgRNA in vitro transcription

Component	Amount per reaction (μL or ng)
Nuclease-free water	Up to 20 μL
ATP solution	2 μL
CTP solution	2 μL
GTP solution	2 μL
UTP solution	2 μL
10× Reaction buffer	2 μL
dsDNA template DNA	200 ng
Enzyme mix	2 μL

9. Add 1 μL TURBO DNase from T7 MEGAscript kit, mix well and incubate at 37 °C for 15 min (optional).
10. Add 115 μL RNase-free water and 15 μL ammonium acetate stop solution, and mix thoroughly.
11. Extract with 150 μL phenol/chloroform/isopropanol (25:24:1, pH > 7.8), and add 300 μL chloroform.
12. Centrifuge at 12,000 × g for 5 min, 4 °C.
13. Transfer aqueous phase to a new RNase-free tube.
14. Add 1 volume of isopropanol to precipitate the RNA and mix well.
15. Chill the mixture for at least 15 min at −20 °C. Centrifuge at 4 °C for 15 min at maximum speed to pellet the RNA.
16. Carefully remove the supernatant solution and resuspend the RNA in 75% ethanol. Centrifuge at maximum speed for 15 min, 4 °C.
17. Carefully remove the supernatant solution and air-dry the RNA pellet for 5–10 min.
18. Add 20–30 μL RNase-free water to dissolve the RNA.
19. Measure the RNA concentration and frozen store at −70 °C.

3.2 Design and Prepare the GFP Repair Template (Fig. 3, See Notes 3 and 4)

1. Design the primers for amplification of donor dsDNA and mix PCR components as Table 4.
2. Run the PCR program in a Thermal cycler (Table 5).
3. Run 2 μL PCR products on a 1% (wt/vol) agarose gel to check the presence of the intended amplicon.
4. Purify the PCR products by an appropriate kit and elute in 20 μL STC buffer.

3.3 Transformation

Protocol for the generation and transformation of protoplasts was previously described by Huang et al. and Thomas Schafhause et al. [10, 11]. It has been modified for *Aspergillus* transformation.

1. Inoculate about 10^9 ZC03 fresh spores in 100 mL LMM and shake at 28 °C, 280 rpm for approximately 14 h.
2. Observe the presence of young germlings under the microscope.
3. Pellet the germlings in 50 mL tube at 13,000 × g for 10 min, 4 °C. Decant the supernatant and wash pellet in 20 mL ddH_2O, centrifuge again, and resuspend in 10 mL filter sterilized OM buffer containing 30 mg/mL Yatalase and 45 mg/mL glucanex. Transfer the mixture into a sterilized 50 mL conical flask (*see* **Note 5**).
4. Shake at 28 °C, 80 rpm for 4.5 h. Check and verify the formation of protoplasts under microscope (*see* **Note 5**).

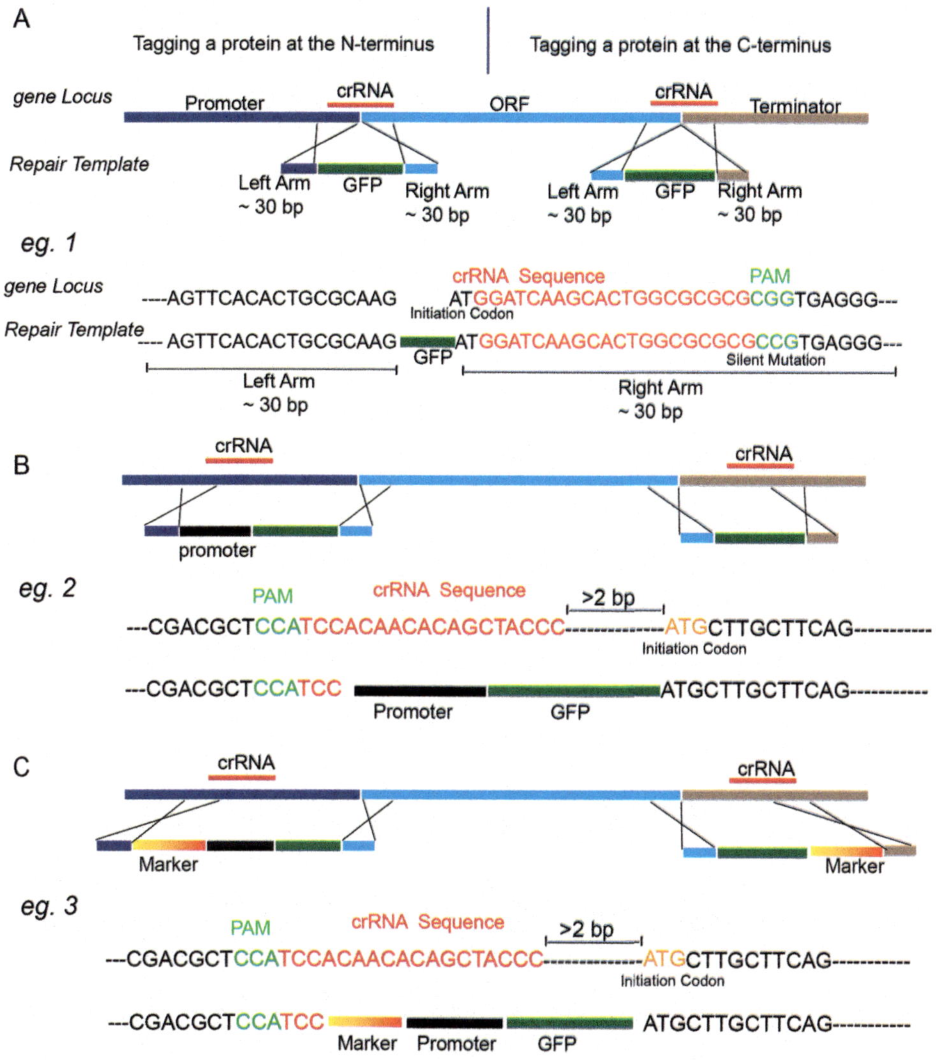

Fig. 3 (**a**) Schematic illustration for design of repair templates for crRNA targets located at the initiation or stop codon region. (**b**, **c**) Schematic illustration of repair templates for crRNA targets located at the promoter or terminator region

Table 4

PCR components for the repair template amplification

Component	Amount per reaction (μL or ng)	Final concentration
PrimeSTAR Max Premix (2×)	25 μL	1×
10 μM primer mixture (F)	2 μL	0.4 μM/μL
10 μM primer mixture (R)	2 μL	0.4 μM/μL
Template (plasmid)	100 ng	2 ng/μL
ddH_2O	Up to 50 μL	

Table 5

PCR program for repair template amplification

Cycle number	Denature	Anneal	Extend
1	98 °C, 2 min		
2–32	98 °C, 10 s	55–60 °C, 20 s	72 °C, (5–10 s/kb)
33			72 °C, 5 min

Table 6

The appropriate quantity of sgRNA and donor for transformation

Component	Amount per reaction (μL or μg)
(a)	
Protoplast	80 μL
sgRNA	≥4 μg
Repair template (containing an integrated selection marker)	≥4 μg
(b)	
Protoplast	80 μL
sgRNA	≥4 μg
Repair template (not containing a selection marker)	≥8 μg
Selection marker	≤4 μg

5. Transfer the protoplasts into a new 50 mL tube, carefully cover the mixture with 10 mL trapping buffer, centrifuge at 11,000 × *g* for 15 min (*see* **Note 5**).
6. Transfer about 6 mL protoplast suspension from the interphase into a sterile 15 mL tube, pellet protoplasts with an equal volume of STC buffer, centrifuge at 12,000 × *g* for 8 min, decant the supernatant, and resuspend the protoplast in about 1 mL STC buffer (*see* **Note 5**).
7. Add sgRNA and GFP repair template as mentioned in Table 6 to 80 μL protoplasts and incubate on ice for 50 min.
8. Add 1.5 mL PEG solution to the mixture, mix gently by turning the tube on its side and rotating it and incubate at RT for 20 min.
9. Add 2 mL STC buffer and 6.5 mL molten SMM (about 45 °C) into the mixture and mix gently (*see* **Note 5**).

10. Quickly plate the 10 mL transformed mixture onto a 10 mL solid SMM in Petri dish, and culture at 37 °C for about 3 days.
11. Purify the candidate transformants on the medium with corresponding selection stress.
12. Extract the genomic DNA of *A. fumigatus* for diagnostic PCR and sequencing (*see* **Note 6**).

4 Notes

1. To avoid affecting functions of the adjacent genes, the location of crRNA target should be close to the target gene ORF.
2. The purity of the dsDNA template is critical for the transcription efficiency. Gel extraction of the intended amplicon is necessary.
3. If the crRNA sequence contains the initiation/stop codon or the distance between the crRNA sequence and initiation/stop codon is less than 3 bp, a precise in-frame integration of a pure GFP tag with microhomology arms at the N- or C-terminus can be carried out. For this case, a selection marker without microhomology arms should be randomly integrated into genome. Design details are described as in Fig. 3-*eg. 1,* where the repair template GFP fragments harbored 39 bp microhomology arms located proximally to the PAM region. In addition, in order to avoid repair-template-editing by Cas9, a silent mutation must be introduced at the PAM site.
4. If there are no suitable crRNA targets described in **Note 3**, selecting a crRNA target sequence, which is closest to the ORF in the promoter or terminator region, will be a compromised alternative strategy. For this case, in order to integrate a GFP tag into the N-terminus of a target protein, an extra-promoter-sequence should be fused into the GFP repair template to complement the disruption of endogenous promoter by Cas9. In addition, the left microhomology arm of the modificatory repair template should be located to the left side of the predicted cleavage site (between the third and the fourth base in the front of the PAM), and the right microhomology arm should be located to ATG region as shown in Fig. 3-*eg. 2.* In order to increase the mutagenesis efficiency, the selection marker can be incorporated into the repair template as shown in Fig. 3-*eg. 3.*
5. For transformation: the superabundant germling pellets will reduce the efficiency of enzymolysis. Check every 30 min under the microscope to see if protoplasts are being formed. If protoplasts have been formed rapidly, reduce the incubation time accordingly. Usually, 3–4 h are sufficient. Protoplasts are

thin-walled and about two times as large as spores. Do not try to mix the trapping buffer and osmotic medium buffer before centrifugation. High quality protoplasts form a white disk in the interphase. Add appropriate supplements for selection markers, such as 150 μg/mL hygromycin B.

6. To verify the integration of exogenous donor in the target protein, PCR fragments (approximately 1 kb) covering the predicted Cas9 cleavage sites were generated from the purified genomic DNA. Then, the perfect seamless conjunction between GFP and target sequence should be confirmed by sequencing and presence of fluorescence.

Acknowledgments

This work was financially supported by the National Natural Science Foundation of China (NSFC81330035, NSFC31370112) to L. Lu; the Priority Academic Program Development (PAPD) of Jiangsu Higher Education Institutions. *A. fumigatus* strain A1160 was obtained from FGSC (http://www.fgsc.net).

References

1. Doudna JA, Charpentier E (2014) Genome editing. The new frontier of genome engineering with CRISPR-Cas9. Science 346:1258096
2. Ran FA, Hsu PD, Wright J, Agarwala V, Scott DA et al (2013) Genome engineering using the CRISPR-Cas9 system. Nat Protoc 8:2281–2308
3. Shalem O, Sanjana NE, Zhang F (2015) High-throughput functional genomics using CRISPR-Cas9. Nat Rev Genet 16:299–311
4. Zhang C, Meng X, Wei X, Lu L (2016) Highly efficient CRISPR mutagenesis by microhomology-mediated end joining in Aspergillus fumigatus. Fungal Genet Biol 86:47–57
5. da Silva Ferreira ME, Kress MR, Savoldi M, Goldman MH, Hartl A et al (2006) The akuB(KU80) mutant deficient for nonhomologous end joining is a powerful tool for analyzing pathogenicity in Aspergillus fumigatus. Eukaryot Cell 5:207–211
6. Wang T, Wei JJ, Sabatini DM, Lander ES (2014) Genetic screens in human cells using the CRISPR-Cas9 system. Science 343:80–84
7. Doench JG, Hartenian E, Graham DB, Tothova Z, Hegde M et al (2014) Rational design of highly active sgRNAs for CRISPR-Cas9-mediated gene inactivation. Nat Biotechnol 32:1262–1267
8. Ren XJ, Yang ZH, Xu J, Sun J, Mao DC et al (2014) Enhanced specificity and efficiency of the CRISPR/Cas9 system with optimized sgRNA parameters in drosophila. Cell Rep 9:1151–1162
9. Fu Y, Sander JD, Reyon D, Cascio VM, Joung JK (2014) Improving CRISPR-Cas nuclease specificity using truncated guide RNAs. Nat Biotechnol 32:279–284
10. Schafhauser T, Kirchner N, Kulik A, Huijbers MM, Flor L et al (2016) The cyclochlorotine mycotoxin is produced by the nonribosomal peptide synthetase CctN in Talaromyces Islandicus ("Penicillium islandicum"). Environ Microbiol 18(11):3728–3741. doi: 10.1111/1462-2920.13294
11. Huang KX, Iwakami N, Fujii I, Ebizuka Y, Sankawa U (1995) Transformations of Penicillium islandicum and Penicillium frequentans that produce anthraquinone-related compounds. Curr Genet 28:580–584

Chapter 18

Endpoint Assessment in Rabbit Models of Invasive Pulmonary Aspergillosis and Mucormycosis

Vidmantas Petraitis, Ruta Petraitiene, William W. Hope, and Thomas J. Walsh

Abstract

Multiple animal models have been developed to study the pathogenesis of invasive pulmonary aspergillosis, as well as to evaluate the efficacy, pharmacokinetics, and pharmacodynamics of various antifungal agents and vaccines. Each model is beneficial depending on the questions that are asked. In this chapter, we will discuss the endpoints assessment of the persistently neutropenic rabbit models of invasive pulmonary aspergillosis and invasive pulmonary mucormycosis.

Keywords Aspergillosis, Mucormycosis, Endpoints, Pulmonary, PCR, Galactomannan, (1 → 3)-β-D-glucan

1 Introduction

Invasive pulmonary aspergillosis (IPA) and invasive pulmonary mucormycosis (IPM) are life-threatening infections in immunosuppressed patients, particularly in those with severe and prolonged neutropenia as a consequence of aplastic anemia, myelotoxic chemotherapy for the treatment of cancer, and in those receiving immunosuppressive medication for rejection prophylaxis after organ transplantation or treatment of graft-versus-host disease in allogeneic bone marrow transplantation [1–4]. Eleven new antifungal agents have been developed in different classes including triazoles, echinocandins, and lipid formulations of amphotericin B through these model systems from bench to bedside. Several new compounds are now in the path of development. These models also provide a platform for the study of antifungal vaccines. Endpoint interpretation allows better understanding of the pathogenesis of IPA and IPM, as well as the evaluation of efficacy, pharmacokinetics, and pharmacodynamics of new antifungal agents and novel vaccines.

Markus Kalkum and Margarita Semis (eds.), *Vaccines for Invasive Fungal Infections: Methods and Protocols*, Methods in Molecular Biology, vol. 1625, DOI 10.1007/978-1-4939-7104-6_18, © Springer Science+Business Media LLC 2017

This chapter herein will describe a panel of endpoint variables in the persistently neutropenic rabbit model of IPA and IPM, including residual fungal burden (quantitative cultures), organism-mediated pulmonary injury (lung weights, pulmonary infarct scores, and ultrafast computerized tomography), survival, serum galactomannan antigenemia [detected by the double sandwich enzyme-linked immunosorbent assay (ELISA)], (1 → 3)-β-D-glucan levels (detected by *Limulus* amebocyte lysate assay), and pharmacokinetic-pharmacodynamic endpoints. Further discussion is provided in describing the use of quantitative real-time PCR as an endpoint in IPM.

2 Materials

2.1 Quantitative Fungal Cultures

1. Sterile polyethylene bag.
2. 0.9% sterile normal saline.
3. Homogenizer (Stomacher 80; Tekmar® Corp., Cincinnati, OH).
4. Sabouraud Glucose Agar (SGA) plates.
5. Incubator 37 °C.

2.2 Organism-Mediated Pulmonary Injury

1. Surgical tools and instruments.
2. Sedation solution: ketamine and xylazine.
3. Ultrafast electron-beam CT scanner (model CE 0459 HiSpeed CT/I; GE Medical Systems, Milwaukee, Wis.).

2.3 (1 → 3)-β-D-Glucan Assay

The assay for the detection of (1 → 3)-β-D-glucan (Fungitell, Associates of Cape Cod).

2.4 Galactomannan Assay

1. Platelia *Aspergillus*, Immunoenzymatic detection of galactomannan antigen of *Aspergillus* in serum (Sanofi Diagnostics Pasteur or now Bio-Rad, Marnes La Coquette, France).
2. Microplate spectrophotometer equipped with 450- and 620 nm filters.

2.5 PCR Studies of IPA and IPM

2.5.1 PCR for Sera

1. MagNA Pure LC system.
2. DNA Isolation Kit III for bacteria and fungi.
3. Bacteria Lysis Buffer.
4. Proteinase K (Sigma Aldrich).
5. Eppendorf thermomixer (Eppendorf).
6. Phosphate-buffered saline (PBS).
7. qPCR LightCycler Instrument (Roche Applied Sciences, Indianapolis, IN).

8. Master mix for MqPCR-1: 0.25 μM of each primer, 1× PCR buffer (Invitrogen Corp., Carlsbad, CA), 3 mM $MgCl_2$, 0.025% BSA (Sigma-Aldrich Corp., St. Louis, MO), 0.025 U Platinum® *Taq* DNA polymerase (Invitrogen Corp., Carlsbad, CA), 0.2 mM PCR Nucleotide Mix^{Plus} (1 dATP, dCTP, dGTP, and 3 dUTP) (Roche Applied Sciences, Indianapolis, IN), 0.1 μM of each fluorescein (FITC) and LC Red-640 probes (RD640) (Idaho Technology, Inc., Salt Lake City, UT), and 0.002 U/μL HK-UNG (uracil *N*-glycosylase) (Epicentre, Madison, WI).
9. Master mix for MqPCR-2: 0.5 μM of each of the primers, 1× PCR buffer (Invitrogen Corp., Carlsbad, CA), 4 mM $MgCl_2$, 0.025% BSA (Sigma-Aldrich Corp., St. Louis, MO), 0.025 U/ml Platinum® Taq DNA polymerase (Invitrogen Corp., Carlsbad, CA), 0.2 mM PCR Nucleotide Mix ^{PLUS} (Roche Applied Sciences, Indianapolis, IN), and 0.2 μM of each FITC and RD640 probes (Idaho Technology, Inc., Salt Lake City, UT).

2.5.2 PCR for BAL

1. Spheroplast buffer: 1.0 M sorbitol, 50.0 mM sodium phosphate monobasic, 0.1% 2-mercaptoethanol, 10 mg of lyticase/mL [Sigma].
2. Rocking platform.
3. AP1 buffer (DNeasy plant kit; Qiagen, Valencia, CA).
4. Lysing matrix D tubes (Fastprep sample preparation system; QBIOgene/MP Biomedical, Irvine, CA).
5. FastPrep instrument (QBIOgene/MP Biomedical).
6. 100 mg/ml RNase A.
7. Eppendorf thermomixer (Eppendorf, Westbury, NY).
8. DNeasy plant kit.
9. AE buffer (Qiagen, Valencia, CA).
10. Sterile water.
11. Oligo software (Molecular Biology Insights, Cascade, CO).
12. Probes (Idaho Technologies, Salt Lake City, UT).
13. Sequencher software package (Gene Codes Corp., Ann Arbor, MI).
14. The NCBI BLAST database search program.
15. The PCR master mix: 0.5 μM of each of the primers, 5 mM $MgCl_2$, 0.025% bovine serum albumin (Sigma-Aldrich Corp., St. Louis, MO), 0.05 U/mL Platinum *Taq* DNA polymerase (Invitrogen Corp., Carlsbad, CA), 10 μL PCR buffer (Invitrogen Corp., Carlsbad, CA), 0.2 mM PCR Nucleotide Mix Plus (dATP, dCTP, and dGTP at 10 mM each and dUTP at 30 mM; Roche Molecular Biochemicals, Indianapolis, IN), and 0.1 μM each of the fluorescein and LC Red-640 probes.
16. HK-UNG thermostable uracil *N*-glycosylase (Epicentre, Madison, WI).

2.6 Histopathology

1. 10% neutral buffered formalin.
2. Paraffin.
3. Periodic acid-Schiff (PAS) stain kit.
4. Grocott-Gomori methenamine silver (GMS) stain kit.
5. Microscope.
   1. Collect the blood via the indwelling Silastic catheter [5] at 24 h post-inoculation, just prior to the initiation of antifungal treatment or vaccine and every other day thereafter for the determination of the serum galactomannan levels.
   2. Determine the concentrations as described above by the one-stage immunoenzymatic sandwich microplate assay method.

2.7 Pharma cokinetics and Pharmacodynamics

1. Indwelling Silastic catheter.
2. Heparinized syringes.
3. HPLC or LC-MS/MS.
4. Pmetrics™ software (v1.3.2, University of Southern CA, Los Angeles, CA, USA).
5. ADAPT 5 (https://bmsr.usc.edu/software/adapt/ Biomedical Simulations Resource, Los Angeles, CA, USA).

3 Methods

3.1 Quantitative Fungal Cultures

Quantitative lung cultures facilitate the determination of the burden of organisms within tissue. Measured in units of colony-forming units per gram of tissue (CFU/g), changes in quantitative lung cultures reflect the growth of organisms in untreated controls or the effect of an antifungal agent or vaccine that may augment pulmonary host defenses.

1. Sample lung tissue from each rabbit and culture by a standard excision of tissue from each lobe.
2. Weigh each fragment individually, place in a sterile polyethylene bag, and homogenize with 0.9% sterile normal saline for 30 s per tissue sample.
3. Prepare lung homogenate dilutions (10^{-1} and 10^{-2}) in 0.9% sterile normal saline.
4. Plate aliquots (100 μL) from homogenates and homogenate dilutions onto SGA plates and incubate at 37 °C for 6-8 h in IPM model and for 24 h in IPA model.
5. Count the number of CFU of *Aspergillus fumigatus* or *Mucorales* for each lobe, and calculate the CFU/g (*see* **Notes 1** and **2**).

3.2 Organism-Mediated Pulmonary Injury

Patients who develop IPA and IPM suffer serious morbidity and high mortality as the result of organism-mediated pulmonary injury. *Aspergillus* spp. and Mucorales mediate pulmonary injury through several mechanisms, the most striking of which is angioinvasion. Through the mechanism of angioinvasion, the damaged blood vessels and endothelium promote vascular thrombosis with ensuing tissue ischemia, infarction, and necrosis. In thrombocytopenic hosts, the infarction is hemorrhagic resulting in impaired ventilation of the damaged lung. Assessment of this process is assessed by pulmonary infarct scores, lung weights, and computerized tomographic scans.

3.2.1 Pulmonary Lesion Scores and Lung Weights

1. For the assessment of pulmonary lesion scores and lung weights, resect carefully the entire heart-lung block at necropsy.
2. Dissect the heart away from lungs, leaving tracheobronchial tree and lungs intact.
3. Weigh the lungs and inspect by at least two observers, who are blinded to the treatment group, and record hemorrhagic infarct lesions (if any) in each individual lobe.
4. Define hemorrhagic infarcts as dark red consolidated lesions that correspond histologically to coagulative necrosis and intra-alveolar hemorrhage.
5. Add the number of positive lobes together, and calculate the mean value of all positive lobes for each treatment group [6–11].

3.2.2 Ultrafast Computerized Tomography (UFCT)

Two-dimensional ultrafast computerized tomography is an accurate tool in measuring pulmonary infiltrates in real time in experimental IPA. Pulmonary infiltrates in neutropenic hosts with invasive pulmonary aspergillosis are caused by vascular invasion, hemorrhagic infarction, and tissue necrosis. Monitoring the dynamics of pulmonary injury of invasive aspergillosis is an important tool for assessing response to antifungal therapy and vaccines. Serial CT scans of the lungs are obtained during all experiments in order to monitor the effects of antifungal or vaccine therapy on organism-mediated pulmonary injury during the course of infection.

1. Sedate the rabbits with ketamine and xylazine and place prone, head first, on the scanning couch.
2. Perform CT with an ultrafast electron-beam CT scanner (*see* **Note 3**).
3. Use a small scan circle and a 9.6-cm-diameter reconstruction circle with a matrix of 512 by 512 (*see* **Note 4**).
4. Scan parameters are 80 kV and 120 mA, and the scan duration is 0.8 s (*see* **Note 5**).
5. Photograph the images by using lung windows with a level of −600 Hounsfield units and a width of 1800 Hounsfield units.
6. Establish a mean 2-dimensional CT scan lesion score by evaluating the infiltrate in each lobe (*see* **Notes 6** and 7).

3.2.3 Multidimensional Volumetric Imaging (MDVI)

We further developed a method for multidimensional volumetric imaging (MDVI) of pulmonary infiltrates for measuring therapeutic response to antifungal or vaccine therapy in IPA in persistently neutropenic rabbits [12]. We developed a semiautomatic method to measure the volume of lung lesions, which is implemented as an extension of the MEDx visualization and analysis software using UFCT. The steps used in the technique are described below. A point is placed within the lung on each CT section.

1. Perform seeded region growing with an inclusion threshold range of (1023–775) to segment the lung.
2. A contour of the segmented lung boundary is automatically created.
3. If necessary, select the option to semiautomatically exclude non-lung tissue or include nonsegmented lung tissue and to re-perform region growing.
4. If necessary, also make fine manual adjustments of the lung boundary contour.
5. Compute the area of all pixels inside the lung boundary contour that are above a threshold of 500 Hounsfield units. This is the lung lesion area. Then determine the sum of the lesion areas from all relevant CT sections and multiply it by the slice thickness. This is the total lesion volume. Implement a common strategy of first segmenting the lung image and then look inside the lung tissue for lesions (*see* **Notes 8** and **9**).
6. Compare volumetric infiltrate measures with UFCT reading, histopathological resolution of lesions, microbiological clearance of *Aspergillus fumigatus*, and galactomannan index (GMI) [12].
7. Perform these steps for each CT section.

3.3 Survival

Although measurement of survival is a time-honored but relatively insensitive endpoint in assessing the effects of antifungal or vaccine therapy, immunomodulation, or virulence in IPA or IPM, a difference in survival provides reassuring data supporting potential clinical efficacy. Survival in IPA or IPM is ultimately determined by organism-mediated pulmonary injury.

1. Record duration of survival in days post-inoculation for each rabbit.
2. Euthanize the rabbits upon reaching prespecified humane endpoints approved by Animal Care and Use Committee by intravenous administration of pentobarbital at the end of each experiment.
3. Euthanize surviving rabbits on day 14 of study.
4. Analyze and plot the data by log-rank test by Kaplan-Meier methods [7, 9, 10, 13].

3.4 (1 → 3)-β-D-Glucan Assay

(1 → 3)-β-D-glucan in serum, bronchoalveolar lavage (BAL) fluid or cerebrospinal fluid (CSF) also is used as a sensitive biomarker for antifungal or vaccine therapeutic response. (1 → 3)-β-D-glucan in serum or BAL fluid also demonstrates a strong correlation between therapeutic outcome and biological outcome variables, including quantitative cultures, organism-mediated pulmonary injury (lung weights, pulmonary infarct score, and CT scan lesion scores), and survival.

1. Collect blood samples from each rabbit every other day for the determination of plasma (1 → 3)-β-D-glucan levels.
2. Use the Fungitell assay for the detection of (1 → 3)-β-D-glucan which is licensed for diagnosis of invasive fungal infections.
3. Detection of (1 → 3)-β-D-glucan is possible using a colorimetric assay read at 405 nm (with 490 nm background subtraction), based upon *para*-nitroanilide absorption at that wavelength. Lipopolysaccharide and (1 → 3)-β-D-glucan initiate the coagulation cascade in the horseshoe crab (*Limulus polyphemus* or *Tachypleus tridentatus*) by activating different serine protease zymogens, factors C and G. Lipopolysaccharide specifically activates factor C, while (1 → 3)-β-D-glucan activates factor G. Specificity of (1 → 3)-β-D-glucan is ensured by using a *Limulus polyphemus* amebocyte lysate that is depleted of factor C. The activated factor G converts the inactive proclotting enzyme to the active clotting enzyme, which in turn cleaves pNA from the chromogenic peptide substrate, Boc-Leu-Gly-Arg-pNA, creating a chromophore that absorbs at 405 nm. The reagent is used in the Fungitell kinetic assay to detect the rate of optical density increase in a sample. This rate is interpreted against a standard curve to produce estimates of (1 → 3)-β-D-glucan levels in the sample.
4. Interpretation of (1 → 3)-β-D-glucan values, according to manufacturer's instructions for use: <60 pg/mL, negative; 60 to 79 pg/mL, indeterminate; ≥ 80 pg/mL, positive. The correlation coefficient of the standard curve is $r \geq 0.9992$ (range from 0.9982 to 0.9998) [10, 14, 15] (*see* **Notes 10** and **11**).

3.5 Galactomannan Assay

Galactomannan is a cell wall carbohydrate found in *Aspergillus* spp. Our studies have consistently demonstrated a strong correlation between therapeutic outcome and biological outcome variables, including quantitative cultures, organism-medicated pulmonary injury (lung weights, pulmonary infarct score, and CT scan lesion scores), and survival [6, 9–11, 14–19].

1. Collect the blood every other day from each rabbit for the determination of serum galactomannan antigen levels.
2. Perform the Platelia *Aspergillus* one-stage immunoenzymatic double-sandwich microplate assay (EIA) to determine galactomannan antigen levels according to manufacturer's directions (*see* **Note 12**).

3. Briefly, mix 300 μL of each sample (serum or BAL fluid) with 100 μL of treatment solution and subsequently heat the mixture at 100 °C for 3 min with a solution of EDTA in order to dissociate the immune complexes and to precipitate serum proteins that could interfere with the ELISA (*see* **Note 13**).
4. Centrifuge the specimens at 28,000 × *g* for 10 min.
5. After centrifugation, use the supernatant for further testing.
6. Add an aliquot of 50 μL of conjugate (horseradish peroxidase-labeled monoclonal antibody EBA-2) to each well of the monoclonal antibody EBA-2-coated microplate, followed by the addition of 50 μL of the supernatant and incubate for 90 min at 37 °C.
7. After incubation wash the plates five times and add 100 μL of substrate-chromogen solution containing tetramethylbenzidine to each well, and incubate the plates for 30 min at room temperature in darkness (*see* **Note 14**).
8. Stop the enzyme reaction by the addition of a 1 N sulfuric acid solution and the blue color in the wells will change to yellow.
9. Determine optical absorbance of specimens and controls with a spectrophotometer set at 450/620 nm wavelengths.
10. Calculate the galactomannan index (GMI) for each test sample by dividing its optical density (OD) by the mean cutoff value of the threshold control serum provided in the test kit (titrated at 1 ng/mL).
11. For validation, each assay contained one negative control (no galactomannan), one positive control containing 5 ng/mL of galactomannan, and a duplicate threshold control serum containing 1 ng/mL galactomannan for the calibration and conversion of the measured absorbances into indexes.
12. The optical density of the threshold control (cut-off control serum) is recommended by the manufacturer to be between 0.300 and 0.800 (≥0.300 and ≤0.800), the ratio between the negative control and the threshold control is recommended to be below 0.40 (<0.40), and that of the positive control and the threshold control is recommended to be greater than 1.50 (>1.50).
13. Calculate the ratio between the optical density of the test sample and that of the threshold control for each sample.
14. According to the manufacturer's recommendations, a ratio of less than 0.50 (<0.50) is considered negative, sera/BAL fluid with an index greater than or equal to 0.50 (≥0.50) is considered positive for galactomannan antigen. For convenience, the term galactomannan index (GMI) simply refers to EIA test results.
15. Plot serial serum or BAL fluid galactomannan levels over time of administration of antifungal compound or vaccine and time of initiation of study drug treatment.

3.6 PCR Studies of IPA and IPM

Genomic DNA of Mucorales or *Aspergillus* spp., which can be detected in BAL fluid and in serum or plasma, can be used as end-point biomarkers for therapeutic response to antifungal agents or vaccines and as indicators of virulence. We will exemplify the utility of fungal PCR through our studies of experimental IPM.

3.6.1 Design of Assays

1. In order to measure circulating Mucorales-derived DNA, apply two previously validated real-time, quantitative PCR (qPCR) assays [20], using fluorescence energy transfer (FRET) technology and targeting the 28S rRNA gene for the following genera: *Rhizopus*, *Mucor*, *Rhizomucor*, and *Cunninghamella*.
2. The amplicons of the first Mucorales qPCR assay (MqPCR-1) from *Rhizopus*, *Mucor*, and *Rhizomucor* species are distinguished through melt curve analysis.
3. The second Mucorales qPCR assay (MqPCR-2) detected *Cunninghamella* species using a different primer/probe set (*see* **Note 15**).

3.6.2 PCR for Sera

Circulating genomic DNA from Mucorales test species is measured in plasma every other day by a quantitative real-time Light Cycler-based PCR assay using primers and probes designed from 28 s rRNA gene sequences.

1. Extract plasma samples (100 μL) using the automated extraction MagNA Pure LC system with the DNA Isolation Kit III for bacteria and fungi.
2. Add 130 μL aliquot of Bacteria Lysis Buffer and 20 μL of Proteinase K to the serum. Vortex the samples and incubate at 65 °C for 10 min in an Eppendorf thermomixer at 400 × *g*.
3. After incubation, centrifuge the samples 1 min at 1000 × *g* and mix gently. Equilibrate the samples (250 μL) to room temperature and subsequently add to the sample cartridge prior to being processed by the MagNA Pure LC instrument.
4. Process an aliquot of 250 μL of PBS as a control. Store the samples at −20 °C until analyzed by qPCR.
5. Perform qPCR assays with a LightCycler. Include a "kit blank" (water processed through extraction protocol) and a negative master mix control (water) in each PCR run.
6. Prepare master mixes in a laminar flow hood that is located in a room separate from that where DNA extractions are performed.
7. For both assays, add 5 μL of extracted plasma to 15 μL of master mix. Just prior to adding 5 μL of extracted specimen to the master mix, briefly vortex all extracted specimens and then centrifuge for 45 s at 4500 × *g*.

8. Uracil is released by incubating at 37 °C for 15 min, followed by enzyme inactivation at 95 °C for 3 min.
9. Perform touch-down PCR cycling as follows: 95 °C denaturation for 0 s, followed by annealing in 1 °C incremental steps between 68 °C and 54 °C for 5 s each with a 72 °C extension of 15 s for each cycle.
10. Follow touchdown cycling with 35 cycles of 95 °C for 0 s, 54 °C for 5 s, and 72 °C for 15 s.
11. Following amplification, perform melt curve analysis by cooling from 96 °C to 40 °C for 30 s, followed by a gradual increase in temperature (2 °C/s) to 75 °C.
12. In case of the second master mix (MqPCR-2), as with qPCR-1, HK-UNG thermostabile uracil *N*-Glycosylase is utilized as recommended by the manufacturer to prevent potential amplicon carryover.
13. The cycling conditions are as follows: uracil activation, 37 °C, 15 min (slope 20 °C/s), uracil heat-inactivation, 95 °C, 3 min (slope 20 °C/s) for 1 cycle.
14. Amplification cycles: denaturation 95 °C, 0 s (slope 20 °C/s), annealing 57 °C, 5 s (slope 10 °C/s), extension 72 °C, 15 s (slope 3 °C/s) for 50 cycles. A melt cycle 96 °C, 0 s (slope 20 °C/s), 40 °C, 30s (slope (2 °C/s), 75 °C, 0 s (slope 0.2 °C/s)) is performed at the end of each run to confirm that the correct amplicon is generated via the PCR product melt temperature analysis.
15. DNA copy number/mL of serum is used for quantification of circulating DNA.
16. The area under the concentration time curve (AUC) is then calculated.
17. The AUC0–∞ is calculated from amplicon plasma concentration profiles over time using the linear trapezoidal rule with extrapolation to infinity by standard techniques.

3.6.3 PCR for BAL

1. Thaw frozen BAL fluid samples before extraction is performed.
2. As previously described [16], vortex the samples for 1 min before a 500 μL aliquot is taken for processing.
3. Following centrifugation for 10 min at 16,000 × *g*, discard the supernatant, and gently resuspend the pellet in 100 μL spheroplast buffer and 10 μL of lysing enzymes and incubate at 37 °C on a rocking platform for 60 min.
4. After centrifugation for 20 min at 400 μg, resuspend the spheroplast-BAL fluid pellet in 400 μL AP1 buffer.
5. Add the sample to lysing matrix D tubes and process using a FastPrep instrument.

6. Centrifuge specimens at 16,000 × *g* for 30–60 s and then vortex gently.
7. Transfer an aliquot of 300 μL of the specimen to a 1.5 mL tube and adjust to a volume of 400 μL with AP1 buffer.
8. Add an aliquot of 4 μL of RNase A (100 mg/ml), vortex vigorously, and incubate for 10 min at 65 °C in an Eppendorf thermomixer at 400 × *g*.
9. Follow the DNeasy plant kit protocol with the following modification: after the 200 μL of preheated (65 °C) AE buffer is applied to the column, heat the entire apparatus (column and collection tube) at 65 °C in an Eppendorf thermomixer for 5 min.
10. Also, process an aliquot of 100 μL of sterile water as described above as a control for any contamination from the DNA extraction kit components.
11. Design a real-time quantitative PCR assay targeting the ITS1, 5.8S, and ITS2 regions of the rRNA gene complex.
12. Design the primers and probes using Oligo software based on a multiple sequence alignment of rRNA sequences from GenBank, utilizing the Sequencher software package. Use the NCBI BLAST database search program to determine the uniqueness of the primers and probes for *A. fumigatus* (*see* **Note 16**).
13. Utilize HK-UNG thermostable uracil *N*-glycosylase as recommended by the manufacturer to prevent potential amplicon carryover.
14. Each reaction mix contains an aliquot of 5 μL of extracted specimen, together with 15 μL of the master mix.
15. The cycling conditions are as follows: uracil activation (37 °C, 180 s), uracil heat inactivation (95 °C, 60 s for 1 cycle), and denaturation (95 °C, 0 s), annealing (58 °C, 5 s), and extension (72 °C, 15 s) for 50 cycles.
16. Perform quantitation standards in conjunction with each set of samples.
17. Screen the BAL fluid samples from each rabbit with the following controls: (a) DNA extracted from normal BAL fluid and (b) a negative control master mix (sterile water).
18. Use tenfold serial dilutions of genomic DNA extracted from *A. fumigatus* isolate 4215 as external quantitation standards for all quantitative PCRs.
19. In order to confirm the lack of PCR inhibitors in BAL fluid samples, perform a separate set of PCR/fluorescent resonance energy transfer reactions that specifically did not target *A. fumigatus* (or mammalian) DNA (*see* **Note 17**).

20. Test the presence of inhibitors, by comparing the amplification efficiency of this reaction with the extracted samples against those performed with sterile water (*see* **Note 18**).

3.7 Histopathology

Histopathology of IPA and IPM provides important insight into the relative burden of organism, morphology of organisms, and degree of organism-mediated pulmonary injury.

1. Excise the lesions and fix in 10% neutral buffered formalin.
2. Stain the paraffin-embedded tissue sections with periodic acid-Schiff (PAS) and Grocott-Gomori methenamine silver stains (GMS).
3. Examine the tissues microscopically for histologic indicators of pulmonary injury [8, 11, 15, 21].

3.8 Pharma cokinetics and Pharmacodynamics

The rabbit models of IPA and IPM are also used to determine the immunopharmacology, pharmacokinetics (PK), and pharmacodynamics (PD) of the exposure-response relationship of antifungal agents and vaccines [7, 8, 10, 19, 21–30]. We will describe herein the use of serum galactomannan suppression to characterize the PK/PD relationship [18].

3.8.1 Blood Collection

1. Collect the blood via the indwelling Silastic catheter [5] at 24 h post-inoculation, just prior to initiation of antifungal treatment or vaccine and every other day thereafter for the determination of the serum galactomannan levels.
2. Determine the concentrations as described above by the one-stage immunoenzymatic sandwich microplate assay method.

3.8.2 Single and Multiple-Dose PK Analyses

1. Conduct single-dose PK analyses in four noninfected rabbits per each dosage group.
2. Time points, depending upon the antifungal agent or vaccine, for example may include pre-dose, 1, 2, 4, 8, 12, 18, 24, and 48 h post-dosing.
3. Determine multiple-dose PKs in infected animals 7 days post-inoculation.
4. Draw blood samples in this population pre-dose and at 1, 4, 8, and 24 h post-dosing.
5. Collect each blood sample for PK assay in heparinized syringes.
6. Separate plasma samples immediately by centrifugation at 400 × *g* and store at −80 °C until assayed.
7. Measure the antifungal agent or vaccine in serum by a validated HPLC or LC-MS/MS assay.

3.8.3 Pharmacokinetic and Pharmacodynamic Mathematical Modeling

Perform mathematical modeling in a step-wise manner as follows.

1. First, construct a population pharmacokinetic (PPK) model using non-parametric estimation in Pmetrics™ software [31] and fitted to the rabbit plasma concentration data [31].
2. Estimate the weighting functions using a combination of ADAPT 5 and Pmetrics error estimation runs. Specifically, in ADAPT 5, estimate slope and intercept values using maximum likelihood estimation for each individual rabbit.
3. In Pmetrics, use the error estimation run script (i.e., ERRrun) to estimate the assay error polynomial coefficients directly from the data.
4. After establishing a model that best describes the PK data, add the galactomannan concentrations to the dataset for each individual rabbit.
5. Build linked PK-PD model using the following set of differential equations:

$$\mathrm{d}XP / \mathrm{d}t(1) = -Ka \cdot X(1) \qquad (1)$$

$$\mathrm{d}XP / \mathrm{d}tXP(2) = K\mathrm{a} \cdot X(1) - \left(\left(\frac{Cl}{V} \right) \cdot X(2) \right) - Kcp \cdot X(2) + Kpc \cdot X(3) \qquad (2)$$

$$\mathrm{d}XP / \mathrm{d}tXP(3) = Kcp \cdot X(2) - Kpc \cdot X(3) \qquad (3)$$

$$\mathrm{d}XP / \mathrm{d}t(4) = K\mathrm{p}_{\mathrm{max}} \cdot \left(1 - \left(\frac{\left(\frac{X(2)}{V} \right)^{Hp}}{\mathrm{C50p}^{Hp} + \left(\frac{X(2)}{V} \right)^{Hp}} \right) \right) \cdot X(4) \qquad (4)$$

$$\left(1 - \left(\frac{X(4)}{\mathrm{popmax}} \right) \right) - ks_{\mathrm{max}} \cdot X(4) \cdot \left(\frac{\left(\frac{X(2)}{V} \right)^{Hs}}{\mathrm{C50s}^{Hs} + \left(\frac{X(2)}{V} \right)^{Hs}} \right)$$

The first three equations describe the pharmacokinetics of the drug, (compartment 1, theoretical absorptive compartment for oral administration; 2, central compartment, and 3, peripheral compartment). Cl is the clearance defined, as the amount of drug being cleared from the central compartment over time and *V* is the volume of the central compartment. *K*a is the first-order absorption constant, *K*cp is the rate of drug moving from the central to peripheral compartment, and *Kpc* is the rate of drug moving from the peripheral to central compartment. Equation 4 describes the rate of change of the serum galactomannan values. Kp_{max} represents the maximum rate of production, *Hp* is the slope function for production, C_{50p} is the amount of drug where there is half maximal production, pop_{max} is the theoretical maximum density of galactomannan, ks_{max} is the maximum rate of galactomannan suppression, C_{50s} is the amount of drug where there is half maximal suppression, and *Hs* is the slope function for the galactomannan suppression.

6. Evaluate an acceptance of the final model by visual inspection of the observed-versus-predicted values plotted over time after the Bayesian step, the coefficient of determination (r^2) from the linear regression of the observed versus predicted values, as well as, evaluation of the estimated bias and precision.
7. After fitting the model to the PK-PD data, use the Bayesian posterior estimates for each rabbit to estimate the concentration-time profiles for antifungal agent or vaccine and GMI for each rabbit. Perform the simulations in ADAPT 5.
8. Calculate area under the plasma concentration-time curves (AUCs) by the linear trapezoidal rule from the simulated concentration-time profiles on the last day of dosing (at steady-state) in ADAPT 5.
9. Using simulated AUC values of the antifungal agent or vaccine and the GMI at the end of the dosing period for each rabbit, construct an inhibitory sigmoid E_{max} model to establish the pharmacodynamic relationship between exposure (AUC) over MIC and response (GMI). Use the model Eq. 5 described below:

$$\text{Effect} = E0 - \left(\frac{E_{\max} \cdot \left(\frac{AUC}{MIC} \right)^H}{EC50^H + \left(\frac{AUC}{MIC} \right)^H} \right) \tag{5}$$

*E*0 is the baseline level of galactomannan prior to exposure to drug, E_{max} is the maximum galactomannan value, EC_{50} is a measure of drug potency, and *H* is the slope factor.

3.8.4 Bridging to Humans

To bridge the exposure-response results from the rabbits to humans, a PPK model may be constructed using the antifungal agent or vaccine plasma concentration data from one or more clinical trials.

1. Develop a PPK model using nonparametric estimation in Pmetrics software [31] (*see* **Note 19**).
2. Use Mean Bayesian parameter estimates from the fitted human model to perform Monte Carlo simulations of 1000 patients using Pmetrics.

3. Use the simulations to calculate steady-state AUCs within Pmetrics by the trapezoidal rule for each simulated patient.
4. Using Eq. 5 above, calculate the effect of AUC/MIC at various MIC values representative of the MIC distribution and epidemiological cutoff value for the investigational antifungal agent for the organism.

3.9 Statistical Analysis

1. Perform the comparisons between the groups by the analysis of variance (ANOVA) with Bonferroni's correction for multiple comparisons or the Mann-Whitney U test, as appropriate. A two-tailed P value of ≤ 0.05 is considered to be statistically significant.
2. Plot survival by Kaplan-Meier analysis. Analyze differences in survival of treatment groups and untreated controls by log-rank test.
3. Express the values as means ± standard errors of the means (SEMs).
4. Compare pharmacokinetic parameters using ANOVA or Student's t test, as appropriate.
5. Perform correlation between AUC_{0-24} and outcome variables using Pearson's correlation method.

4 Notes

1. A finding of one colony of *Aspergillus fumigatus* or Mucorales is considered positive culture.
2. Before implementing these comparative experiments, we conducted preliminary studies of the methodology of quantitative cultures of infected tissues [6–11]. Among the methods studied are cultures of lung sections, minced tissue, and gently homogenized tissue. No loss of viability is found using these techniques. As there are no significant differences among these methods, the aforementioned method is selected for all subsequent experiments.
3. With the high-resolution, table-incremented, volume acquisition mode, 3-mm-thick ultrafast CT scans are obtained every 4 s.
4. These parameters resulted in a pixel size of less than 1 mm.
5. In virtually all cases, 30 slices are sufficient to scan the entire thorax of the rabbit.
6. The pulmonary lesion score in each lobe is initially 0. Each lobe is evaluated and scored independently. If the pulmonary infiltrate within the lobe demonstrated worsening, stabilization, or improvement, a score of −1, 0, or +1, respectively, is added at that time to the previous score.

7. The mean pulmonary lesion score for that day represents the mean of all lobes of all rabbits in each treatment group [32].
8. The use of an automatic method to segment the lung, such as seeded region growing, provides for a robust technique with less inter/intraoperator variability than manual tracing. The threshold range (1023 to 775) is determined empirically. If it is necessary to include/exclude tissue that is not properly segmented in the region-growing step, an option exists for the operator to trace the targeted tissue to include/exclude. For inclusion, the pixel values within the targeted tissue will be modified to be within the threshold range. For exclusion, the pixel values will be modified to be outside the threshold range. Perform the region-growing algorithm again, and the targeted tissue is now included/excluded as desired.
9. The threshold value of 500 Hounsfield units for lesion determination is based on previous literature and empirical evidence. Selecting a threshold value of 500 Hounsfield units excludes the air in the lungs but might include blood vessels, which have similar density to the lung lesions. Inclusion of these small vessels may reduce the sensitivity of detecting a lesion volume change over time.
10. Common human fungal pathogens are *Candida* spp. and *Aspergillus* spp., opportunistic fungal pathogens, including *Fusarium* spp., *Trichosporon* spp., *Saccharomyces cerevisiae, Acremonium, Coccidioides immitis, Histoplasma capsulatum, Sporothrix schenckii, Blastomyces dermatitidis*, and *Pneumocystis carinii*. The (1 → 3)-β-D-glucan produced by these organisms can be detected by the Fungitell assay.
11. Certain fungal species produce very low levels of (1 → 3)-β-D-glucan and are not usually detected by the Fungitell assay. These include *Cryptococcus, Zygomycetes* such as *Absidia, Mucor*, and *Rhizopus*.
12. The assay uses the rat monoclonal antibody EB-A2, which is directed against *Aspergillus* galactomannan and recognizes the (1 → 5)-β-D-galactofuranoside side chain of the galactomannan molecule. The monoclonal antibody is used: (a) to sensitize the wells of the microplate and to bind the antigen, and (b) as the detector antibody in the conjugate reagent (peroxidase-linked monoclonal antibody).
13. A monoclonal antibody-galactomannan-monoclonal antibody/peroxidase complex is formed in the presence of *Aspergillus* galactomannan antigen.
14. The substrate solution will react with the complexes bound to the well to form a blue color reaction.

15. The assays are specific for the target genera and did not amplify mammalian genes or those found in other fungal genera, including *Candida* spp. and *Aspergillus* spp. that are likely to be present in the same host [13, 16, 20, 33].
16. The amplicon generated is 253 bp long.
17. The primers and probes are designed to target the common plasmid cloning vector pBR322. The PCR master mix included a specific amount of target DNA (pBR322).
18. Equivalent amplification efficiencies compared to reactions performed with water reflected the lack of inhibitors.
19. The model fitting process includes evaluating both two- and three-compartment models with and without lag-time and oral bioavailability terms.

References

1. Kontoyiannis DP, Marr KA, Park BJ, Alexander BD, Anaissie EJ, Walsh TJ, Ito J, Andes DR, Baddley JW, Brown JM, Brumble LM, Freifeld AG, Hadley S, Herwaldt LA, Kauffman CA, Knapp K, Lyon GM, Morrison VA, Papanicolaou G, Patterson TF, Perl TM, Schuster MG, Walker R, Wannemuehler KA, Wingard JR, Chiller TM, Pappas PG (2010) Prospective surveillance for invasive fungal infections in hematopoietic stem cell transplant recipients, 2001-2006: overview of the transplant-associated infection surveillance network (TRANSNET) database. Clin Infect Dis 50(8):1091–1100. doi:10.1086/651263
2. Kosmidis C, Denning DW (2015) The clinical spectrum of pulmonary aspergillosis. Thorax 70(3):270–277. doi:10.1136/thoraxjnl-2014-206291
3. Patterson TF (2009) Risk stratification for invasive aspergillosis: early assessment of host susceptibility. Med Mycol 47(Suppl 1):S255–S260. doi:10.1080/13693780902718339
4. Rubio PM, Sevilla J, Gonzalez-Vicent M, Lassaletta A, Cuenca-Estrella M, Diaz MA, Riesco S, Madero L (2009) Increasing incidence of invasive aspergillosis in pediatric hematology oncology patients over the last decade: a retrospective single centre study. J Pediatr Hematol Oncol 31(9):642–646. doi:10.1097/MPH.0b013e3181acd956
5. Walsh TJ, Bacher J, Pizzo PA (1988) Chronic Silastic central venous catheterization for induction, maintenance and support of persistent granulocytopenia in rabbits. Lab Anim Sci 38(4):467–471
6. Francis P, Lee JW, Hoffman A, Peter J, Francesconi A, Bacher J, Shelhamer J, Pizzo PA, Walsh TJ (1994) Efficacy of unilamellar liposomal amphotericin B in treatment of pulmonary aspergillosis in persistently granulocytopenic rabbits: the potential role of bronchoalveolar D-mannitol and serum galactomannan as markers of infection. J Infect Dis 169(2):356–368
7. Petraitiene R, Petraitis V, Groll AH, Sein T, Piscitelli S, Candelario M, Field-Ridley A, Avila N, Bacher J, Walsh TJ (2001) Antifungal activity and pharmacokinetics of posaconazole (SCH 56592) in treatment and prevention of experimental invasive pulmonary aspergillosis: correlation with galactomannan antigenemia. Antimicrob Agents Chemother 45(3):857–869. doi:10.1128/AAC.45.3.857-869.2001
8. Petraitis V, Petraitiene R, Groll AH, Bell A, Callender DP, Sein T, Schaufele RL, McMillian CL, Bacher J, Walsh TJ (1998) Antifungal efficacy, safety, and single-dose pharmacokinetics of LY303366, a novel echinocandin B, in experimental pulmonary aspergillosis in persistently neutropenic rabbits. Antimicrob Agents Chemother 42(11):2898–2905
9. Petraitis V, Petraitiene R, Hope WW, Meletiadis J, Mickiene D, Hughes JE, Cotton MP, Stergiopoulou T, Kasai M, Francesconi A, Schaufele RL, Sein T, Avila NA, Bacher J, Walsh TJ (2009) Combination therapy in treatment of experimental pulmonary aspergillosis: in vitro and in vivo correlations of the concentration- and dose-dependent interactions between anidulafungin and voriconazole by Bliss independence drug interaction analysis. Antimicrob Agents Chemother 53(6):2382–2391. doi:10.1128/AAC.00329-09

10. Petraitis V, Petraitiene R, Moradi PW, Strauss GE, Katragkou A, Kovanda LL, Hope WW, Walsh TJ (2016) Pharmacokinetics and concentration-dependent efficacy of isavuconazole for treatment of experimental invasive pulmonary aspergillosis. Antimicrob Agents Chemother 60(5):2718–2726. doi:10.1128/AAC.02665-15
11. Petraitis V, Petraitiene R, Sarafandi AA, Kelaher AM, Lyman CA, Casler HE, Sein T, Groll AH, Bacher J, Avila NA, Walsh TJ (2003) Combination therapy in treatment of experimental pulmonary aspergillosis: synergistic interaction between an antifungal triazole and an echinocandin. J Infect Dis 187(12):1834–1843. doi:10.1086/375420
12. Petraitis V, Petraitiene R, Solomon J, Kelaher AM, Murray HA, Mya-San C, Bhandary AK, Sein T, Avila NA, Basevicius A, Bacher J, Walsh TJ (2006) Multidimensional volumetric imaging of pulmonary infiltrates for measuring therapeutic response to antifungal therapy in experimental invasive pulmonary aspergillosis. Antimicrob Agents Chemother 50(4):1510–1517. doi:10.1128/AAC.50.4.1510-1517.2006
13. Petraitis V, Petraitiene R, Antachopoulos C, Hughes JE, Cotton MP, Kasai M, Harrington S, Gamaletsou MN, Bacher JD, Kontoyiannis DP, Roilides E, Walsh TJ (2013) Increased virulence of Cunninghamella bertholletiae in experimental pulmonary mucormycosis: correlation with circulating molecular biomarkers, sporangiospore germination and hyphal metabolism. Med Mycol 51(1):72–82. doi:10.3109/13693786.2012.690107
14. Hope WW, Petraitis V, Petraitiene R, Aghamolla T, Bacher J, Walsh TJ (2010) The initial 96 hours of invasive pulmonary aspergillosis: histopathology, comparative kinetics of galactomannan and (1→3) beta-d-glucan and consequences of delayed antifungal therapy. Antimicrob Agents Chemother 54(11):4879–4886. doi:10.1128/AAC.00673-10
15. Petraitiene R, Petraitis V, Bacher JD, Finkelman MA, Walsh TJ (2015) Effects of host response and antifungal therapy on serum and BAL levels of galactomannan and (1→3)-beta-D-glucan in experimental invasive pulmonary aspergillosis. Med Mycol 53(6):558–568. doi:10.1093/mmy/myv034
16. Francesconi A, Kasai M, Petraitiene R, Petraitis V, Kelaher AM, Schaufele R, Hope WW, Shea YR, Bacher J, Walsh TJ (2006) Characterization and comparison of galactomannan enzyme immunoassay and quantitative real-time PCR assay for detection of Aspergillus fumigatus in bronchoalveolar lavage fluid from experimental invasive pulmonary aspergillosis. J Clin Microbiol 44(7):2475–2480. doi:10.1128/JCM.02693-05
17. Hope WW, Kruhlak MJ, Lyman CA, Petraitiene R, Petraitis V, Francesconi A, Kasai M, Mickiene D, Sein T, Peter J, Kelaher AM, Hughes JE, Cotton MP, Cotten CJ, Bacher J, Tripathi S, Bermudez L, Maugel TK, Zerfas PM, Wingard JR, Drusano GL, Walsh TJ (2007) Pathogenesis of Aspergillus fumigatus and the kinetics of galactomannan in an in vitro model of early invasive pulmonary aspergillosis: implications for antifungal therapy. J Infect Dis 195(3):455–466. doi:10.1086/510535
18. Kovanda LL, Petraitiene R, Petraitis V, Walsh TJ, Desai A, Bonate P, Hope WW (2016) Pharmacodynamics of isavuconazole in experimental invasive pulmonary aspergillosis: implications for clinical breakpoints. J Antimicrob Chemother 71(7):1885–1891. doi:10.1093/jac/dkw098
19. Petraitiene R, Petraitis V, Lyman CA, Groll AH, Mickiene D, Peter J, Bacher J, Roussillon K, Hemmings M, Armstrong D, Avila NA, Walsh TJ (2004) Efficacy, safety, and plasma pharmacokinetics of escalating dosages of intravenously administered ravuconazole lysine phosphoester for treatment of experimental pulmonary aspergillosis in persistently neutropenic rabbits. Antimicrob Agents Chemother 48(4):1188–1196
20. Kasai M, Harrington SM, Francesconi A, Petraitis V, Petraitiene R, Beveridge MG, Knudsen T, Milanovich J, Cotton MP, Hughes J, Schaufele RL, Sein T, Bacher J, Murray PR, Kontoyiannis DP, Walsh TJ (2008) Detection of a molecular biomarker for zygomycetes by quantitative PCR assays of plasma, bronchoalveolar lavage, and lung tissue in a rabbit model of experimental pulmonary zygomycosis. J Clin Microbiol 46(11):3690–3702. doi:10.1128/JCM.00917-08
21. Petraitis V, Petraitiene R, Groll AH, Roussillon K, Hemmings M, Lyman CA, Sein T, Bacher J, Bekersky I, Walsh TJ (2002) Comparative antifungal activities and plasma pharmacokinetics of micafungin (FK463) against disseminated candidiasis and invasive pulmonary aspergillosis in persistently neutropenic rabbits. Antimicrob Agents Chemother 46(6):1857–1869
22. Groll AH, Gullick BM, Petraitiene R, Petraitis V, Candelario M, Piscitelli SC, Walsh TJ (2001) Compartmental pharmacokinetics of the antifungal echinocandin caspofungin (MK-0991) in rabbits. Antimicrob Agents Chemother 45(2):596–600. doi:10.1128/AAC.45.2.596-600.2001
23. Groll AH, Lyman CA, Petraitis V, Petraitiene R, Armstrong D, Mickiene D, Alfaro RM, Schaufele RL, Sein T, Bacher J, Walsh TJ

(2006) Compartmentalized intrapulmonary pharmacokinetics of amphotericin B and its lipid formulations. Antimicrob Agents Chemother 50(10):3418–3423. doi:10.1128/AAC.00241-06

24. Groll AH, Mickiene D, Petraitis V, Petraitiene R, Kelaher A, Sarafandi A, Wuerthwein G, Bacher J, Walsh TJ (2005) Compartmental pharmacokinetics and tissue distribution of the antifungal triazole ravuconazole following intravenous administration of its di-lysine phosphoester prodrug (BMS-379224) in rabbits. J Antimicrob Chemother 56(5):899–907. doi:10.1093/jac/dki287
25. Groll AH, Mickiene D, Piscitelli SC, Walsh TJ (2000) Distribution of lipid formulations of amphotericin B into bone marrow and fat tissue in rabbits. Antimicrob Agents Chemother 44(2):408–410
26. Groll AH, Mickiene D, Werner K, Piscitelli SC, Walsh TJ (1999) High-performance liquid chromatographic determination of liposomal nystatin in plasma and tissues for pharmacokinetic and tissue distribution studies. J Chromatogr B Biomed Sci Appl 735(1):51–62
27. Groll AH, Sein T, Petraitis V, Petraitiene R, Callender D, Gonzalez CE, Giri N, Bacher J, Piscitelli S, Walsh TJ (1998) Compartmental pharmacokinetics and tissue drug distribution of the pradimicin derivative BMS 181184 in rabbits. Antimicrob Agents Chemother 42(10):2700–2705
28. Lee JW, Amantea MA, Francis PA, Navarro EE, Bacher J, Pizzo PA, Walsh TJ (1994) Pharmacokinetics and safety of a unilamellar liposomal formulation of amphotericin B (AmBisome) in rabbits. Antimicrob Agents Chemother 38(4):713–718
29. Walsh TJ, Foulds G, Pizzo PA (1989) Pharmacokinetics and tissue penetration of fluconazole in rabbits. Antimicrob Agents Chemother 33(4):467–469
30. Walsh TJ, Jackson AJ, Lee JW, Amantea M, Sein T, Bacher J, Zech L (2000) Dose-dependent pharmacokinetics of amphotericin B lipid complex in rabbits. Antimicrob Agents Chemother 44(8):2068–2076
31. Neely MN, van Guilder MG, Yamada WM, Schumitzky A, Jelliffe RW (2012) Accurate detection of outliers and subpopulations with Pmetrics, a nonparametric and parametric pharmacometric modeling and simulation package for R. Ther Drug Monit 34(4):467–476. doi:10.1097/FTD.0b013e31825c4ba6
32. Walsh TJ, Garrett K, Feurerstein E, Girton M, Allende M, Bacher J, Francesconi A, Schaufele R, Pizzo PA (1995) Therapeutic monitoring of experimental invasive pulmonary aspergillosis by ultrafast computerized tomography, a novel, noninvasive method for measuring responses to antifungal therapy. Antimicrob Agents Chemother 39(5):1065–1069
33. Walsh TJ, Wissel MC, Grantham KJ, Petraitiene R, Petraitis V, Kasai M, Francesconi A, Cotton MP, Hughes JE, Greene L, Bacher JD, Manna P, Salomoni M, Kleiboeker SB, Reddy SK (2011) Molecular detection and species-specific identification of medically important Aspergillus species by real-time PCR in experimental invasive pulmonary aspergillosis. J Clin Microbiol 49(12):4150–4157. doi:10.1128/JCM.00570-11

Part IV

Mechanism of Vaccine Protection

Chapter 19

$CD4^+$ T Cells Mediate Aspergillosis Vaccine Protection

Diana Diaz-Arevalo and Markus Kalkum

Abstract

Adaptive effector $CD4^+$ T cells play essential roles in the defense against fungal infections, especially against invasive aspergillosis (IA). Such protective $CD4^+$ T cells can be generated through immunization with specialized antifungal vaccines, as has been demonstrated for pulmonary *Aspergillus fumigatus* infections in mouse experiments. Adaptive transfer of fungal antigen-specific $CD4^+$ T cells conferred protection onto non-immunized naive mice, an experimental approach that could potentially become a future treatment option for immunosuppressed IA patients, focusing on the ultimate goal to improve their otherwise dim chances for survival. Here, we describe the different techniques to analyze $CD4^+$ T cell immune responses after immunization with a recombinant fungal protein. We present three major methods that are used to analyze the role of $CD4^+$ T cells in protection against *A. fumigatus* challenge. They include (1) transplantation of $CD4^+$ T cells from vaccinated mice into immunosuppressed naive mice, observing increasing protection of the cell recipients, (2) depletion of $CD4^+$ T cells from vaccinated mice, which abolishes vaccine protection, and (3) T cell proliferation studies following stimulation with overlapping synthetic peptides or an intact protein vaccine. The latter can be used to validate immunization status and to identify protective T cell epitopes in vaccine antigens. In the methods detailed here, we used versions of the well-studied Asp f3 protein expressed in a bacterial host, either as the intact full length protein or its N-terminally truncated version, comprised of residues 15–168. However, these methods are generally applicable and can well be adapted to study other protein-based subunit vaccines.

Key words $CD4^+$ T cells, Isolation by negative selection, Magnetic microbeads, Synthetic peptide, Vaccine, *A. fumigatus*, T cell depletion

1 Introduction

$CD4^+$ T cells are known as helper T cells that become activated after interaction of their T cell receptor (TCR) with peptide antigens displayed by MHC class II molecules, presented on the surface of antigen-presenting cells (APCs) [1]. After activation, T cells can differentiate into one of different subtypes, TH1, TH2, Treg, TH17, TFH, or TH9, which secrete cytokines to drive distinct types of immune responses that eliminate the pathogens [2–4].

It has been demonstrated in human and murine studies that antigen-specific $CD4^+$ T cells coincide with the protection against

Markus Kalkum and Margarita Semis (eds.), *Vaccines for Invasive Fungal Infections: Methods and Protocols*, Methods in Molecular Biology, vol. 1625, DOI 10.1007/978-1-4939-7104-6_19, © Springer Science+Business Media LLC 2017

or regression of *Aspergillus*-inflicted lesions [5–8]. Hence, the protective mechanism mediated by successful antifungal vaccines can be driven by antigen-specific primed $CD4^+$ T cells. Accordingly, there is substantial interest in characterizing the in vivo and in vitro $CD4^+$ T cell immune responses to test novel anti-aspergillosis vaccines [7, 9–12].

In recent years, several studies reported that $CD8^+$ T cells can also mediate protection against fungi. For *Histoplasma capsulatum* vaccinated mice, it was demonstrated that $CD8^+$T cells play a protective role in the absence of $CD4^+$ T cells, and antifungal memory $CD8^+$ T cells were maintained in the absence of $CD4^+$ T cells. Likewise for *A. fumigatus*, $CD8^+$ T cell immunity contributed to the protection of $CD4^+$ T cell depleted mice, and it was shown that the absence of $CD8^+$ T cells is associated with susceptibility to infection [13–15].

Animal models to study innate and acquired host-responses as well as therapeutic strategies against aspergillosis have been pursued extensively. For the most part murine, and to some extent avian models, have been used to study aspergillosis vaccine candidates. Mouse models are particularly popular among researchers, due to the wide availability strains with various genetic backgrounds that can be managed at ease and under affordable costs. Thereby, immunocompetent and immunosuppressed animals have been used to study susceptibility to the infection, to compare virulence to various strains of *Aspergillus*, to test preventive vaccines, and to study the protection after transplantation of adaptive T and B cells [16]. The mouse model with its established cell biological techniques is most adequate to study depletion or transplantation of adaptive immune cells and to elucidate their role in protection against the disease.

In this chapter, we describe three methods to analyze the functionality of $CD4^+$ T cells. The first method uses the transplantation of adaptive $CD4^+$ T cells to transfer protection against aspergillosis from vaccinated to naive mice. Isolation of adaptive $CD4^+$ T cells is required for this study, while maintaining their functionality for protection. The cells are isolated using a negative selection method [17], which relies on magnetic beads with crosslinked antibodies specific for certain membrane proteins of non-$CD4^+$ T cells. This method can be used to gently isolate the cells without perturbing their functional capacity.

The second method, depletion of $CD4^+$ T cells, is used to confirm the ability of vaccine-primed $CD4^+$ T cells to drive the immune response and to confer protection against aspergillosis. Complete depletion is achieved by the systemic treatment of mice with a $CD4^+$ T cell-specific antibody (GK1.5) for 3 days [7, 18–21]; and the efficiency of $CD4^+$ T cell depletion in the spleens and blood is assessed by flow cytometry. Treatment with the GK1.5 antibodies efficiently depletes >98% of the $CD4^+$ T cells, which suppresses vaccine protection to a low ~10% level [7].

The third method described here measures the vaccine-dependent proliferation of primed $CD4^+$ and $CD8^+$ T cells using the CellTiter-Glo luminescent cell viability assay [22], instead of using radioactive ^3H thymidine. In addition, this assay does not require prior isolation of T cells or radiation of antigen-presenting cells. The assay utilizes magnetic beads crosslinked to GK1.5 antibody and Ly-2 antibody (anti-CD8a) to enrich T cells following the stimulation with antigens (peptides or proteins) and controls.

2 Materials

2.1 Materials for Adaptive Transfer and Depletion of $CD4^+$ T Cells

2.1.1 Mouse Immunization, Antigens-Adjuvant

Mice: Female CF-1 mice 6–8 weeks of age (Charles River Laboratories).

Antigens: 15 μg full length or N-terminally truncated rAsp f3, the latter encompassing residues 15–168 (rAsp f3(15–168) expressed in *E- coli*, TiterMax adjuvant (TiterMax USA, Inc., Norcross, GA USA).

2.1.2 Negative Selection of $CD4^+$ T Cells

1. $CD4^+$ T Cell Isolation Kit, mouse (Cat # 130-104-454, Miltenyi Biotec).
2. Separation Buffer: phosphate buffered saline (PBS), pH 7.2, 0.5% bovine serum albumin (BSA), and 2 mM EDTA.
3. LS Column for max 1×10^8 labeled cells and max. 2×10^9 total cells (Miltenyi Biotec).
4. MidiMACS Separator (Miltenyi Biotec).
5. Labeled antibodies by fluorescence-activated cell sorter (FACS) analysis: Anti-Mouse CD4 FITC, Clone: RM4–4, Isotype Rat IgG2b, κ, and Anti-Mouse CD3ε PE, Clone: 145-2C11.
6. FACS Buffer (PBS, 0.5–1% BSA).
7. FACS tubes (Corning Falcon Round-Bottom Polystyrene Tubes, 12 × 75 mm size).
8. Sterile surgical instruments (forceps and scissors), petri dishes, sterile cell-strainer (40 μm), ethanol beaker, centrifuge (medium speed), and Flow Cytometer.

2.1.3 Immuno-suppression of Mice

2.5 mg/mouse cortisone acetate (CA), methylcellulose (0.5%) and Tween 80 (0.1%), PBS, Levofloxacin (Levaquin; Ortho-McNeil).

2.2 Depletion of $CD4^+$ T Cells

Monoclonal anti-CD4 IgG,GK1.5 antibody or alternatively, GK1.5 hybridoma cells (TIB-207; ATCC, Manassas, VA) to produce the mAb. The latter also requires Iscove's Modified Dulbecco's Medium (IMDM), Fetal bovine serum (FBS), BD Cell™ MAb Medium (BD

Biosciences, San Jose, CA), Corning CELLine Disposable Bioreactor, Sterile (CELLine), HiTrap protein G column (GE Healthcare Biosciences, Pittsburgh, PA), standard CO2 incubator, Binding buffer: 20 mM sodium phosphate, pH 7.0, Elution buffer: 0.1 M glycine-HCl, pH 2.7, 1 M Tris–HCl, pH 9.0, Ultrafiltration devices such as Amicon® Pro Purification System-100K (EMD Millipore, Billerica, MA), rat isotype control, Pierce Bicinchoninic acid (BCA) Protein Assay Kit, sodium citrate (3.8%), IMDM, and complete IMDM, 900 mL of IMDM +100 mL FBS + 10 mL of 100 × Penicillin-Streptomycin (10,000 U/mL) (Pen/Strep).

2.3 Challenge of Immunosuppressed Mice with A. fumigatus Conidia

Acidified water containing sulfamethoxazole (0.8 mg/mL) and trimethoprim (0.16 mg/mL), three million viable conidia in suspension in PBS (30 μL).

2.3.1 Culturing of A. fumigatus to Produce Conidia

A. fumigatus strain, potato dextrose (PD) agar (BD/Difco, Franklin Lakes, NJ), PBS, pH 7.2- Tween 80 (0.1%), PBS, 260 mL-vented tissue culture flasks, loops.

2.4 T Cell Proliferation Assay

2.4.1 Overlapping Peptides and Controls

Ten consecutive 20 amino acid containing peptides that cover the compete sequence of rAsp f3(15–168), each peptide overlapped five amino acids at the beginning and the end of the sequence (Peptide 2.0, Inc. Chantilly, VA) (Table 1), Sep-Pak C18 column (Waters Corporation, Milford, MA), DMSO (100%), 10 ng/mL phorbol myristate acetate (PMA) and 500 ng/mL Ionomycin, RPMI 1640–10% FBS.

2.4.2 Magnetic Beads

CD4 (L3T4 or GK1.5) MicroBeads, mouse (Cat # 130-049-201), CD8a (Ly-2) MicroBeads, mouse (Cat # 130-049-401) (Miltenyi Biotec, Inc., Bergisch Gladbach, Germany), 96-well plate magnetic separation rack and separation buffer.

1. CellTiter-Glo luminescent cell viability assay (Promega Corporation, Madison, WI), plate shaker for mixing 96-well plates, luminometer, CCD camera, or spectrophotometer.
2. Opaque 96-microwell Plates, 96-well plate centrifuge adapter, complete RPMI: 900 mL RPMI-1640 Medium plus 100 mL of FBS plus Pen/Strep.

3 Methods

3.1 Adaptive Transfer and Depletion of CD4⁺ T Cells

3.1.1 Immunization (Fig. 1)

1. Prepare the vaccine by emulsifying a solution of rAsp f3 [or rAsp f3 (15–168)] in PBS by combining it with an equal volume of TiterMax, followed by vortexing in the presence of glass beads (final rAsp f3 concentration should be 0.3 mg/mL).
2. Vaccinate the CF1 mice with TiterMax emulsified rAsp f3 [or rAsp f3 (15–168)] by subcutaneous injections at the base of the

Table 1

Synthetic overlapping Asp f3(15–168) peptides used for T cell proliferation assay

Peptide residue positions	Peptide sequence
P1 (15–34)	VFSYIPWSEDKGEITACGIP
P2 (30–49)	ACGIPINYNASKEWADKKVI
P3 (45–64)	DKKVILFALPGAFTPVCSAR
P4 (60–79)	VCSARHVPEYIEKLPEIRAK
P5 (75–94)	EIRAKGVDVVAVLAYNDAYV
P6 (90–109)	NDAYVMSAWGKANQVTGDDI
P7 (105–124)	TGDDILFLSDPDARFSKSIG
P8 (120–139)	SKSIGWADEEGRTKRYALVI
P9 (135–154)	YALVIDHGKITYAALEPAKN
P10 (150–168)	EPAKNHLEFSSAETVLKHL

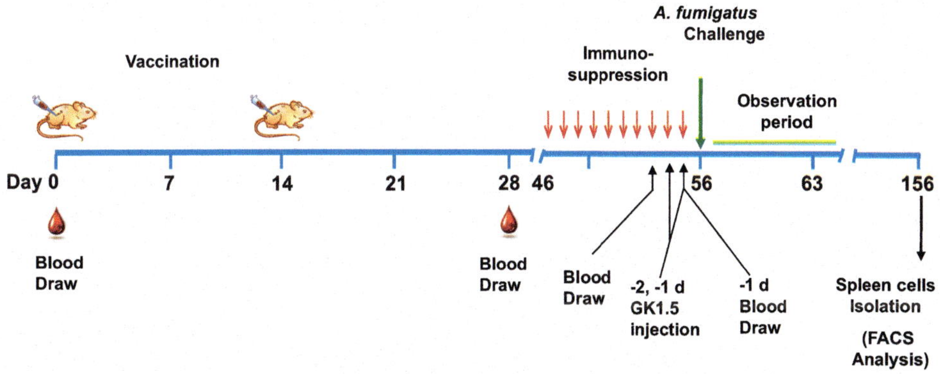

Fig. 1 Workflow of vaccination, cortisone acetate immunosuppression, *A. fumigatus* challenge, and T cell depletion with anti-CD4-IgG (GK1.5 mAb). The time points for blood draws on days 0, 14, and 28 days for antibody titer determination are indicated

tail. Per mouse 50 μL should be injected, corresponding to 15 μg rAsp f3. To avoid leakage of the emulsion, keep the needle inserted into the subcutaneous space for 10–15 s after each injection.

3. 14 days after the first immunization, vaccinate a second time with freshly prepared rAspf3 emulsified in TiterMax as described in **steps 1** and **2** above.
4. Obtain blood serum 2 weeks after the second immunization. Blood should be taken from the tail (small incision into one of the lateral veins after warming the animal up under a heat lamp). Determine the titer of anti-rAspf3 antibodies using ELISA and/or Western blot.

3.1.2 Isolation of CD4+ T Cells

1. Euthanize ten vaccinated and ten mock-vaccinated mice humanely with carbon dioxide.
2. Dip the entire mouse into 70% ethanol, held in a beaker. With sterile surgical instruments carefully cut an incision through the peritoneal layer and remove the entire spleen.
3. Pool the spleens of vaccinated mice and place them into RPMI-FBS (10%) medium at room temperature and continue the procedure in a sterile tissue culture hood.
4. Place sterile cell-strainers (40 μm) onto a petri dish with 10 mL of RPMI-FBS (10%) medium and transfer the spleens to these cell-strainers. With the plunger from a 5 mL syringe, smash the spleens and pass them through the strainer.
5. Transfer the spleen cell suspension to a 50 mL centrifuge tube. Wash the cells twice with separation buffer and count the cells after Trypan blue (0.4%) staining.
6. Repeat the same procedure (**steps 3–5**) with mock-vaccinated mice.
7. Resuspend the cell pellet, transfer 4×10^8 cells into 1600 μL of separation buffer and mix with 400 μL of Biotin-Antibody Cocktail from the $CD4^+$ T cell purification kit. Incubate for 5 min at 4 °C.
8. Add 1200 μL of separation buffer and mix with 800 μL of Anti-Biotin MicroBeads, incubate for 10 min at 4 °C.
9. Place the LS Column into the magnetic field of the MidiMACS separator and rinse the column with 5 mL separation buffer.
10. Add the cell suspension onto the column and collect the flow-through containing unlabeled cells (enriched $CD4^+$ T cells).
11. Wash column with 3 mL of separation buffer, collect the eluting $CD4^+$ T cells and combine with the flow-through from the previous step (*see* **Note 1**).
12. Wash the unlabeled cells twice with PBS, resuspend the cells in 30 mL of PBS, analyze the viability of the cells by counting the cells after Trypan blue staining. Separate an aliquot of 2×10^6 cells for FACS analysis and keep the rest for transplantation.

3.1.3 FACS Analysis

1. Adjust the cell suspension to a concentration of 2×10^6 unlabeled cells/1 mL in ice-cold FACS Buffer. Add 100 μL of cell suspension to each of five FACS tubes (2×10^5 cells/tube). Add 0.05 to 0.1 μg/mL of: Isotype control to tube #1, anti-Mouse CD4 FITC (Clone: RM4–4) and anti-Mouse CD3ε PE (Clone: 145-2C11) to tube #2, anti-Mouse CD4 FITC (Clone: RM4–4) to tube #3, anti-Mouse CD3ε PE (Clone: 145-2C11) to tube #4 and FACS buffer to tube #5.

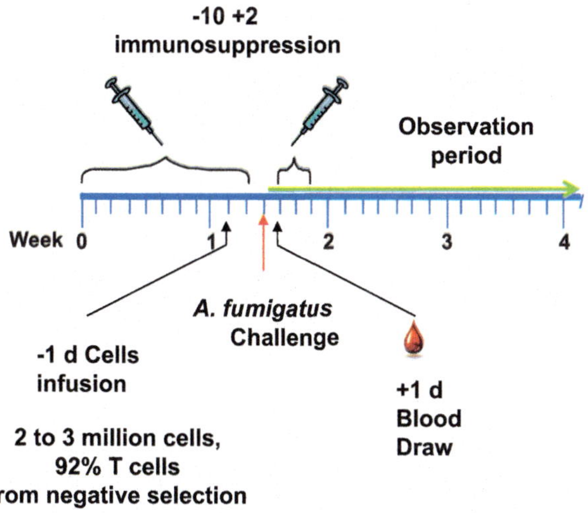

Fig. 2 Workflow: experimental transplantation of enriched CD4⁺ T cells into cortisone acetate-immunosuppressed naive CF-1 mice (10 day treatment), on the day before *A. fumigatus* challenge

2. Incubate for 30 min at 4 °C in the dark.
3. Wash the cells twice with cold FACS buffer by centrifugation at 350 × *g* for 5 min, following resuspension of the cells in 400 μL ice-cold FACS buffer, repeat. Keep the cells in the dark on ice or at 4 °C. Analyze the labeled cells with the flow cytometer.

3.1.4 Immuno-suppression of Naive and Immunized Mice (Fig. 1)

1. The immunosuppressive cortisone acetate suspension is injected subcutaneously at the base of the tail. Typically, 100 μL of a suspension of 2.5-mg of CA with methylcellulose (0.5%)-Tween 80 (0.1%), in PBS (sterilized by autoclaving) are injected each day for ten consecutive days prior to challenge and/or $CD4^+$ T cell transplantation.
2. To reduce the risk of bacterial infection, change the drinking water to acidified water containing Sulfamethoxazole (0.8 mg/mL) and Trimethoprim (0.16 mg/mL). Inject 200 μg of Levofloxacin subcutaneously 1 h prior to fungal challenge.

3.1.5 Transfer of CD4⁺ T Cells from rAspf3 Vaccinated and Mock Vaccinated into Naive Immunosuppressed Mice (Fig. 2)

1. Transplant 2.5×10^6 enriched $CD4^+$ T cells (in 100 μL of PBS, from Subheading 3.1.2) per recipient (naive immunosuppressed CF-1mice) one day before *A. fumigatus* challenge (day −1) and 1 day after the last injection of the immunosuppressant (day +1) by tail vein injection [7, 23].
2. Challenge with *A. fumigatus* spores (*see* Subheading 3.3).

3.2 Depletion of CD4 T Cells in Vaccinated and Mock-Vaccinated Mice

3.2.1 Production of Monoclonal Anti-Mouse CD4 IgG from GK1.5 Hybridoma Cells

1. Thaw the vial with GK1.5 hybridoma cells in a 37 °C water bath. Thawing should be performed rapidly (approximately 2 min). Decontaminate the vial's outside surface by dipping it into 70% ethanol.
2. Transfer the cells to a centrifuge tube containing 9.0 mL complete IMDM and centrifuge at 300 × *g* for 5 min.
3. Discard the supernatant and resuspend the cell pellet with complete IMDM.
4. Count the cell suspension and adjust cell density to 2–5 × 10^5 viable cells/mL and dispense into a 25 cm^2 cell culture flask. Incubate the culture at 37 °C in an incubator with 5% CO_2.
5. Grow the cells to a density of 30 × 10^6 (*see* **Note 2**).
6. Transfer the cells to a centrifuge tube and spin down at 300 × *g* for 5 min.
7. Resuspend the cells in 15 mL BD Cell™ MAb medium.
8. At the same time, add 50 mL of BD Cell™ MAb medium into the medium compartment of CELLine reactor and let it stand for 5 min.
9. Loosen the front cap of medium compartment, open the cell compartment and add 15 mL cell suspension using a serological pipette into the cone (*see* **Note 3**).
10. Close the cell compartment and add 975 mL of BD Cell™ MAb medium into the medium compartment.
11. Tighten both caps and place the CELLine reactor into a standard CO_2 incubator.
12. After 7 days of culture, loosen the front cap and open the cell compartment and transfer the 65 mL of the cell suspension into a centrifuge tube.
13. Spin down at 300 × *g* for 5–7 min, collect the supernatant (contained the monoclonal antibody), keep it at −20 °C.
14. Resuspend the cell pellet in 30 mL IMDM and count the viable cells using Trypan blue.
15. Collect 30 × 10^6 cells and add to 15 mL fresh medium.
16. Return 15 mL of cell suspension back into the cell compartment and place the CELLine into a standard CO_2 incubator.
17. Repeat the **steps 12–16** on days 14 and 21.
18. On the 28th day collect and keep the supernatant of the cell compartment and discard the CELLine reactor.

3.2.2 Monoclonal Anti-Mouse CD4 IgG Purification

1. Thaw the supernatant of the GK1.5 mAb and dilute it 1:1 with binding buffer (*see* **Note 4**).
2. Add 200 μL 1 M Tris–HCl, pH 8.0, per 1 mL of elution to collection tubes.

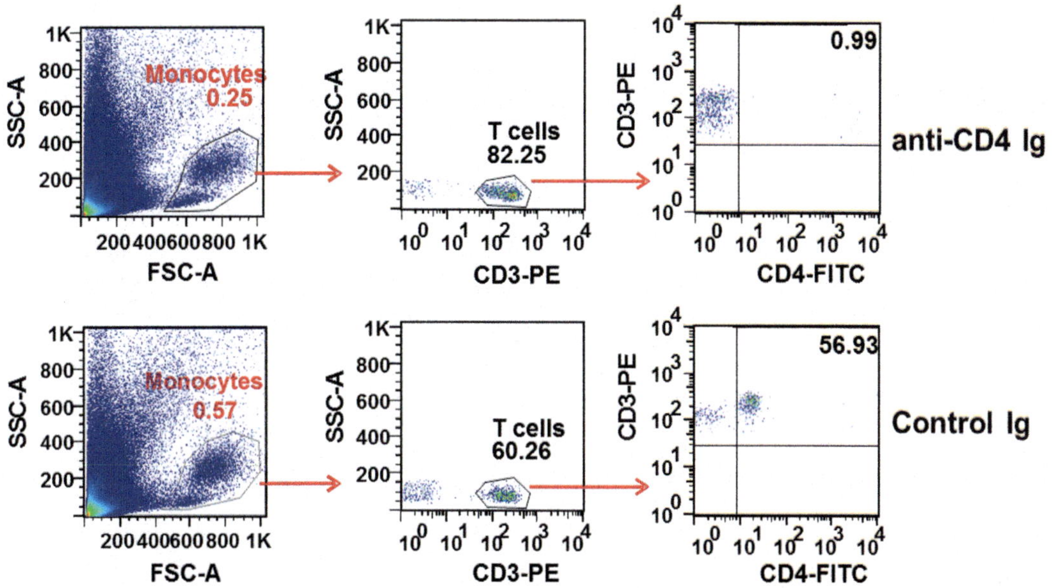

Fig. 3 FACS analysis of CD3⁺ CD4⁺ T cells in tail vein blood (taken at day −1) from mice that were depleted of CD4⁺ T cells in vivo by i.v. treatment with rat GK1.5 antibody (anti-CD4 IgG). Nonspecific rat IgG (control IgG) was used as a control. Relative frequencies of CD3⁺CD4⁺ T cells are indicated in the upper right quadrants

3. Wash the column with 10 column volumes of binding buffer at 1 mL/min.
4. Apply the sample onto the column at 0.7 mL/min. Collect the flow-through to measure antibody concentration by the BCA assay.
5. Wash with 7–10 column volumes of binding buffer.
6. Elute with 3–5 column volumes of elution buffer.
7. Analyze the purity of the mAb by SDS-GEL electrophoresis.
8. Collect all positive fractions and dialyze against PBS for 12 h or exchange and concentrate the eluted fractions with an Amicon 100 K MWCO ultrafiltration device.

3.2.3 Depletion of CD4⁺ T Cells (Fig. 1)

1. Inject GK1.5 mAb or rat isotype control (1.0 mg per mouse) via intravenous injection into the tail vein on days −2 and −1 prior to fungal challenge (*see* **Note 5**).
2. Monitor the depletion of the CD4⁺ T cells by FACS analysis (Fig. 3), using tail vein blood (50 μL samples) collected with 6.25 μL of sodium citrate (3.8%). Use the same procedure as in Subheading 3.1.3 (FACS analysis) (*see* **Note 6**).

3.3 *A. fumigatus* Infection and Evaluation

3.3.1 *A. fumigatus* Culture and Collection of Conidia (Spores)

1. Pour 50 mL of PD agar into a 260 mL tissue flat culture flask and leave it to set for 30 min.
2. Place 5 μL of a spore suspension from an *A. fumigatus* stock culture into the culture flask. Add 200 μL of PBS and spread the spores on the surface of the PD agar.
3. Incubate at 37 °C for 5–10 days with periodic monitoring.
4. Place 15 mL of PBS-0.1% Tween 80 into the flask and pipette it up and down until most of the spores have been dislodged.
5. Collect the spores using a 25 mL plastic pipette.
6. Wash the spores twice with PBS-0.1% Tween 80 and resuspend them in 10 mL of sterile PBS.
7. Count the spores with a hemocytometer and keep them at −80 °C in 15% glycerol-PD broth (*see* **Note 7**).

3.3.2 *A. fumigatus* Challenge

1. Administer 200 μg of levofloxacin subcutaneously 1 h prior to infection.
2. Anesthetize the mice with ketamine-xylazine (100 mg/kg to 10 mg/kg, respectively). To confirm that animals are deeply anesthetized, test for absence of reflexes by gently squeezing the footpad.
3. Inoculate the mice intranasally with 30 μL of conidial suspension containing 3×10^6 viable conidia by depositing the suspension onto the nostrils while holding the mouse in a vertical position. Hold the mouse for a few seconds to minutes until its breathing rhythm returns to normal.
4. Placed mice on their backs during recovery from anesthesia. Keep the mice warm using a heat pad (37 °C) under the mouse cage/enclosure.
5. Observe the mice twice a day for up to10 days, measure their weight on a scale, and determine their body temperature using an infrared noncontact thermometer (e.g., MiniTemp MT4 IR Thermometer, Raytek, Santa Cruz, CA). For this, restrain each mouse manually, expose the ventral side of the body, and point the thermometer to three different test areas on the animal's abdomen. Calculate and record the average of all three measurements.

3.4 T Cell Proliferation Assay

3.4.1 Lympho-proliferation Assay

1. Collect splenocytes from rAspf3 (15–168) immunized mice and mock-vaccinated mice following the protocol Subheading 3.1.2 (Isolation of $CD4^+$ T cells) from **steps 1** to **5**, but do not pool the spleens for this assay.
2. Suspend 2.5×10^6 cells/mL in RPMI-10% FBS with antibiotic/anti-mycotic and distribute 100 μL per well onto a round-bottom 96-well microtiter plate. Each antigen should be tested in three wells.

3. Dilute the stimulants (or antigens) inside of 1.5 mL microcentrifuge tubes at room temperature as follows: for peptides create a solution of 20 μg peptide/mL, for positive controls a solution of 200 ng/mL PMA with 1 μg/mL ionomycin, and 10 μg/mL of rAsp f3 from 1 mg/mL stock solutions.
4. Add 100 μL of stimulants to be tested to triplicates of wells with cells. Include a negative control (non-stimulated cells) with 100 μL of complete RPMI medium.
5. Place the 96 microtiter plates into a humidified incubator at 37 °C, 5% CO_2, for 3 days.

3.4.2 Purification of T Cells with CD4/CD8-Specific Magnetic Beads

1. Centrifuge the cells with a 96-well plate centrifuge adapter for 5 min at 350 × *g* and discard the supernatant.
2. Add separation buffer and centrifuge for 5 min at 350 × *g*. Remove the supernatant. Repeat this wash twice.
3. Resuspend the cells in 50 μL separation buffer.
4. Add 10 μL of CD4-microBeads, and 10 μL of CD8a-microBeads, incubate at 4 °C for 30 min.
5. Place the plate onto the microtiter plate magnetic separation rack and allow the CD4/CD8 microbeads to bind to the magnet (it takes approximately 10 min).
6. Remove the nonbinding cells and separation buffer.
7. Add 200 μL of separation buffer and repeat **steps 5** and **6**.
8. Reconstitute the CellTiter-Glo® Substrate (lyophilized) with the CellTiter-Glo® Buffer and leave it at room temperature for 30 min. Transfer the CellTiter-Glo® buffer-substrate mix into opaque 96-microwell plates, and keep the plate in a dark container.
9. Resuspend the CD4/CD8-magnetic beads with 100 μL of separation buffer, and transfer them well-by-well into the opaque 96-microwell plate with the reconstituted Cell Titer-Glo reagents from **step 8** and mix.
10. Add separation buffer into three separate wells with the CellTiter-Glo luminescent substrate that are free from cells and beads. Use these wells as controls to determine the bioluminescent background signal.
11. Place the plates onto an orbital shaker at 200 RPM for 2 min to lyze the cells.
12. Analyze the ATP content by measuring the bioluminescence with a plate-reading luminometer.
13. Calculate the stimulation indices by dividing the mean of relative luminescent units of stimulated cells by the mean relative luminescence of non-stimulated controls:

RLU(stimulated cells − background)/RLU(non-stimulated control − background) = Stimulation Index

4 Notes

1. The labeled non-CD4+ T cells can also be removed from the column and frozen for future analysis. To do so, remove the column from the separator and place it onto a fitting centrifuge tube and add separation buffer (5 mL) onto the column. Immediately flush out the cells by pushing the plunger into the column.
2. Most of the hybridoma cells will require a brief period of adaptation to BD Cell™ MAb medium. Seed the cells from the existing culture into the 75% of complete IMDM medium combined with 25% of BD Cell™ MAb medium. The cells will produce growth factors that will help them to adapt to the new medium. Every other day, split the cell population from one onto two separate flasks with BD Cell™ MAb medium. After five splits, spin down the cells at 300 × *g* for 5–7 min, resuspend the cells in 100% BD Cell™ MAb medium, place them in a humidified 37 °C, 5% CO_2 incubator for 2 days, and transfer the 30 × 10^6 to the CELLine reactor.
3. Minimize the introduction of air bubbles into the cell compartment of the CELLine reactor during seeding. If air gets trapped within the cell compartment, try to remove the big bubbles by aspirating them back into the pipette.
4. The sample should be completely solubilized. We recommend filtration immediately before loading the supernatant on the column (0.45 μm filter).
5. The vaccinated mice use for CD4+ T cell depletion is immunosuppressed with CA. Do not forget other controls as group of mock-vaccinated (PBS) mice and a group of mice vaccinated and CA immunosuppressed.
6. Only use two mice per group to prevent stress in all mice.
7. Spores should be collected fresh to challenge the mice.

Acknowledgment

This work was supported by the Hermann Foundation.

References

1. Jenkins MK, Khoruts A, Ingulli E, Mueller DL, McSorley SJ et al (2001) In vivo activation of antigen-specific CD4 T cells. Annu Rev Immunol 19:23–45
2. Dong C (2010) Helper T-cell heterogeneity: a complex developmental issue in the immune system. Cell Mol Immunol 7:163
3. Read KA, Powell MD, McDonald PW, Oestreich KJ (2016) IL-2, IL-7, and IL-15: multistage regulators of CD4+ T helper cell differentiation. Exp Hematol 44:799–808
4. Kanno Y, Vahedi G, Hirahara K, Singleton K, O'Shea JJ (2012) Transcriptional and epigenetic control of T cell lineage specification:

molecular mechanisms underlying commitment and plasticity. Annu Rev Immunol 30:707

5. Jolink H, Hagedoorn RS, Lagendijk EL, Drijfhout JW, van Dissel JT et al (2014) Induction of *A. fumigatus*-specific CD4-positive T cells in patients recovering from invasive aspergillosis. Haematologica 99:1255–1263
6. Bozza S, Gaziano R, Lipford GB, Montagnoli C, Bacci A et al (2002) Vaccination of mice against invasive aspergillosis with recombinant Aspergillus proteins and CpG oligodeoxynucleotides as adjuvants. Microbes Infect 4:1281–1290
7. Diaz-Arevalo D, Bagramyan K, Hong TB, Ito JI, Kalkum M (2011) CD4+ T cells mediate the protective effect of the recombinant Asp f3-based anti-aspergillosis vaccine. Infect Immun 79:2257–2266
8. Hebart H, Bollinger C, Fisch P, Sarfati J, Meisner C et al (2002) Analysis of T-cell responses to Aspergillus fumigatus antigens in healthy individuals and patients with hematologic malignancies. Blood 100:4521–4528
9. Chaudhary N, Staab JF, Marr KA (2010) Healthy human T-cell responses to Aspergillus fumigatus antigens. PLoS One 5:e9036
10. Hernández-Santos N, Huppler AR, Peterson AC, Khader SA, McKenna KC et al (2013) Th17 cells confer long-term adaptive immunity to oral mucosal *Candida albicans* infections. Mucosal Immunol 6:900–910
11. Fierer J, Waters C, Walls L (2006) Both CD4+ and CD8+ T cells can mediate vaccine-induced protection against Coccidioides immitis infection in mice. J Infect Dis 193:1323–1331
12. Specht CA, Lee CK, Huang H, Tipper DJ, Shen ZT et al (2015) Protection against experimental cryptococcosis following vaccination with glucan particles containing Cryptococcus alkaline extracts. MBio 6:e01905–e01915
13. Nanjappa SG, Heninger E, Wüthrich M, Sullivan T, Klein B (2012) Protective antifungal memory CD8+ T cells are maintained in the absence of CD4+ T cell help and cognate antigen in mice. J Clin Invest 122:987–999
14. Carvalho A, De Luca A, Bozza S, Cunha C, D'Angelo C et al (2012) TLR3 essentially promotes protective class I–restricted memory CD8+ T-cell responses to Aspergillus fumigatus in hematopoietic transplanted patients. Blood 119:967–977
15. Wüthrich M, Filutowicz HI, Warner T, Deepe GS, Klein BS (2003) Vaccine immunity to pathogenic fungi overcomes the requirement for CD4 help in exogenous antigen presentation to CD8+ T cells implications for vaccine development in immune-deficient hosts. J Exp Med 197:1405–1416
16. Clemons K, Stevens D (2005) The contribution of animal models of aspergillosis to understanding pathogenesis, therapy and virulence. Med Mycol 43:101–110
17. Manyonda IT, Soltys AJ, Hay FC (1992) A critical evaluation of the magnetic cell sorter and its use in the positive and negative selection of CD45RO+ cells. J Immunol Methods 149:1–10
18. Alters S, Sakai K, Steinman L, Oi V (1990) Mechanisms of anti-CD4-mediated depletion and immunotherapy. A study using a set of chimeric anti-CD4 antibodies. J Immunol 144:4587–4592
19. Wofsy D, Seaman WE (1986) Analysis of the function of L3T4+ T cells by in vivo treatment with monoclonal antibody to L3T4. Immunol Res 5:97–105
20. Rashid A, Auchincloss H, Sharon J (1992) Comparison of GK1. 5 and chimeric rat/mouse GK1. 5 anti-CD4 antibodies for prolongation of skin allograft survival and suppression of alloantibody production in mice. J Immunol 148:1382–1388
21. Arora S, McDonald RA, Toews GB, Huffnagle GB (2006) Effect of a CD4-depleting antibody on the development of Cryptococcus Neoformans-induced allergic bronchopulmonary mycosis in mice. Infect Immun 74: 4339–4348
22. Crouch S, Kozlowski R, Slater K, Fletcher J (1993) The use of ATP bioluminescence as a measure of cell proliferation and cytotoxicity. J Immunol Methods 160:81–88
23. Yi T, Zhao D, Lin C-L, Zhang C, Chen Y et al (2008) Absence of donor Th17 leads to augmented Th1 differentiation and exacerbated acute graft-versus-host disease. Blood 112:2101–2110

Chapter 20

T-Cell-Mediated Cross-Protective Immunity

Nina Khanna and Claudia Stuehler

Abstract

Human invasive fungal infections are caused by different mold and yeast species. Hence, cross-reactive T cells that recognize conserved epitopes of various fungal pathogens are of special interest for vaccination protocols or adoptive T cell transfer. Here, we describe an ELISpot-based method to test cross-reactivity of T cell lines or clones to different molds and yeasts.

Key words Cross-reactive T cells, ELISpot, Heat-inactivated fungi, Dendritic cells, T cell lines, T cell clones

1 Introduction

Invasive fungal infections are caused by a variety of different molds and yeasts [1, 2]. Hence, cross-reactive T cells that recognize conserved epitopes of various fungal pathogens are of special interest for vaccination protocols or adoptive T cell transfer. We have previously shown that *Aspergillus* (*A.*) *fumigatus*-specific T cell lines and clones were able to respond to *Candida albicans* and to other *Aspergillus* species including *A. flavus, A. terreus, A. niger*, and some *Mucorales* species such as *Rhizopus microspores* and *Lichtheimia corymbifera* [3, 4].

T cell cross-reactivity is inherent in the way T cells recognize antigen [5–8]. T cells are activated after recognizing a pathogen-derived peptide epitope bound to major histocompatibility complex (MHC) molecules on antigen-presenting cells (APC). MHC class I or class II molecules can accommodate 9 or 11 amino acids in their antigen binding grove, respectively. Each MHC molecule can bind a great variety of different peptides as only some amino acids of the peptide serve as so-called anchor residues that make intimate contact with the MHC molecule, whereas the other amino acids can vary freely. Similarly, not all amino acids of the peptide presented in peptide-MHC complexes make contact to the T cell receptor (TCR). In general, only three to four amino acids

Markus Kalkum and Margarita Semis (eds.), *Vaccines for Invasive Fungal Infections: Methods and Protocols*, Methods in Molecular Biology, vol. 1625, DOI 10.1007/978-1-4939-7104-6_20, © Springer Science+Business Media LLC 2017

of the peptide are exposed on the surface of the peptide-MHC complex and recognized by the TCR. Therefore, one specific TCR can recognize a great variety of peptides that share common motives. Depending on their phylogenetic relationship, the different fungal species show certain degrees of protein sequence homology (Table 1). Hence, there is a reasonable likelihood that T cells generated against one particular fungus might be cross-reactive to other phylogenetically related fungi.

Often in in vitro experiments a certain degree of cross-reactivity can be observed if T cells are stimulated with unphysiologically high peptide concentrations. However, these cells would not respond in vivo during an infection and it is therefore of importance to assess genuine cross-reactivity under more physiologic conditions. In vitro challenge of T cell lines or clones with autologous dendritic cells exposed to inactivated fungal pathogens can provide a good estimate of potential protective cross-reactivity in vivo. To definitely proof cross-reactivity of a single antigen-specific T cell/TCR to different fungal pathogens, the experimental work has to be conducted with T cell clones. However, cross-reactivity can also be assessed on the population level with oligo- or polyclonal T cell lines. Antigen-specific T cell lines can be generated within 2 weeks for instance via CD154- or CD137-based enrichment of antigen-specific cells.

Here, we describe an ELISpot-based assay to analyze antigen-specific T cell lines or clones for potential cross-reactivity to various clinically relevant molds and yeasts.

2 Materials

2.1 Fungal Cultivation and Inactivation

1. Liquid culture medium: Potato Dextrose Broth, prepared according to manufacturers' instructions (*see* **Note 1**). Suspend 24 g of powder in 1 L of distilled water. Mix thoroughly. Heat to completely dissolve the powder. Autoclave at 121 °C for 20 min. Store at 4 °C after cooling.
2. Culture plates: Prepare Potato Dextrose Broth with 15 g Agar per liter. Autoclave at 121 °C for 20 min, let the agar medium cool down to approximately 50 °C, and pour 20 ml per plate into 90 mm petri dishes. Let the plates dry in a laminar flow cabinet. Store at 4 °C.
3. Incubator at 25 °C (*see* **Note 2**).
4. Starting cultures of the different fungal strains (*see* **Note 3**).
5. Sterile 0.9% NaCl.
6. NaCl/Tween: Sterile 0.9% NaCl with 0.05% Tween 80 (*see* **Note 4**).
7. Sterile petri dish spatulae, cotton swaps, or similar devices to harvest spores.

Table 1
Sequence identity and similarity of various pathogenic molds and yeasts to immunogenic *A. fumigatus* proteins (NCBI blastp January 2016)

	Crf1		Gel1		Pep1		Pmp20		Cat1		SHMT		DppV		Mep		Sod1		Pep2	
	Identity	Similarity	Identity	Similarity	Identity	Similarity	Identity	Similarity	Identity	Similarity	Identity	Similarity	Identity	Similarity	Identity	Similarity	Identity	Similarity	Identity	Similarity
Aspergillus flavus	72	81	82	89	71	79	86	92	84	90	90	94	78	88	78	87	87	93	86	93
Aspergillus terreus	76	86	85	90	69	84	92	97	80	87	92	96	73	86	67	78	90	96	82	91
Aspergillus niger	65	78	84	89	71	82	90	95	80	87	92	95	65	78	64	77	89	97	88	95
Scedosporium apiospermum	46	62	55	69	–	–	54	69	61	73	84	91	43	59	–	–	74	86	70	81
Fusarium oxysporum	60	73	55	68	51	66	54	70	57	71	80	89	42	60	64	76	75	86	71	82
Lichtheimia corymbifera	36	56	49	64	37	49	37	57	48	62	67	80	35	52	–	–	45	60	50	68
Candida albicans	48	64	52	68	30	45	38	61	41	56	75	85	–	–	–	–	75	86	57	73
Candida glabrata	48	64	56	69	–	–	32	50	39	57	74	84	–	–	–	–	70	83	55	70
Rhizopus microsporus	30	49	43	59	40	52	37	57	49	64	64	77	36	51	42	57	58	70	51	67
Rhizopus oryzae	–	–	–	–	39	51	–	–	–	–	–	–	–	–	–	–	–	–	52	69
Scedosporium prolificans	–	–	–	–	–	–	–	–	–	–	–	–	–	–	–	–	–	–	–	–
Fusarium solani	–	–	–	–	–	–	–	–	–	–	–	–	–	–	–	–	–	–	–	–

Only data >30% sequence identity were included in the table

Crf1, extracellular cell wall glucanase Crf1 (Afu 1g16190); Gel1, 1,3-β-glucanosyl-transferase Gel1 (Afu 2g01170); Pep1, aspartic protease Pep1 (Afu 5g13300); Pmp20, cytosolic peroxisomal peroxiredoxin Pmp20 (Asp f3; Afu 6g02280); Cat1, mycelial Catalase 1 (Afu 3g02270); SHMT, serine hdroxymethyltransferase (Afu 3g09320); DppV, dipeptidyl-peptidase V (Afu 2g09030); Mep, metalloprotease (Afu 8g07080); Sod 1, superoxide dismutase (Afu 5g09240); Pep2, aspartic protease (Afu 3g11400)

8. Sterile needles or similar devices for the transfer of fungal hyphae to fresh plates.
9. Sterile cell strainers (40 μm), cotton wool, or tissue paper for filtration of spore solutions (*see* **Note 5**).
10. 250 ml conical flasks or similar culture vessels.
11. Orbital shaker for 250 ml conical flasks (optional, *see* **Note 6**).
12. Heating block for 1.5 or 2 ml tubes.

2.2 Generation of Antigen-Specific T Cell Lines or Clones

1. Peripheral blood drawn in the presence of an anticoagulant like heparin or EDTA or isolated peripheral blood mononuclear cells (PBMC). From 10 ml of whole blood you can expect around 1–2 × 10^7 PBMC.
2. Sterile Dulbecco's phosphate-buffered saline (DPBS).
3. For isolation of PBMC from whole blood: Ficoll-Paque (ρ = 1.077 g/ml) and sterile DPBS/EDTA: Dulbecco's phosphate-buffered saline with 2 mM EDTA.
4. Culture medium: RPMI 1640 with 5% pooled human serum, sterile filtered (*see* **Note 7**).
5. Specific antigen (e.g., peptide, peptide pool, recombinant protein, lysate). In this protocol, we used commercially available peptide pools of *A. fumigatus* Crf1, Pmp20, and Gel1 (Miltenyi Biotec).
6. Incubator with 5% CO_2 at 37 °C.
7. Human CD154 MicroBead Kit (Miltenyi Biotec; *see* **Note 8**).
8. MACS Separator for MS Columns (Miltenyi Biotec).
9. Purified anti-CD40 blocking antibody (optional according to the manufacturers' instructions but highly recommended for longer incubation times).
10. MACS buffer: PBS pH 7.2 with 0.5% bovine serum albumin and 2 mM EDTA.
11. Gamma-irradiation device.
12. Interleukin (IL)-2, IL-7, and IL-15 (*see* **Note 9**).
13. For T cell expansion or generation of T cell clones: purified anti-CD3 antibody (OKT-3), allogeneic PBMCs, T2 feeder cells.

2.3 Assessment of Cross-Reactivity by ELISpot

1. Inactivated fungi (*see* Subheading 2.1).
2. Expanded antigen-specific T cell lines or clones (*see* Subheading 2.2).
3. Autologous PBMC for the generation of dendritic cells (DC) and as control for the T cell lines or clones (fresh or frozen).

4. Optional: anti-CD14 microbeads (Miltenyi Biotec) for DC generation.
5. Culture medium RPMI/HS: RPMI 1640 with 5% pooled human serum, sterile filtered (*see* **Note 7**).
6. Dulbecco's phosphate-buffered saline (DPBS).
7. Optional: DPBS with $CaCl_2$ and $MgCl_2$ (*see* **Note 10**).
8. Recombinant human IL-4 (1000 U/μl), GM-CSF (800 U/μl), IL-6 (1000 U/μl), IL-1β (10 ng/μl), TNF-α (10 ng/μl) and prostaglandin E2 (PGE2, 1 μg/μl).
9. Positive control antigen (e.g., Staphylococcal enterotoxin B, SEB).
10. Optional: Irrelevant antigen (e.g., viral peptide pools, tetanus toxoid).
11. Multiscreen Filter Plates (e.g., Millipore MSIPN4W50).
12. Anti-human IFN-γ and IL-17 ELISpot reagents (e.g., from Mabtech) including purified coating antibodies (1-D1K for IFN-γ and MT44.6 for IL-17), biotinylated detection antibodies (7-B6-1 for IFN-γ and MT504 for IL-17), Streptavidin-ALP and BCIP/NBT substrate solution (*see* **Notes 11** and **12**).
13. PBS/Tween: PBS with 0.05% Tween 20.

3 Methods

3.1 Fungal Cultivation and Inactivation

All preparations should be done in a laminar flow cabinet under sterile conditions. Culture media and culture plates should be prewarmed to room temperature before use. Keep inoculated culture plates sealed with parafilm to avoid release of spores. Check regularly for the contamination of the plates, especially when simultaneously working with different fungal strains.

1. Transfer hyphae or spores from the starting culture to 2–5 fresh culture plates, depending on the amount of fungal spores needed and the growth properties of the fungal strain (Table 2). Fungal spores can be transferred with a sterile cotton swap moistened with sterile 0.9% NaCl. Actively growing hyphae can be transferred by cutting out small pieces of agar from the edge of the growing fungus with sterile needles and placing them on fresh culture plates. Seal the plates with parafilm.
2. Incubate the plates at 25 °C for 1–4 weeks until the fungi sporulate (*see* **Note 2** and Table 2). Check regularly.
3. To harvest the spores, carefully open the lid of the petri dish and flood the surface with 10 ml sterile NaCl/Tween (*see* **Note 4**). Bring the spores into solution by carefully detaching the spores for instance with a sterile petri dish spatula or cotton swap.

Table 2
Culture conditions for different pathogenic molds and yeasts recommended by the American Type Culture Collection (ATCC) and approximate data on growth rates and spore numbers based on our experience[a]

	Recommended culture medium (ATCC)[b]	Recommended growth temperature (ATCC)	Time to sporulation on PDA plates at 25 °C[a]	Number of spores/plate ($\times 10^8$)[a]	Time to germination in liquid culture[a]	Comments[a]
Molds						
Aspergillus flavus	PDA	25 °C	3–4 weeks (1–2 weeks at 37 °C)	2–10	10–20 h, accelerated at 37 °C	Increased growth rate at 37 °C
Aspergillus fumigatus	PDA	25 °C	3–4 weeks (1–2 weeks at 37 °C)	2–10	10–20 h, accelerated at 37 °C	Increased growth rate at 37 °C
Aspergillus niger	PDA	24–26 °C	3–4 weeks (1–2 weeks at 37 °C)	2–10	10–20 h, accelerated at 37 °C	Increased growth rate at 37 °C
Aspergillus terreus	YM, PDA	24–26 °C	3–4 weeks (1–2 weeks at 37 °C)	2–10	10–20 h, accelerated at 37 °C	Increased growth rate at 37 °C
Fusarium oxysporum	PDA	24–26 °C	3–4 weeks	0.2–1	10–20 h	
Lichtheimia corymbifera	YM, PDA	24–26 °C	1–2 weeks	1–10	12–24 h, accelerated at 37 °C	Increased growth rate at 37 °C
Rhizomucor	PDA	37 °C	1–2 weeks	1–10	12–24 h, accelerated at 37 °C	Increased growth rate at 37 °C

Rhizopus oryzae	PDA	24 °C	1–2 weeks	2–10	10–15 h, accelarated at 37 °C	Increased growth rate at 37 °C
Scedosporium apiospermum	YM, PDA	20–25 °C	2–3 weeks	0.2–1	12–24 h, accelerated at 37 °C	Increased growth rate at 37 °C
Scedosporium prolificans	PDA	24 °C	2–3 weeks	0.2–1	12–24 h	
Yeasts						
Candida albicans	YM, YEPD	24–26 °C	–	–	4–6 h at 37 °C	Development of pseudohyphae strongly strain-dependent; increased in YEPD with 10% FBS at 37 °C
Candida glabrata	YM, YEPD	24–26 °C	–	–	4–6 h at 37 °C	No development of pseudohyphae
Candida krusei	YM	24 °C	–	–	4–6 h at 37 °C	Growth predominately as pseudohyphae
Candida parapsilosis	YM, PDA	30–35 °C	–	–	4–6 h at 37 °C	Increased development of pseudohyphae in YEPD with 10% FBS at 37 °C

[a]The given data are only approximate values from our experience and can vary considerably depending on the fungal strain and the specific culture conditions

[b]Not all recommended culture media are included in this table; *PDA* potato dextrose agar, *YEPD* yeast extract peptone dextrose, *YM* yeast mold agar

4. Filter the spore solution through a sterile cell strainer, cotton wool, or tissue paper to remove hyphae and pieces of agar (*see* **Note 5**).
5. Spin down (400 × *g*, 5 min), decant the supernatant, and wash with 0.9% NaCl.
6. Determine the concentration of the spores with a hemocytometer.
7. To obtain germinating spores or hyphae for T cell stimulation inoculate 100 ml of liquid culture medium in 250 ml conical flasks with up to 1×10^8 fungal spores (*see* **Notes 6**, **13**, and **14**). Incubate the cultures at 25 or 37 °C with or without shaking for several hours to days depending on the fungal strain and the growth stage needed (Table 2). Check regularly under a microscope for the desired growth state.
8. Transfer the liquid cultures to 50 ml tubes and spin them down (400 × *g*, 5 min). If possible decant the supernatant or transfer the hyphal structures to fresh tubes with disposable sterile plastic pasteur pipettes (*see* **Note 15**). Wash with 0.9% NaCl.
9. Prepare stock solutions in distilled water and aliquot them in 1.5 ml or 2 ml tubes.
10. Heat-inactivate the fungal preparations at 96 °C for 2–4 h in a heating block.
11. All aliquots should be tested individually for surviving spores by plating a small volume on culture plates and culturing them for 7 days at 25 °C. If necessary, repeat the heat-inactivation step.
12. The concentration of germinating spores can be determined with a hemocytometer.
13. Large hyphal structures can be mechanically fragmented to smaller pieces for instance by repeatedly forcing the hyphal solution through a thin needle. As quantification of hyphal structures is difficult, we recommend titrating the optimal amount of antigen for stimulation of dendritic cells in preliminary experiments (*see* **Note 16**).

3.2 Generation of Antigen-Specific T Cell Lines and T Cell Clones

Various protocols for the generation of antigen-specific T cell lines and T cell clones are published. This protocol describes the generation of antigen-specific T cell lines within 14 days by CD154-based MicroBead selection. For generation of T cell lines by repeated restimulation and generation of T cell clones from T cell lines, *see* **Notes 17** and **18**, respectively.

1. PBMC isolation from blood: Mix blood 1:1 with DPBS. Carefully layer 20–35 ml of diluted blood over 15 ml of Ficoll-Paque in a 50 ml conical tube. Spin down at 700 × *g* for 15 min at 20 °C with reduced brake. Carefully transfer the

interphase containing the lymphocytes and monocytes to a fresh 50 ml conical tube (for instance with a disposable sterile plastic pasteur pipette). Fill the tube with DPBS/EDTA and spin down at 400 × *g* for 5 min at 20 °C. Wash a second time with DPBS. Resuspend cells in RPMI/HS and count with a hemocytometer.

2. For CD154-based selection transfer 5–8 × 10^7 PBMC in 5 ml of RPMI/HS to one well of a 6-well plate for each condition.
3. Add antigen to each well (e.g., peptide, peptide pool, recombinant protein, lysate). In this protocol, we used a combination of *A. fumigatus* Crf1, Pmp20 and Gel1 peptide pools at a final concentration of 1 μg/peptide/ml (*see* **Note 19**).
4. Add purified anti-CD40 blocking antibody at a final concentration of 1 μg/ml to prevent downregulation of CD154 (optional according to the manufacturers' instructions but strongly recommended for longer incubation times).
5. Incubated the cells at 37 °C with 5% CO_2 for 12–14 h.
6. Optional: Store a small aliquot of each sample at 4 °C to determine expression of the activation marker before isolation.
7. CD154 selection is performed according to the manufacturers' instructions as described below.
8. Count the cells, spin them down (300 × *g*, 10 min), and resuspend the cells in MACS buffer (40 μl per 10^7 cells). Add 10 μl of CD154-Biotin per 10^7 cells. Mix well and incubate for 15 min at 2–8 °C.
9. Wash the cells by adding 0.5–1 ml MACS buffer per 10^7 cells and centrifuge (300 × *g*, 10 min). Aspirate the supernatant completely.
10. Resuspend the cell pellet in 80 μl of MACS buffer per 10^7 cells. Add 20 μl of Anti-Biotin Microbeads per 10^7 cells. Mix well and incubate for 15 min at 2–8 °C.
11. Wash the cells by adding 1–2 ml MACS buffer per 10^7 cells and centrifuge (300 × *g*, 10 min). Aspirate the supernatant completely.
12. Resuspend up to 10^8 cells in 500 μl of MACS buffer.
13. Place a MS MACS Column in the magnetic field (sufficient for up to 1 × 10^7 labeled cells and 2 × 10^8 total cells). Rinse the column with 500 μl MACS buffer.
14. Apply cell suspension onto the column. Wash 3× with 500 μl MACS buffer. The flow through containing the unlabeled cells is also collected for each sample and used later as feeder cells.
15. Remove the column from the magnet and place it on a suitable collection tube. Pipette 1 ml of MACS buffer onto the column and immediately flush out the cells by firmly pushing the plunger into the column.

16. To increase the cell purity, the eluted positive fraction can be passed over a second column.
17. Count the positive and negative fractions in a hemocytometer. In our experience, 5–8 × 10^7 PBMC will yield 1–5 × 10^5 *A. fumigatus* peptide-specific cells.
18. Optional: Analyze small aliquots of the positive and negative fractions (as well as the aliquots retrieved before isolation) on a flow cytometer for cell types and purity (e.g., CD3, CD4, CD8, CD56, CD154).
19. The positive fractions can be either expanded as polyclonal T cell lines as described below or used for T cell cloning (*see* **Note 18**).
20. Gamma-irradiate all negative fractions at 35 Gy.
21. Transfer up to 4 × 10^5 cells of each positive fraction together with cells of the respective gamma-irradiated negative fraction in a ratio of 1:50 to one well of a 48-well plate in a final volume of 1 ml.
22. Add 5 U/ml IL-2 at days 0, 2, 4, and 6. Replenish 50% of the medium if it turns orange to yellow (*see* **Note 9**).
23. Add 10 ng/ml IL-7 and IL-15 at days 7, 9, and 11. Replenish 50% of the medium if it turns orange to yellow. As soon as the medium has to be replenished every day and microscopic inspection shows a dense layer of growing cells, split the culture to two wells (*see* **Note 20**).
24. Determine the specificity of the cell lines by ELISpot, intracellular cytokine assay, ELISA, or other (*see* **Note 11** and Subheading 3.3).
25. If the cell number of the T cell lines is not sufficient for further characterization, we recommend expanding the T cell lines with the rapid expansion protocol from Beck et al. [9] as described below.
26. Incubate 1–3 × 10^5 antigen-specific T cells together with 2.5 × 10^7 35 Gy-irradiated allogeneic PBMC and 5 × 10^6 60 Gy-irradiated T2 feeder cells in 25 ml RPMI/HS containing 30 ng/ml OKT-3 in 25 cm^2 cell culture flasks.
27. On day 1, add 50 U/ml IL-2.
28. On day 4, transfer the cultures to 50 ml conical tubes, spin down (400 × *g*, 5 min), and resuspend the cell pellet in RPMI/HS. Transfer the cells to fresh 25 cm^2 cell culture flasks with 25 ml PRMI/HS with 50 U/ml IL-2.
29. On days 7 and 10 add 50 U/ml IL-2. If the medium turns yellow, exchange 10 ml of the culture medium. If the medium turns yellow every day, split the culture to two flasks.
30. Cells can be used for experiments after 12–15 days.

3.3 Assessment of Cross-Reactivity by ELISpot

As expanded T cell lines or clones are devoid of antigen-presenting cells (APC), additional APCs are needed to process and present fungal antigens. In this protocol, we use autologous dendritic cells (DC) generated within 3–4 days [10, 11] (*see* **Note 21**).

T cell clones are preferred to test cross-reactivity due to their purity. In contrast, T cell lines are only enriched for antigen-specific cells and may contain T cells with other specificities. To confirm that the antigen-specific T cells mediate cross-reactivity to different fungal pathogens and that the response is not due to other cells contained in the T cell line, we compare the response to PBMC of the same donor (Fig. 1).

1. The optimal amount of fungal antigen for feeding immature DC should be titrated in preliminary experiments, especially when working with larger hyphal structures. For germinating spores a multiplicity of infection (MOI) of 1–2 spores per APC in most cases works well. For stimulation with hyphal structures it is essential to properly titrate the optimal amount of antigen (*see* **Note 16**).
2. Twelve to fifteen days before the cross-reactivity assay expansion of the antigen-specific T cell lines or clones has to be started (*see* Subheading 3.2, **steps 25–30**).
3. Generation of autologous monocyte-derived DC is started 3–4 days before the cross-reactivity assay. For monocyte enrichment by adherence, 2–3 × 10^7 freshly isolated or frozen PBMC

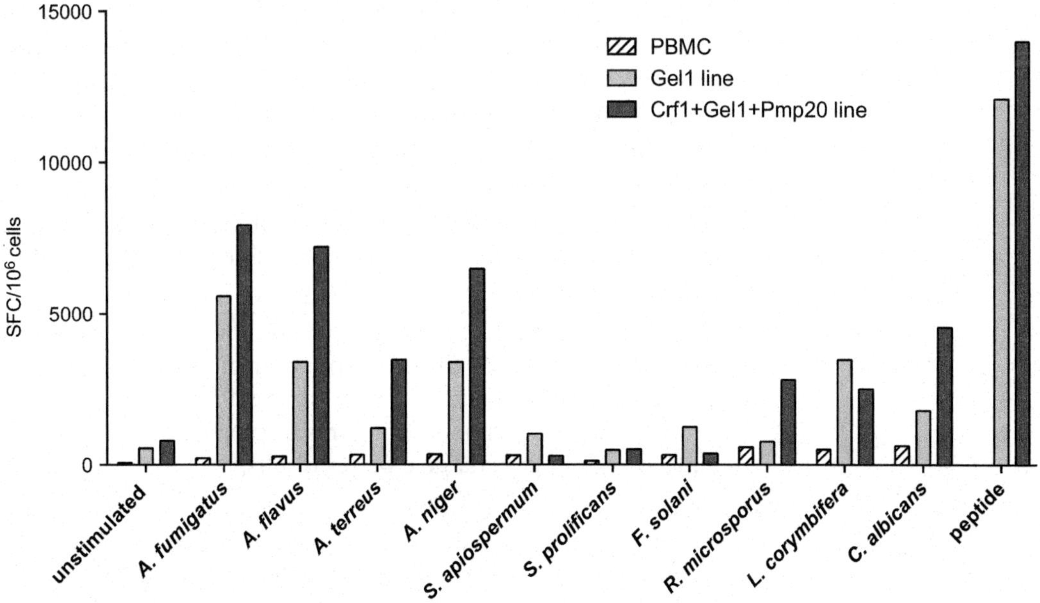

Fig. 1 IFN-γ secretion of PBMC, an A. fumigatus Gel1-specific and an A. fumigatus Crf1 + Gel1 + Pmp20-specific T cell line of the same donor after stimulation with different fungal pathogens determined by ELISpot

per well are incubated in tissue culture-treated 6-well plates for 2–3 h at 37 °C and 5% CO_2 (*see* **Note 22**). For each fungal pathogen, a separate well is needed plus additional wells for control DC. For the cross-reactivity assay we recommend a DC:T cell ratio of 1:10. For the total number of cells needed *see* **Note 23** and Table 3.

4. After 2–3 h when the monocytes have attached to the culture plate, carefully aspirate the non-adherent cells and repeatedly wash the layer of adherent cells with culture medium or DPBS with $CaCl_2$ and $MgCl_2$ (*see* **Note 10**). Check microscopically for the removal of non-adherent cells.
5. Add RPMI/HS with 1000 U/ml IL-4 and 800 U/ml GM-CSF and incubate for 2–3 days at 37 °C and 5% CO_2 to let the cells differentiate to immature DC.
6. One day prior to the stimulation experiment coat ELISpot plates with IFN-γ and IL-17 coating antibody (*see* **Notes 11** and **12**). Pretreat the plates with ethanol if necessary (pretreatment is dependent on the type of plate used, for instance Millipore PVDF plates type MSIP plates should be pretreated with 15 μl sterile 35% ethanol for maximally 1 min at RT). Wash the plates 3× with sterile PBS and add IFN-γ or IL-17 coating antibody in the concentration recommended by the manufacturer. We suggest preparing at least duplicates for each condition and titrating the cell number of antigen-specific T cells (Table 3). Store the plates at 4 °C.
7. The evening before the stimulation experiment the immature DC are stimulated with heat-inactivated fungi overnight with the amount of antigen determined in preliminary experiments. Control DC or DC that will be used for peptide stimulation are matured overnight by addition of a maturation cocktail containing 1000 U/ml IL-6, 10 ng/ml IL-1β, 10 ng/ml TNF-α, and 1 μg/ml PGE2.
8. At the day of stimulation, wash the ELISpot plates 3× with PBS and block the membrane by the addition of 200 μl RPMI/HS per well for at least 90 min.
9. Preparation of control PBMC (optional, if working with T cell clones): For isolation of PBMC from fresh blood *see* Subheading 3.2, **step 1**. Alternatively, cryopreserved PBMC can be used. However, we recommend using freshly prepared PBMC if possible as they in general give better results.
10. Detach the DC by gentle scraping with a cell scraper (mature DC adhere only weakly to the cell culture plate) and transfer them to 15 ml conical tubes. Rinse the wells with RPMI/HS or DPBS to recover any left cells. Spin down (400 × *g*, 5 min) and resuspend the pellet in RPMI/HS. Count the cells with a hemocytometer.

Table 3
Number of samples and cell numbers needed for a hypothetical cross-reactivity assay with three different T cell lines and PBMC from the same donor

Sample	Number of wells	Number of PBMC/T cells	Number of DC
Control DC and fungus-pulsed DC only (background control)	11 × 2 wells	–	2× 3 × 10^4 of control DC and each fungus-pulsed DC population
PBMC only (background control, optional)	1 × 2 wells (optional)	2× 3 × 10^5	–
PBMC + unpulsed mature DC (negative control)	1 × 2 wells	2× 3 × 10^5	2× 3 × 10^4 control DC
PBMC + SEB (positive control)	1 × 2 wells	2× 3 × 10^5	–
PBMC + fungus-pulsed DC	10 × 2 wells	20× 3 × 10^5	2× 3 × 10^4 of each fungus-pulsed DC population
T-cell lines only (background control, optional)	3 × 2 wells (optional)	2× 5 × 10^4 of each line	–
T-cell lines + unpulsed mature DC or DC pulsed with irrelevant antigen (I)	3 × 2 wells	2× 5 × 10^3 of each line	6× 5×10^2 control DC
T-cell lines + unpulsed mature DC or DC pulsed with irrelevant antigen (II)	3 × 2 wells	2× 5 × 10^4 of each line	6× 5×10^3 control DC
T-cell lines + DC pulsed with specific antigen (positive control) (I)	3 × 2 wells	2× 5 × 10^3 of each line	2× 5×10^2 of each antigen-pulsed DC population
T-cell lines + DC pulsed with specific antigen (positive control) (II)	3 × 2 wells	2× 5 × 10^4 of each line	2× 5 × 10^3 of each antigen-pulsed DC population
T-cell lines + fungus-pulsed DC (I)	3 × 10 × 2 wells	20× 5 × 10^3 of each line	6× 5 × 10^2 of each fungus-pulsed DC population
T-cell lines + fungus-pulsed DC (II)	3 × 10 × 2 wells	20× 5 × 10^4 of each line	6× 5 × 10^3 of each fungus-pulsed DC population
Total numbers	198 wells	PBMC: 26× 3 × 10^5 (7.8 × 10^6) T-cell lines (3×): 26× 5 × 10^4 + 24× 5 × 10^3 (1.42 × 10^6)	Control DC: 4× 3 × 10^4 + 6× 5 × 10^3 + 6× 5 × 10^2 (1.53 × 10^5) Antigen-pulsed DC (3×): 2× 5 × 10^3 + 2× 5 × 10^2 (1.1 × 10^4) Fungus-pulsed DC (10×): 4× 3 × 10^4 + 6× 5 × 10^3 + 6× 5 × 10^2 (1.53 × 10^5)

Cross-reactivity to ten different fungal pathogens is analyzed in duplicates using two different cell numbers (5 × 10^3 and 5 × 10^4 cells/well) and a DC:T-cell ratio of 1:10. If two different cytokines are tested (e.g., IFN-γ and IL-17) the double amount of cells is needed

11. Preparation of T cell lines or clones: Spin the cells down, wash with RPMI/HS or DPBS, resuspended in RPMI/HS, and count them with a hemocytometer.
12. Prepare dilutions for the T cell lines, PBMC, and DC according to the number of cells needed for restimulation (Table 3). To facilitate the assay procedure, we recommend preparing tenfold concentrations for each sample. For example, if the final number per well is 5×10^4 cells, the cells should be adjusted to 5×10^5 cells/ml. The optimal number of cells per well in the ELISpot assay strongly depends on the specificity of the T cell line. For highly specific T cell lines or T cell clones cell numbers $<10^4$ per well should be used, for lines with lower specificity the cell number can be increased to 10^5 cells per well. We recommend titrating the optimal cell number in preliminary experiments or using at least two different cell numbers (Table 3). For stimulation of whole PBMC a cell number of 3×10^5 per well works well in our hands.
13. Discard the blocking medium from the ELISpot plates.
14. To each well add 100 μl of the respective tenfold T-cell/PBMC suspension and 100 μl of the respective tenfold DC suspension.
15. 24–72 h after stimulation, the ELISpot can be developed. IFN-γ secretion is usually faster and the plates can be developed after 24 h. For the IL-17 ELISpot we recommend stimulating the cells for 48–72 h.
16. Shake out the cell suspension and wash the plates 5× with PBS/Tween. Add biotinylated IFN-γ or IL-17 detection antibody in the concentration recommended by the manufacturer. Incubate for 2 h at RT. Wash the plates 5× with PBS/Tween and add streptavidin-ALP in the concentration recommended by the manufacturer. Incubate for 1 h at RT. Wash the plates 5× with PBS/Tween, peel off the underdrain, and rinse the plates from both sides with tap water. Add to each well 50 μl of BCIP/NBT solution. After the appearance of spots, rinse the plates from both sides with tap water and let the plates dry overnight.
17. The number of spot forming cells (SFC) is determined with an ELISpot reader.

4 Notes

1. Different fungal species need different culture media for optimal growth. However, Potato Dextrose Broth worked well for all fungal species used in this protocol (*see* Table 2).

2. Different fungal species need different temperatures for optimal growth. However, 25 °C worked well for all fungal species used in this protocol. If possible, some species can be incubated at 37 °C to accelerate growth (*see* Table 2).
3. Starting cultures can be obtained on petri dishes, agar slants, cryopreserved, freeze-dried, or others. Please follow the instructions of the provider on how to start the culture.
4. Other protocols suggest varying concentrations of other detergents such as Tween 20 or Triton X-100 in 0.9% NaCl, PBS, or distilled water. All detergent solutions should work similarly.
5. Removal of hyphal structures and agar from spore suspensions can be achieved by different methods. A very convenient way is the use of sterile 40 μm cell strainers that fit on top of 50 ml conical tubes. Further options can be filtration of the spore suspensions through sterile filter paper or several layers of sterile lens tissue or filtration through cotton wool or glass wool inserted into 5 ml pipet tips or syringes.
6. In our experience, spores germinate faster and more uniformly in conical flasks on an orbital shaker at low speed. However, if there is no orbital shaker available, the spore solutions can also be incubated without shaking.
7. Pooled human serum can be either purchased or prepared from at least five different healthy volunteers. For long-term expansion of very rare populations of antigen-specific cells, we strongly recommend the use of human serum instead of fetal calf serum to avoid background due to T cell responses to bovine proteins. For short-term experiments with T cell lines or clones fetal calf serum might also work.
8. Alternatively, antigen-specific T cells can be enriched with CD137 MicroBeads or by weekly restimulation with antigen for several weeks (*see* **Note 16**).
9. Instead of IL-2/IL-7/IL-15, also other cytokine combinations such as IL-4/IL-7 can be used for T cell expansion [12].
10. Monocyte adhesion is dependent on the presence of divalent cations. To avoid monocyte detachment during the wash steps we recommend using either cell culture medium or DPBS supplemented with $CaCl_2$ and $MgCl_2$ for washing.
11. ELISpot allows an estimation of the number of cells that secrete the specific cytokine of interest. Other methods for the detection of responding cells such as intracellular cytokine (ICC) assays, ELISA or Multiplex Cytokine detection assays can be used alternatively or in addition to the ELISpot assay. ICC assays also allow quantification of responding cells, can detect several cytokines simultaneously, and can provide additional

information about the phenotype of responding cells. However, the sensitivity is in our experience often lower than in ELISpot. ELISA and Multiplex Cytokine detection assays are very sensitive, but only provide information about the total amount of cytokines secreted by a whole cell population and do not give information about the frequency of responding cells.

12. In this protocol we analyzed IFN-γ and IL-17 secretion to estimate cross-reactivity of the T cell lines. IFN-γ and IL-17 are signature cytokines for T_H1 and T_H17 cells, respectively, which have been shown to be protective in anti-fungal immunity. Depending on the fungal pathogen, the importance of a T_H1 or T_H17 response can differ, for instance T_H17 immunity seems to be of minor importance in protection against *A. fumigatus*, but of great importance in protection against *C. albicans* infections.

13. Resting spores are in general only little immunogenic and do not induce proper maturation of antigen-presenting cells and T cell stimulation.

14. If the spore suspension is too concentrated, often only a part of the spores germinate. If the spores do not germinate uniformly, dilution of the spore solution might help.

15. Longer hyphae often do not form compact pellets during centrifugation. We suggest either centrifuging the cultures without brake or letting the hyphal structures settle for some time after centrifugation and transfer them with disposable sterile plastic pasteur pipettes to fresh tubes.

16. Small hyphal fragments might be counted with a hemocytometer. For hyphal preparations with larger fragments, we generally titrate the optimal amount of antigen in preliminary experiments. It is often also helpful to estimate the ratio of fungal structures to immune cells by visual inspection in flat-bottom 96-well plates under a microscope.

17. For the generation of T cell lines by repeated restimulation, around 2×10^7 PBMC per well are cultured in 6-well plates for several weeks. The cells are restimulated weekly with antigen-pulsed antigen-presenting cells (for the generation of dendritic cells, *see* Subheading 3.3). The cultures are supplemented with 5 U/ml IL-2 every second day and the medium replenished as needed.

18. For limiting dilution cloning, 300 cells of the T cell lines are mixed with 1×10^8 gamma-irradiated (35 Gy) allogeneic PBMC and 7.5×10^6 gamma-irradiated (60 Gy) T2 feeder cells in 200 ml RPMI/HS. The medium is supplemented with 30 ng/ml purified anti-CD3 antibody (OKT-3) and 50 U/ml IL-2. The cell suspension is then distributed to ten 96-well U-bottom plates (200 μl/well). Wrap the plates in aluminum

foil to reduce evaporation and incubate them at 37 °C and 5% CO_2 for 14 days. Wells that contain a growing T cell clone can be recognized by a dense cell pellet.

19. If antigen is limited, PBMC can be stimulated with antigen in a 15 ml conical tube in 100–200 μl of RPMI/HS for 1 h at 37 °C and afterward transferred to the 6-well plate and the culture medium filled up to 5 ml.
20. In our experience, the cells grow better in dense conditions. If the cells are split too early, growth might be slowed down. Microscopic estimation of the density of viable cells is only possible during the second week of expansion, after the feeder cells start to degenerate.
21. Instead of DC, also macrophages can be used as APC for stimulation of the T cell lines. However, DC have in general a higher potency to stimulate T cells. If macrophages are used, the APC:T cell ratio should be increased from 1:10 to 1:5.
22. Alternatively to monocyte isolation by adherence, $CD14^+$ cells can be isolated by $CD14^+$ microbeads. The initial cell number is around 20% of PBMC, but in our experience the final number of dendritic cells is comparable to the number obtained by monocyte adherence.
23. PBMC contain approximately 5% monocytes. In our experience the amount of monocyte-derived DC after 3 days is approximately 1–2% of PBMC. To reduce cell manipulation and cell loss, we generally do not detach and count the immature DC prior to stimulation but assume a cell number equivalent to 1–2% of the PBMC per well at the start of the culture. If you want to count the DC prior to stimulation, we suggest setting up a separate well.

References

1. Brown GD, Denning DW, Gow NA, Levitz SM, Netea MG, White TC (2012) Hidden killers: human fungal infections. Sci Transl Med 4(165):165rv113. doi:10.1126/scitranslmed.3004404
2. Marr KA (2008) Fungal infections in hematopoietic stem cell transplant recipients. Med Mycol 46(4):293–302. [pii] 791304420. doi:10.1080/13693780701885552
3. Stuehler C, Khanna N, Bozza S, Zelante T, Moretti S, Kruhm M, Lurati S, Conrad B, Worschech E, Stevanovic S, Krappmann S, Einsele H, Latge JP, Loeffler J, Romani L, Topp MS (2011) Cross-protective TH1 immunity against Aspergillus fumigatus and *Candida albicans*. Blood 117(22):5881–5891. [pii] blood-2010-12-325084. doi:10.1182/blood-2010-12-325084
4. Stuehler C, Nowakowska J, Bernardini C, Topp MS, Battegay M, Passweg J, Khanna N (2015) Multispecific Aspergillus T cells selected by CD137 or CD154 induce protective immune responses against the most relevant mold infections. J Infect Dis 211(8):1251–1261. doi:10.1093/infdis/jiu607
5. Birnbaum ME, Mendoza JL, Sethi DK, Dong S, Glanville J, Dobbins J, Ozkan E, Davis MM, Wucherpfennig KW, Garcia KC (2014) Deconstructing the peptide-MHC specificity of T cell recognition. Cell 157(5):1073–1087. doi:10.1016/j.cell.2014.03.047
6. Degauque N, Brouard S, Soulillou JP (2016) Cross-reactivity of TCR repertoire: current concepts, challenges, and implication for allotransplantation. Front Immunol 7:89. doi:10.3389/fimmu.2016.00089

7. Nikolich-Zugich J, Slifka MK, Messaoudi I (2004) The many important facets of T-cell repertoire diversity. Nat Rev Immunol 4(2):123–132. doi:10.1038/nri1292
8. Sewell AK (2012) Why must T cells be cross-reactive? Nat Rev Immunol 12(9):669–677. doi:10.1038/nri3279
9. Beck O, Topp MS, Koehl U, Roilides E, Simitsopoulou M, Hanisch M, Sarfati J, Latge JP, Klingebiel T, Einsele H, Lehrnbecher T (2006) Generation of highly purified and functionally active human TH1 cells against Aspergillus fumigatus. Blood 107(6):2562–2569
10. Ramadan G (2014) Fast monocyte-derived dendritic cell-based immunotherapy. Methods Mol Biol 1139:131–144. doi:10.1007/978-1-4939-0345-0_12
11. Ramadan G, Konings S, Kurup VP, Keever-Taylor CA (2004) Generation of Aspergillus- and CMV-specific T-cell responses using autologous fast DC. Cytotherapy 6(3):223–234. doi:10.1080/14653240410006040
12. Gerdemann U, Keirnan JM, Katari UL, Yanagisawa R, Christin AS, Huye LE, Perna SK, Ennamuri S, Gottschalk S, Brenner MK, Heslop HE, Rooney CM, Leen AM (2012) Rapidly generated multivirus-specific cytotoxic T lymphocytes for the prophylaxis and treatment of viral infections. Mol Ther 20(8):1622–1632. doi:10.1038/mt.2012.130

Chapter 21

Assessment of Post-Vaccination Phagocytic Activation Using *Candida albicans* Killing Assays

Wenqing Li and Yan Hu

Abstract

Candida albicans is an important opportunistic fungal pathogen. It is now the fourth leading cause of nosocomial bloodstream infections and a great threat to the immuncompromised patients attributed to the disseminated candidiasis with the mortality up to 40%. Phagocytic cells are the first line of defense against *Candida* infections. Antibodies induced by vaccination can effectively enhance the capacities of phagocytosis and killing of neutrophils and macrophages. In this chapter, flow cytometric analysis (FACS) and killing assay by plate culture methods are introduced to evaluate the phagocytosis and killing of strains of *Candida albicans* opsonized with immune serum obtained from mice vaccinated with yeast and recombinant enolase.

Key words Neutrophils, Macrophage, Phagocytosis, Killing, Flow cytometric analysis, Antibody

1 Introduction

Candida albicans is a widespread opportunistic pathogen that continues to be a leading cause of mucocutaneous and disseminated infections in immunocompromised hosts. It is now the fourth most common cause of nosocomial bloodstream infections, with an associated mortality rate of up to 40–50%, even with modern antifungal therapy [1, 2]. Until now, one of the main concerns has been focused on the preventive or therapeutic use of vaccines against candidiasis.

Phagocytic cells are the first line of defense against systemic and mucocutaneous *Candida* infections. The efficiency of phagocytosis and killing of various *Candida* isolates by neutrophils and macrophages is closely related to the susceptibility of host to candidiasis. The antibodies induced by the live yeasts, attenuated yeasts, recombinant cell wall polysaccharides, proteins and peptides of *Candida* species can effectively protect host against *Candida* infections with enhancing phagocytosis and killing of yeasts through opsonization and neutralization of antigens [3]. Therefore,

Markus Kalkum and Margarita Semis (eds.), *Vaccines for Invasive Fungal Infections: Methods and Protocols*, Methods in Molecular Biology, vol. 1625, DOI 10.1007/978-1-4939-7104-6_21, © Springer Science+Business Media LLC 2017

the assessment of the capacities of phagocytosis and killing of neutrophils and macrophages is essential to evaluate the protective efficiency of vaccines against *Candida* infection.

In this chapter, flow cytometric analysis (FACS) and killing assay by plate culture method were mainly introduced to evaluate the phagocytosis and killing of strains of *Candida albicans* which were opsonized with immune serum obtained from mice vaccinated with yeast and recombinant enolase.

2 Materials

2.1 Immunization

2.1.1 Live Candida albicans

1. *Candida albicans* isolate 3630 was obtained from the Australian Medical Mycology Reference Laboratory (AMMRL) at the Royal North Shore Hospital, Sydney. The strain 3630 was isolated from the nail of a patient with cutaneous candidiasis.
2. *Candida albicans* isolate 3683 was obtained from the Austral ian Medical Mycology Reference Laboratory (AMMRL) at the Royal North Shore Hospital, Sydney. The strain 3683 was isolated from the mouth of a patient at Fairfield Hospital, Victoria, Australia in 1991.
3. *C. albicans* SC5314 (ATCC Catalogue number MYA-2876) was a gift from Dr. P. Sundstrom, Ohio State University. SC5314 is described in the ATCC catalogue as a clinical specimen submitted by Dr. Y.R. Thorstenson, and has been described as an isolate from a patient with disseminated candidiasis [4].
4. Glycerol.
5. Sabouraud broth.
6. Shaker.
7. Phosphate Buffered Saline (PBS): NaCl 40 g, KCl 1 g, Na_2HPO_4 7.2 g, KH_2PO_4 1.2 g dissolved in 4 L distilled water. Adjust pH to 7.4, add distilled water till 5 L. Autoclave and store at room temperature.

2.1.2 Heat-Killed Yeast [5]

1. The high virulence *Candida albicans* ATCC 26555 was used for vaccination with the heat-killed yeast.

2.1.3 Preparation of Recombinant Protein of Candida albicans (See Note 1) (Cloning, Expression, Purification, and Immunological Identification Recombinant Enolase) [6]

1. Coding sequence of enolase.
2. 5′primer (5′-GGGCATATGATGTCTTACGCCACTAAA ATC-3′) and 3′ primer (5′-AAACTCGAGCAATTGAGAAG CCTTTTGG-3′) with NdeI/XhoI restriction enzyme sites.
3. Prokaryotic expression vector pET30a (+) (Novagen).
4. *Escherichia coli* BL21 (DE3) (Promega).
5. 1.0 mM isopropyl-β-d-thiogalactopyranoside (IPTG).

6. Centrifuge and sonicator.
7. His Bind Purification Kit (Novagen).
8. ToxinEraserTM endotoxin removal resin (Genmed).
9. Limulus Amebocyte Lysate (LAL) assay (Genmed).
10. Bradford reagent.
11. Bovine serum albumin (BSA) standard.
12. SDS-PAGE (12% gel).
13. Polyvinylidene difluoride (PVDF) membrane.
14. Blocking buffer: PBS, 0.05% Tween 20 (PBS-T, pH 7.4) and 1% bovine serum albumin (BSA).
15. Horseradish peroxidase (HRP)-conjugated anti-mouse immunoglobulin G (Fab specific, 1:2000 dilutions).
16. Dilution buffer: 0.1% BSA in PBS-T.
17. Diaminobenzidine solution (Dako Denmark A/S, Denmark): 1 mL Reagent A solution and 50 μL Reagent B solution well mixed.
18. Complete Freund's adjuvant.
19. Incomplete Freund's adjuvant.

2.2 Mice (See Note 2)

Inbred mice (BALB/c, CBA/CaH, and C57BL/6J) are the widely used strains in the study. Mice are suggested to be kept in filter top cages in a PC2 facility, and given food and water ad libitum. All the animal experiments should be done in the environment with PC2 facility and approved by the Animal Experimentation Ethics Committee.

2.3 Enzyme Linked Immunosorbent Assay (ELISA)

1. Microtiter plates.
2. 0.1 M carbonate/bicarbonate buffer (pH 9.5): Na_2CO_3 1.59 g and $NaHCO_3$ 2.94 g mixed in 1000 mL distilled water and stored at 4 °C.
3. PBS-T (pH 7.4): 0.5 mL Tween-20 in 1000 mL PBS, mixed together and store at room temperature.
4. Blocking buffer: 5% skim milk in PBS-T.
5. Dilution buffer: 0.1% BSA in PBS-T.
6. (HRP)-conjugated goat anti-mouse immunoglobulin G (1:20,000 dilution).
7. 1 mg/mL 3,3-,5,5-tetramethylbenzidine.
8. 2 M H_2SO_4.
9. Microplate spectrophotometer.

2.4 Isolation of Phagocytic Neutrophils and Monocytes

1. RPMI-1640 medium.
2. Centrifuge.
3. Bone marrow culture medium (BMM): Glutamine 0.292 g, Pyruvic acid 0.11 g, HEPES 2.383 g, $NaHCO_3$ 2 g, Monothioglycerol 10 μL, Hydrocortisone 21-hemisuccinate 0.462 mol, FCS (fetal calf serum) 150 mL. Add RPMI-1640 w/o l-glutamine and $NaHCO_3$ to 1 L.
4. 75 cm^2 cell culture flask.
5. Cell culture incubator, 5% CO_2 at 37 °C with 95% humidity.

2.5 Percoll Density Gradient

1. Percoll.
2. 10× Hanks' balanced salt solution without Ca^{2+} and Mg^{2+} (HBSS).
3. 10 mM HEPES.
4. Pasteur pipettes μ.
5. RPMI-1640 medium.
6. Mouse-osmolality phosphate-buffered saline (MPBS): Na_2HPO_4 0.92 g, KH_2PO_4 0.2 g, KCl 0.2 g, NaCl 9.83 g. Dissolved in 1 L distilled water and filtered with 0.2-mm filter.

2.6 Differentiation of Macrophages In Vitro

1. RPMI-1640 medium.
2. Medium nylon mesh (diameter at 0.2 mm).
3. Red cell lysis solution (Sigma, USA. 100 mL ready-to-use solution, store at 2–8 °C).
4. Cell counter.
5. Macrophage culture medium (MCM): 10% FCS, 20% L-cell supernatant in RPMI-1640 with l-glutamine and $NaHCO_3$.
6. L-cell supernatant: Supernatant collected from 3 to 4 day L-cell cultures (1 × 10^7 cells set up in 150 cm^2 flask).
7. L-cell Medium (for AIC L929 cells). 5% FCS in RPMI-1640 with l-glutamine and $NaHCO_3$.
8. 95 × 15 mm bacterial culture dishes.
9. Cell scraper.

2.7 Opsonization of Yeasts with Normal or Immune Serum

1. Sterile PBS.
2. 37 °C water bath.

2.8 Phagocytosis of Yeasts by Phagocytic Cells

1. Microscopic slides.
2. Giemsa stain.
3. Ethanol.
4. 0.1 mg/mL FITC in 0.5 M carbonate/bicarbonate buffer (pH 9.5).

5. 10× Hanks' balanced salt solution without Ca^{2+} and Mg^{2+} (HBSS).
6. PBS.
7. 1.5 mL microcentrifuge tube.
8. 37 °C water bath with horizontal shaking at 90 rpm.
9. Stop solution: 0.02% ethylenediaminetetraacetic acid (EDTA) in PBS.
10. 10 μg/mL ethidium bromide (EB).
11. Flow Cytometer with CellQuest Version 3.1, FACS Calibur.
12. 0.1 mg/mL FITC-rat IgG2a/PE-rat IgG2a.

2.9 Candida Killing Assays

2.9.1 Assessment of Killing with FACS

1. *C. albicans* cells.
2. 0.3 mg/mL FITC in HBSS (pH 7.2).
3. PBS.
4. 1.5 mL microcentrifuge tube.
5. 37 °C water bath with horizontal shaking at 90 rpm.
6. Distilled water.
7. 0.02% (w/v) DNAse solution.
8. 100 μg/mL propidium iodide (PI).

2.9.2 Assessment of Killing of Yeast by Plating

1. *C. albicans* cells.
2. PBS.
3. Distilled water.
4. YPD medium.
5. Incubator 37 °C.

3 Methods

3.1 Immunization Protocol

3.1.1 Immunization with Live Yeast

1. Store yeasts at −70 °C in 15% (v/v) glycerol in Sabouraud's broth and grow in Sabouraud's broth for 48 h at room temperature with continuous agitation.
2. Inject mice with 3 × 10^5 *C. albicans* 3630 and 3683, but 4 × 10^4 SC5314, in 200 μL PBS via the tail vein [6, 7] (*see* **Note 4**).

3.1.2 Immunization with Heat-Killed Yeast

1. Incubate *C. albicans* ATCC 26555 at 37 °C for 48 h.
2. Collect the cells by centrifugation and wash with PBS prior to the inactivating treatment.
3. Heat-kill the cells (20 × 10^6 cells/mL in PBS) by incubating at 100 °C for 1 h.
4. Inject 2 × 10^7 cells via the tail vein.

3.1.3 Preparation of Recombinant Cell-Wall Protein Enolase of Candida albicans (Cloning, Expression, Purification, and Immunological Identification Recombinant Enolase) and Immunization (See Notes 5 and 6).

1. Amplify the coding sequence of enolase by polymerase chain reaction (PCR) using 5′primer (5′-GGGCATATGATGTCTTACGCCACTAAAATC-3′) and 3′primer (5′-AAACTCGAGCAATTGAGAAGCCTTTTGG-3′) with NdeI/XhoI restriction enzyme sites (underlined), respectively.
2. Purify the PCR product and clone into the corresponding restriction sites of a prokaryotic expression vector pET30a (+) and confirm the recombinant vector by double-enzyme digestion and sequencing.
3. Transform the recombinant plasmid into *Escherichia coli* BL21 (DE3) and induce protein expression by IPTG at a final concentration of 1.0 mM for 5 h at 37 °C.
4. Collect the induced bacterial cells by centrifugation and disrupt by ultrasonication.
5. Purify of the recombinant enolase from the supernatant by affinity column chromatography using His Bind Purification Kit. Remove endotoxin by ToxinEraserTM endotoxin removal resin, resulting in levels <0.1endotoxin units/mL as indicated by the LAL assay, following the manufacturer's protocol.
6. Determine the protein concentration using the Bradford method, with BSA as a standard.
7. Subject the purified rEnolase (5 μg) to SDS-PAGE (12% gel) and then electro-transfer to PVDF membrane.
8. Block the membranes with the blocking buffer overnight at 4 °C and then incubate with either immune or normal serum from C57BL/6J mice at 1:100 dilutions for 2 h at room temperature (RT).
9. After washing five times with PBS-T, probe the membranes with HRP-conjugated anti-mouse immunoglobulin G for 1 h at RT. Dilute both primary and secondary antibodies with 0.1% BSA in PBS-T. After further washing, develop the membranes with diaminobenzidine solution as a substrate.
10. Vaccinate ten (6-week) female C57BL/6 mice subcutaneously with 100 μg of purified recombinant enolase (rEno1p) in complete Freund's adjuvant, then boost twice, at 2 week intervals, with 50 μg of rEno1p in incomplete Freund's adjuvant, and infect systemically 2 weeks after the final boost. Ten female C57BL/6 mice of the same age received adjuvant alone mixed with PBS as a control group, and a further ten of the same age mice received PBS alone (without adjuvant) as a negative control group.

3.2 Obtain Immune Serum

1. Obtain the blood from immunized mice by direct heart puncture on weeks 2, 5, and 8 after systemic immunization.
2. Collect the sera by centrifugation of blood at 30,705 × *g* for 15 min at 4 °C. Store pooled sera at −20 °C until used.

3.3 Antibody Assay—ELISA

Antibody isotypes and titers in serum were measured by an enzyme linked immunosorbent assay (ELISA).

1. Coat microtiter plates with 0.5 μg purified rENO1 antigen in 0.1 M carbonate-bicarbonate buffer (pH 9.6) per well and incubate at 4 °C overnight.
2. Block with blocking buffer for 2 h at 37 °C.
3. Add 100 μL serum samples diluted 1:100 with PBS-T containing 0.1% BSA per well and incubate at 37 °C for 2 h.
4. Add 100 μL HRP-conjugated goat antimouse IgG to each well and incubate the plate for 0.5 h at 37 °C.
5. Develop with substrate 3,3-,5,5-tetramethylbenzidine.
6. Stop the reaction by adding 2 M H_2SO_4 (50 μL per well).
7. Measure the microtiter plates with microplate spectrophotometer at 450 nm.

3.4 Isolation of Phagocytic Neutrophils and Monocytes

Long-term bone marrow cultures for the production of neutrophils and monocytes were established as follows [8, 9].

1. Flush bone marrow cells from femurs and tibias using RPMI-1640 medium, centrifuge at 626 × *g* for 10 min.
2. Resuspend in BMM.
3. Inoculate 3.3 × 10^7 cells into a 75 cm^2 cell culture flask in 20 mL BMM, incubate in 5% CO_2, at 37 °C with 95% humidity for 3 weeks, replacing half of the medium with fresh medium every week.
4. On week 4, remove the culture medium and add an equal volume of freshly isolated bone marrow cells into the flasks, after that culture them for a further week.
5. Collect the total supernatant on week 5 for the isolation of neutrophils and monocytes.
6. Harvest the cells weekly.

3.5 Obtain Phagocytic Cell with Percoll [8, 10] (See Note 3)

1. Prepare Percoll density solutions by mixing nine volumes Percoll with one volume of 10× PBS. Dilute this solution to 1× HBSS (pH 7.2) with 10 mM HEPES to the following working concentrations: 81% (1.1002 g/mL); 65% (1.0812 g/mL); and 55% (1.0693 g/mL) (*see* **Note 3**).
2. Isolate neutrophils and monocytes on a discontinuous Percoll density gradient. Harvest the non-adherent cells from the cultures and resuspend in 3 mL 1× HBSS with 10 mM HEPES. Layer the cells onto the gradients and centrifuge at 2143 × *g* for 40 min at 10 °C. Harvest the cells in the third layer with Pasteur pipettes as neutrophils and others as monocytes (Fig. 1). Wash the cells twice with MPBS and suspend in RPMI-1640 for use.

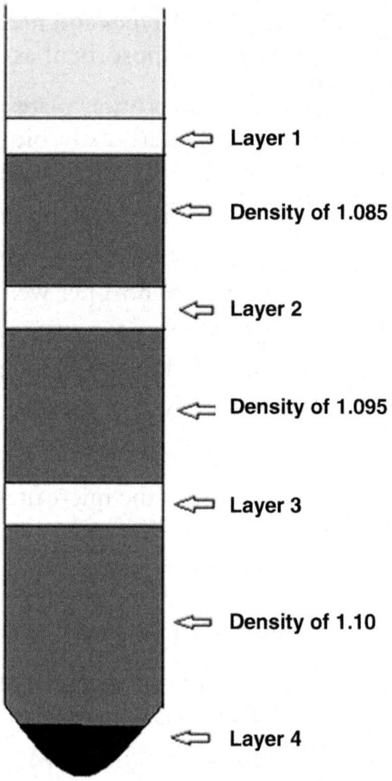

Fig. 1 Layering of cells after centrifugation on Percoll density gradients. According to the density, the third layer containing neutrophils, and the second containing monocytes

3.6 Differentiation of Macrophages In Vitro

1. Flush mouse bone marrow cells from femurs and tibias with RPMI-1640, pass through medium nylon mesh to remove clumps.
2. Centrifuge at 626 x *g* for 10 min and resuspend in red cell lysis solution for 5 min at 37 °C.
3. Wash the cell suspension twice with RPMI-1640, count, and dispense 1 × 10^7cells in 15 mL MCM into 95 × 15 mm bacterial culture dishes.
4. Incubate the plates in 5% CO_2, 95% humanity at 37 °C for 7 days. Replace the medium on days 4 and 6 with an equal volume of MCM.
5. Harvest the macrophages using a cell scraper, wash once with RPMI-1640, and resuspend at the appropriate concentration for use.

3.7 Opsonization of Yeasts with Normal or Immune Serum

Incubate the yeasts with 20% normal mouse serum, or immune serum from systemically immunized mice, in PBS, in a 37 °C water bath for 30 min and wash twice with PBS before use.

3.8 Phagocytosis of Yeasts by Phagocytic Cells

1. Place functional neutrophils, monocytes, and macrophages on slides, stain with Giemsa, and examine their morphology.
2. Fix the yeasts with 75% ethanol for 1 h at room temperature and label with 0.1 mg/mL FITC in 0.5 M carbonate/bicarbonate buffer (pH 9.5) for an hour in the dark with continuous agitation. After washing twice with PBS, resuspend *Candida* in HBSS and store at −70 °C for use.
3. Wash the fixed yeast cells, with or without opsonization, twice with PBS and incubate with phagocytic cells (1×10^6) in 1 mL PBS in a 1.5 mL microcentrifuge tube at ratios of effector to yeast of 1:1, 1:2, and 1:4 for 30 min in a 37 °C water bath with horizontal shaking at 90 rpm.
4. After incubation, spin down the cells, and add 1 mL of stop solution to stop phagocytosis. Finally, add 500 μL EB followed by flow cytometric analysis (FACS). Preliminary experiments demonstrated that a 30 min incubation at a ratio of effector to yeast of 1:1 was optimal for comparison of phagocytosis (Fig. 2a) (*see* **Note 7**).
5. Perform FACS using two-color fluorescence. Typical FACS dot-plots for phagocytosis and killing of *C. albicans* by mouse neutrophils are shown in Fig. 3.
6. Adjust detector/Amps and color compensation using phagocytic cells incubated with FITC-rat IgG2a/PE-rat IgG2a. Yeasts labeled with FITC lose their green fluorescence and acquire red fluorescence after staining with EB, unless they are internalized by phagocytic cells. Thus, after staining with EB, a single positive (green) population represents cells with ingested yeasts, and a double positive population represents cells with both ingested and adherent yeasts. Thus, phagocytosis was calculated as the percentage of single positive (green) plus double positive (green and red) fluorescent cells. A representative result from a quantitative assay of neutrophil phagocytosis of *C. albicans* is shown in Fig. 3.

3.9 Candida Killing (See Note 8)

3.9.1 Assessment of Killing with FACS [11, 12]

1. Label live *C. albicans* with 0.3 mg/mL FITC in HBSS (pH 7.2) for 1 h by agitation in the dark at room temperature.
2. Wash the yeasts twice with PBS, and resuspend in PBS for use. Incubate the labeled yeasts, with or without opsonization, with phagocytic cells (1×10^6) in 1 mL PBS in a 1.5 mL microcentrifuge tube at an effector-to-yeast ratio of 1:1, 2:1, 4:1 for 90 min in a 37 °C water bath with horizontal shaking.
3. After incubation, lyze the cells by hypotonic shock (1 mL distilled water added for 10 min). Remove extracellular DNA by adding 0.02% (w/v) DNAse solution for 5 min at 37 °C.

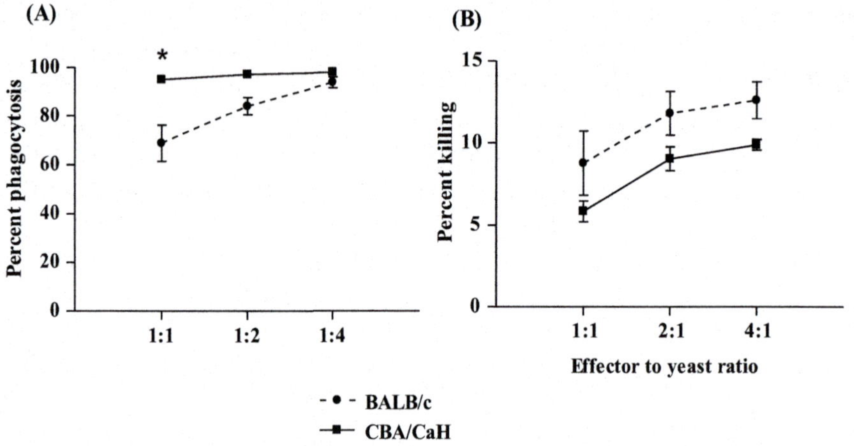

Fig. 2 Comparison of different ratios of effector to yeast for phagocytosis (**a**) and killing (**b**) assays for BALB/c and CBA/CaH mice. Phagocytosis and killing were performed with neutrophils and strain 3630 without opsonization. "*" denotes a significant difference between BALB/c and CBA/CaH mice ($p < 0.05$)

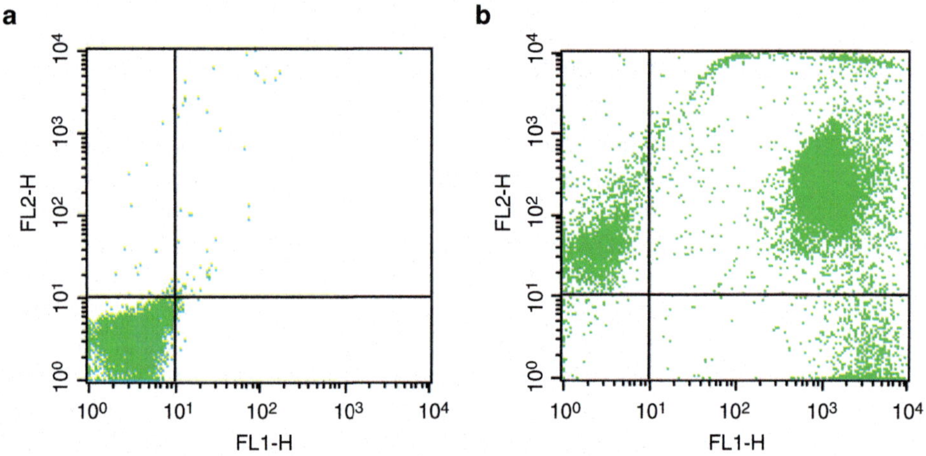

Fig. 3 A representative FACS dot-plot showing phagocytosis of *C. albicans* by mouse neutrophils. (**a**) Neutrophils labeled with IgG as control. (**b**) Neutrophils after phagocytosis of yeasts labeled with FITC and the addition of ethidium bromide (EB). Double positive cells in the top-right quadrant represent phagocytic cells with ingested and adherent yeasts, single positive cells in the bottom right quadrant represent cells with ingested yeasts only. In the top-left quadrant are cells with adherent *Candida* only

4. After washing twice with PBS, add 200 μL PI at 100 μg/mL to the tube for 30 min at 4 °C in the dark before FACS analysis. Killing of yeasts showed a direct correlation with increased effector: target (E:T) ratio, and 1:1 was chosen for a comparison of killing by effectors from the two strains of inbred mice (Fig. 2b) (*see* **Note 9**). After staining with FITC, the dye PI is able to penetrate dead yeasts and stain the DNA, yielding red fluorescence, while the yeasts retain their green membrane fluorescence. Therefore, the number of yeasts showing both

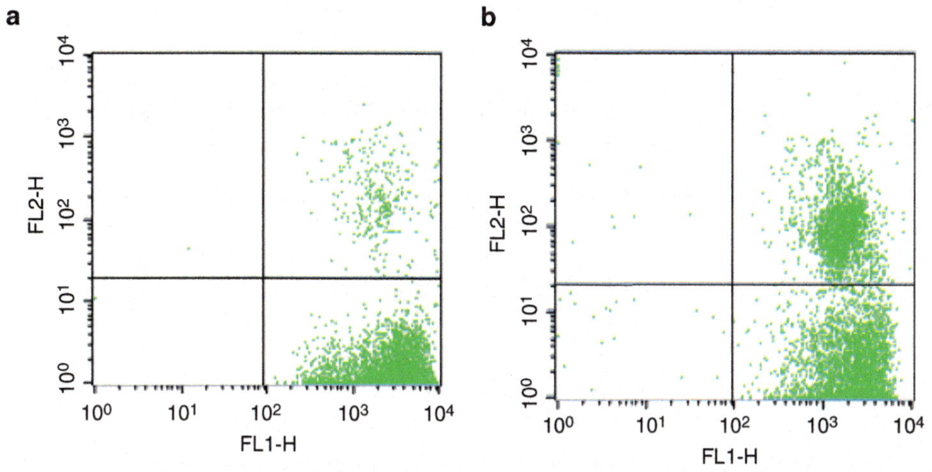

Fig. 4 A representative FACS dot-plot showing killing of *Candida albicans* by mouse neutrophils. Double positive cells in the top-right quadrant represent dead yeasts, and those in the bottom-right quadrant represent live yeasts. (**a**) Shows yeasts only as a control, while (**b**) represents phagocytic cells cocultured with live yeasts

green and red fluorescence reflects the number of dead yeasts in the sample.

5. Use the FITC-labeled yeasts without the addition of cells as a control, to adjust Detector/Amps and color compensation. Calculate the percentage of killed *Candida* as follows: Percentage of killed yeasts = Percentage of double positive yeasts in sample—percentage of double positive yeasts in control. A quantitative assay of killing of *C. albicans* by mouse neutrophils is presented in Fig. 4.

3.9.2 Assessment of Killing of Yeast by Plating [13, 14]

1. Coculture 4×10^4 neutrophils with 2×10^4 *C. albicans* cells (2:1 ratio) for 2 h at 37 °C in PBS.
2. After incubation, lyse the cells by hypotonic shock (1 mL distilled water added for 10 min).
3. Serially dilute yeasts, overlay with YPD, and incubate 48 h at 37 °C.
4. Count CFU and calculate percentage of killing as follows: (1-CFU from the plates of yeasts with cells/CFU from the plates of yeasts only) × 100%.

4 Notes

1. The vaccine targets against Candida infection are mainly cell-wall polysaccharides, proteins, and peptides of Candida species. Recombinant β-1,2-mannotriose, the secreted aspartic proteases family (rSap2), the agglutination-like sequence 1 (rAls1), and enolase can enhance mouse resistance to

Candidiasis. Here, we choose recombinant enolase as an example of vaccine target since it is located on the cell wall of *C. albicans* and plays an important role in energy metabolism. According to our study, enolase is highly immunogenic and the antibody titer in the immune serum of mice can reach up to 1:51,200.

2. The inbred mice BALB/c, CBA/CaH, and C57BL/6J have different genetic background. According to previous studies, BALB/c mice are resistant to systemic Candida infection, whereas CBA/CaH mice are susceptible to systemic Candida infection and C57BL/6J mice are the widely used strain in animal experiments. For other objectives of studies, special gene knockout mice should be considered.

3. Percoll density gradient preparation varies between laboratories. However, a simple method to prepare Percoll is as follows.

   Dilute Percoll with 10× PBS at 9:1 (Percoll:PBS) first, and then make required densities with diluted Percoll and 1× HBSS (pH 7.2) with 10 mM HEPES.

   Always layer the gradient solutions from bottom of tube starting with the most dense solution, followed by the second and third dense, and finally carefully place the sample on the top. Always make fresh gradient density Percoll within 1 week of the experiment.

4. The concentration of *Candida albicans* used in systemic immunization is different from strain to strain, and very important. In this protocol, 3×10^5 *C. albicans* 3630 and 3683, but 4×10^4 SC5314, in 200 μL PBS was injected via the tail vein. The reduced concentration for SC5314 was necessary because the higher dose resulted in the death of the mice within 1 week after injection. Where necessary for comparisons between yeasts, the dose for 3630 and 3683 was also reduced to 4×10^4.

5. In the immunization protocol, the dose of recombinant protein should be considered. For the first time of immunization, the same dose of recombinant enolase (100 μg) and complete Freund's adjuvant (CFA) were mixed together. For the boost immunization, a half dose of recombinant enolase (50 μg) was mixed together with incomplete Freund's adjuvant (IFA). The dose of recombinant protein should be decided by the purified protein concentration. The dose 100 μg of the recombinant protein has been proved to be the ideal dose, because of the high antibody titer after the immunization and the better protective effect against infection.

6. In the immunization protocol, in order to avoid the influence of Freund's adjuvant in the immune response, mice that received adjuvant alone mixed with PBS were used as a control group, and a further group of mice received PBS alone (without adjuvant) as a negative control group. With the two

control groups, the protective effect against Candida infection of recombinant proteins can be more convincing.

7. In the phagocytosis assay, the ratios of effectors to yeasts have been evaluated at 1:1, 1:2, and 1:4. According to the results (Fig. 2a), a ratio of effector to yeast of 1:1 was optimal for comparison of phagocytosis.
8. Both FACS and killing assay by plate culture methods can be used for the killing assay of neutrophils and macrophages. The FACS method is quick and accurate, and the results are more intuitive. However, there are more procedures and a little bit hard to master. The plate culture method is easy to operate, and results are more stable and repeatable. But the amount of work is more than the FACS method, since plenty of plates need to be overlaid with Candida. And more time is needed, since the plates are required to be cultured 48 h at 37 °C. Therefore, researchers can choose from the two methods according to their own conditions.
9. In the killing assay, the ratios of effectors to yeasts have been evaluated at 1:1, 2:1, and 4:1. According to the results (Fig. 2b), a ratio of effector to yeast of 1:1 was optimal for comparison of killing.

Acknowledgments

This work was supported by the National Natural Science of Foundation of China (No. 81170969).

References

1. Schaberg DR, Culver DH, Gaynes RP (1991) Major trends in the microbial etiology of nosocomial infection. Am J Med 91:72S–75S
2. Spellberg BJ, Filler SG, Edwards JE Jr (2006) Current treatment strategies for disseminated candidiasis. Clin Infect Dis 42:244–251
3. Cutler JE, Deepe GS Jr, Klein BS (2007) Advances in combating fungal diseases: vaccines on the threshold. Nat Rev Microbiol 5:13–28
4. Gillum AM, Tsay EY, Kirsch DR (1984) Isolation of the *Candida albicans* gene for orotidine-5′-phosphate decarboxylase by complementation of *S. cerevisiae* ura3 and *E. coli* pyrF mutations. Mol Gen Genet 198:179–182
5. Murciano C, Yanez A, Gil ML, Gozalbo D (2007) Both viable and killed *Candida albicans* cells induce in vitro production of TNF-alpha and IFN-gamma in murine cells through a TLR2-dependent signalling. Eur Cytokine Netw 18:38–43
6. Li W, Hu X, Zhang X, Ge Y, Zhao S, Hu Y et al (2011) Immunisation with the glycolytic enzyme enolase confers effective protection against *Candida albicans* infection in mice. Vaccine 29:5526–5533
7. Farah CS, Hu Y, Riminton S, Ashman RB (2006) Distinct roles for interleukin-12p40 and tumour necrosis factor in resistance to oral candidiasis defined by gene-targeting. Oral Microbiol Immunol 21:252–255
8. Giudicelli J, Philip PJ, Delque P, Sudaka P (1982) A single-step centrifugation method for separation of granulocytes and mononuclear cells from blood using discontinuous density gradient of Percoll. J Immunol Methods 54:43–46

9. Hart PH, Spencer LK, Kenny PA, Lopez AF, McDonald PJ, Finlay-Jones JJ (1987) Functional neutrophils from long-term murine bone marrow cell cultures. J Immunol Methods 100:223–233
10. Cowland JB, Borregaard N (1999) Isolation of neutrophil precursors from bone marrow for biochemical and transcriptional analysis. J Immunol Methods 232:191–200
11. Saresella M, Roda K, Speciale L, Taramelli D, Mendozzi E, Guerini F et al (1997) A rapid evaluation of phagocytosis and killing of *Candida albicans* by CD13+ leukocytes. J Immunol Methods 210:227–234
12. Vassiloyanakopoulos AP, Okamoto S, Fierer J (1998) The crucial role of polymorphonuclear leukocytes in resistance to Salmonella dublin infections in genetically susceptible and resistant mice. Proc Natl Acad Sci U S A 95:7676–7681
13. Fu Y, Luo G, Spellberg BJ, Edwards JE Jr, Ibrahim AS (2008) Gene overexpression/suppression analysis of candidate virulence factors of *Candida albicans*. Eukaryot Cell 7:483–492
14. Luo G, Ibrahim AS, Spellberg B, Nobile CJ, Mitchell AP, Fu Y (2010) *Candida albicans* Hyr1p confers resistance to neutrophil killing and is a potential vaccine target. J Infect Dis 201:1718–1728

Chapter 22

Immunization with Antigen-Pulsed Dendritic Cells Against Highly Virulent *Cryptococcus gattii* Infection: Analysis of Cytokine-Producing T Cells

Keigo Ueno, Makoto Urai, Shogo Takatsuka, Masahiro Abe, Yoshitsugu Miyazaki, and Yuki Kinjo

Abstract

Cryptococcosis caused by highly virulent *Cryptococcus gattii* (Hv-*Cg*) is an emerging infectious disease that affects immunocompetent individuals. The Hv-*Cg* outbreak began in 1999, but the mechanisms responsible for its hyper-virulence as well as protective immunity against Hv-*Cg* infection remain to be elucidated. To better understand the protective immunity against Hv-*Cg* infection, we developed a novel immunization method using antigen-pulsed dendritic cells (DCs). We constructed a capsule-deficient *Cg* strain (Δ*cap60*) and used it as a vaccine antigen. Mouse bone marrow-derived DCs were pulsed with Δ*cap60* and transferred into mice twice before pulmonary infection with Hv-*Cg* strain R265. This DC-based immunization strongly induced cell-mediated immunity, including Th1 cells, Th17 cells, and multinucleated giant cells enclosing fungal cells in lungs. This vaccination significantly ameliorated the fungal burden and the survival rate after pulmonary infection with R265. The efficacy of DC-based immunization was significantly but partially reduced in IFNγ-deficient mice, thereby suggesting that the Th1 and Th17 responses play roles in vaccine-induced protection against Hv-*Cg* infection. This approach might provide new insights into overcoming Hv-*Cg* infections in immunocompetent subjects. In this chapter, we describe the procedures for DC-vaccine preparation and the analysis of cytokine-producing $CD4^+$ T cells.

Key words Adoptive transfer, Bone marrow-derived dendritic cell, *Cryptococcus gattii*, DC vaccine, Pulmonary infection, Th17 cell

1 Introduction

Cryptococcus gattii (*Cg*) and *C. neoformans* (*Cn*) are encapsulated fungi that cause cryptococcosis, a life-threatening infectious disease with lesions in the lungs and central nervous system. An outbreak of *Cg* infection started on Vancouver Island and in the surrounding area during 1999, and cryptococcosis caused by *Cg* is perceived as an emerging infectious disease. The highly virulent *C. gattii* (Hv-*Cg*) isolated in the outbreak can infect healthy

Markus Kalkum and Margarita Semis (eds.), *Vaccines for Invasive Fungal Infections: Methods and Protocols*, Methods in Molecular Biology, vol. 1625, DOI 10.1007/978-1-4939-7104-6_22, © Springer Science+Business Media LLC 2017

individuals, and the mortality rate due to *Cg* infection has been estimated to be 8–20% [1–3]. The public health authorities in British Columbia and the USA have brought this situation to the public's attention [4, 5].

Previous studies have detected a weaker migration of leukocytes and lower amounts of cytokines in the lungs and cerebrospinal fluid of hosts infected with Hv-*Cg* compared with those in hosts infected with the conventional *Cn* strain H99, which has been analyzed frequently [6–10]. These studies also indicate that Hv-*Cg* is less likely to be recognized by the immune system. Because Hv-*Cg* induces a weaker inflammatory response after infection, some studies have shown that Hv-*Cg* can infect immunocompetent and immunocompromised subjects in the same manner. For example, a comparison of immunocompetent and $CD4^+$ T cell-depleted mice showed that they had equal fungal burdens of Hv-*Cg* in their lungs and comparable survival rates [11]. Similar results were obtained in immunodeficient $CD4C/HIV^{MutA}$ transgenic mice expressing proteins of human immunodeficiency virus and exhibiting severely atrophied lymphoid organs [12]. By contrast, these immunodeficient mice were more susceptible than immunocompetent mice to infection by *Cn* strain H99, and it is generally considered that $CD4^+$ T cells play a crucial role in protection against *Cn* infection [13]. However, it has not been determined whether a $CD4^+$ T cell response is required for the protection against Hv-*Cg* infection. Studies have demonstrated that granulocyte–macrophage colony-stimulating factor (GM-CSF) and complement factor C3 are key factors for the protection against Hv-*Cg* infection [14, 15]. Thus, the protective immunity against Hv-*Cg* infection still remains unclear [13].

Several experimental vaccines have been developed to analyze the protective immunity against cryptococcosis, which have been evaluated in a murine infection model based on "gain-of-function analysis" [16]. These studies have provided insights into protective immunity against cryptococcosis, which includes T cell-mediated immunity (CMI) and antibody-mediated immunity (AMI) [16]. Two experimental vaccines have been developed against Hv-*Cg* infection [17, 18]. In the first study, an intranasal vaccine was used based on crude protein-antigens that are expressed in Hv-*Cg* strain R265. This intranasal vaccine induced an Hv-*Cg*-specific antibody referred to as AMI, but there have been no evaluations of the efficacy of the passive transfer of serum from immunized mice and the vaccine's efficacy in B cell-deficient mice. This previous study also identified immunodominant proteins by two-dimensional gel electrophoresis using immune sera from immunized mice [17]. In the second study, we proposed an immunization method using antigen-pulsed dendritic cells (DCs) [18], where we constructed a capsule-deficient mutant (Δ*cap60*) and used heat-inactivated Δ*cap60* cells as the vaccine antigens. The antigen-pulsed DCs (DC vaccine) were adoptively transferred into mice before pulmonary infection with R265. This immunization markedly activated CMI, including Thl cells, Th17 cells, and the multinucleated giant cells (MGCs) that enclose fungal cells in the lungs. Furthermore, this vaccination could significantly ameliorate the lung pathology, fungal burden, and mortality following infection with R265. The DC vaccine-induced protective effect decreased significantly, but partially, in an interferon gamma (IFN-γ)-deficient mouse. These results suggest that an IFNγ-independent response is also involved in vaccine-induced protection against Hv-*Cg* infection [18]. The role of interleukin (IL)-17A in cryptococcosis is controversial, but a previous study showed that IL-17A-deficient mice are susceptible to *Cn* infection [19], and it was also demonstrated that IL-17A is required for the development of the MGCs that engulf fungal cells [19].

MGCs develop by fusing macrophages to enclose foreign substances, such as pathogens that cannot be eliminated, and they are key players in CMI for controlling cryptococcal cells in lesions [20, 21]. In addition, cytokine-producing T cells such as Thl and Th17 are required for MGC formation [19, 22, 23]. In this chapter, we describe an experimental DC vaccine that is available for analyzing CMI in Hv-*Cg* infection. In particular, we focus on the analysis of the cytokine-producing T cells involved in MGC formation.

2 Materials

2.1 Isolation of Bone Marrow (BM) Cells

1. C57BL/6J mice.
2. Complete medium: RPMI 1640 medium supplemented with 10% fetal bovine serum (FBS), 1% streptomycin–penicillin solution (10,000 units of penicillin and 10 mg/mL of streptomycin), and 44 μM 2-mercaptoethanol.
3. 10 cm diameter Petri dishes, untreated for cell culture.
4. 26 G × 13 mm needle.
5. 2.5 mL syringe.
6. 70 μm cell strainer.
7. 10× Red blood cell (RBC) lysis buffer: 150 mM ammonium chloride, 10 mM sodium bicarbonate, and 1 mM ethylenediaminetetraacetic acid (EDTA)/2Na, sterilized by filtering through a sterile 0.2 μm membrane after adjusting the pH to 7.4. Working solution prepared by mixing nine volumes of 10× RBC lysis buffer and one volume of sterile distilled water.
8. Hemocytometer.
9. Trypan blue solution, 0.4% (w/v), sterile-filtered.

2.2 Differentiation Culture for BM-Derived DCs (BMDCs)

1. Complete medium: RPMI 1640 medium supplemented with 10% FBS, 1% streptomycin–penicillin solution (10,000 units of penicillin and 10 mg/mL of streptomycin), and 44 μM 2-mercaptoethanol.
2. Murine GM-CSF.
3. 10 cm diameter Petri dishes, untreated for cell culture.
4. Hemocytometer.
5. Trypan blue solution, 0.4% (w/v), sterile-filtered.

2.3 Immunization with Antigen-Pulsed BMDCs

1. Heat-killed Δ*cap60* cells (1×10^9 cells/mL).
2. Complete medium: RPMI 1640 medium supplemented with 10% FBS, 1% streptomycin–penicillin solution (10,000 units of penicillin and 10 mg/mL of streptomycin), and 44 μM 2-mercaptoethanol.
3. Murine GM-CSF.
4. 10 cm diameter Petri dishes, untreated for cell culture.
5. Sterile and endotoxin-free Dulbecco's phosphate buffered saline (DPBS).
6. Hemocytometer.
7. Trypan blue solution, 0.4% (w/v), sterile-filtered.
8. C57BL/6J mice.
9. 27 G × 19 mm needle and 1 mL syringe.

2.4 Preparation of Lung Leukocytes

1. Ophthalmic scissors with two sharp tips.
2. Sterile DPBS.
3. 2R medium: RPMI 1640 medium supplemented with 2% FBS.
4. Collagenase-D: 100 mg/mL stock solution prepared with DPBS containing magnesium and calcium.
5. Hyaluronidase: 100 mg/mL stock solution prepared with DPBS containing magnesium and calcium.
6. DNase I: 10 mg/mL stock solution prepared with DPBS containing magnesium and calcium.
7. EDTA: 500 mM EDTA (pH 8.0) solution prepared with distilled water and then diluted to 100 mM with DPBS.
8. 70 μm cell strainer and 2.5 mL syringe.
9. 14 mL round-bottom tube with snap cap.
10. 18 G × 51 mm SURFLO® indwelling needle and 20 mL syringe.
11. Percoll.
12. Complete medium: RPMI 1640 medium supplemented with 10% FBS, 1% streptomycin–penicillin solution (10,000 units of penicillin and 10 mg/mL of streptomycin), and 44 μM 2-mercaptoethanol.

2.5 Induction of Cytokine-Producing T Cells by Polyclonal Stimulation

1. Complete medium: RPMI 1640 medium supplemented with 10% FBS, 1% streptomycin–penicillin solution (10,000 units of penicillin and 10 mg/mL of streptomycin), and 44 μM 2-mercaptoethanol.
2. Phorbol 12-myristate 13-acetate (PMA): 50 μg/mL stock solution prepared with dimethyl sulfoxide (DMSO).
3. Ionomycin: 1 mM stock solution prepared with DMSO.
4. 2× PMA/ionomycin medium: complete medium containing 100 ng/mL PMA and 1 mM ionomycin.
5. Brefeldin: ready-to-use reagent, 1000× solution with DMSO.
6. Monensin: 72 mM stock solution prepared with methanol.
7. 10× BrefeldinA/monensin medium: complete medium containing 10× brefeldin and 20 μM monensin.
8. Cell staining buffer: DPBS containing 0.5% (w/v) bovine serum albumin and 0.1% (w/v) sodium azide.

3 Methods

This protocol and representative results are shown in Figs. 1 and 2, respectively.

3.1 Isolation of BM Cells

1. Prepare two sterile 50 mL conical tubes. Add 10 mL of RPMI 1640 complete medium to one tube and 40 mL of 70% ethanol to the other. Keep the tube containing medium in crushed ice.
2. Sterilize the forceps and scissors by soaking in 70% ethanol.
3. Euthanize three mice with carbon dioxide gas, and isolate the femurs and tibias from both legs with forceps and scissors. Remove any surrounding tissues manually using paper towels. Sterilize by soaking the bones in 70% ethanol for 10 s and aseptically transfer the bones into the complete medium. Keep the conical tube containing bones in crushed ice (*see* **Note 1**).
4. Prepare three sterile 10 cm diameter dishes. Transfer the medium and bones from the conical tube into the first dish. This medium includes a small amount of ethanol used for sterilization, as described above, so it should be discarded. Place the bones in the second dish and add 30 mL of complete medium to the dish (*see* **Note 2**).
5. Hold a bone with forceps above the second dish and cut off both ends of each bone using scissors. Place the bone shafts in the second dish containing the complete medium. Flush out marrow clumps from the shafts using the complete medium from the second dish with a 26 G needle and 2.5 mL syringe. Receive the marrow clumps in the third dish (*see* **Note 3**).

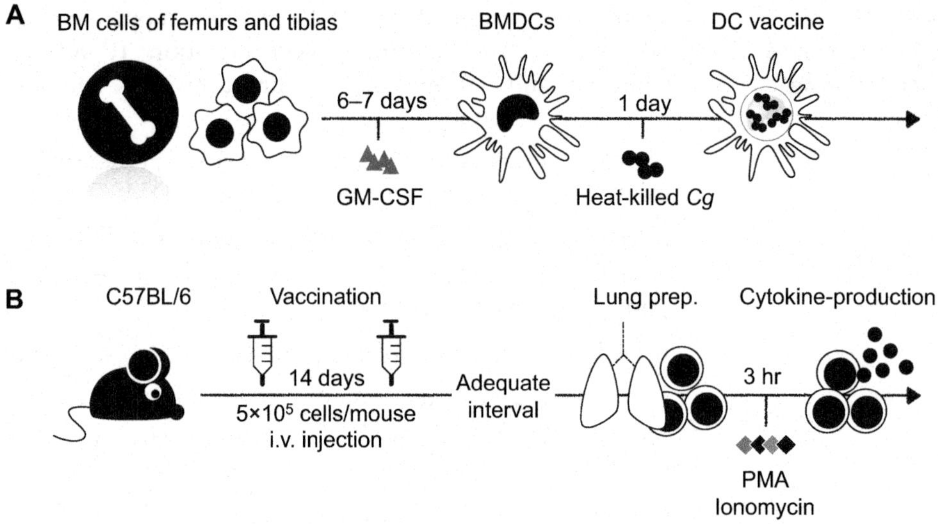

Fig. 1 Illustration of the protocol. (**a**) Preparation of DC vaccine. BM cells are cultured in RPMI medium containing 10-ng/mL GM-CSF for 6–7 days. Non-adherent cells are harvested as BMDCs. BMDCs are then pulsed overnight with 10 ng/mL GM-CSF and heat-killed acapsular C. gattii (Δcap60: "Heat-killed Cg" in the figure). BMDCs engulfing several Δcap60 cells are observed by microscopy after cultivation. The collected cells are used for DC-based vaccination. (**b**) Analysis of cytokine-producing T cells after vaccination. The DC vaccine is intravenously injected twice every 2 weeks. Lung leukocytes are isolated at appropriate times and are stimulated with PMA and ionomycin for 3 h to induce cytokine-producing T cells

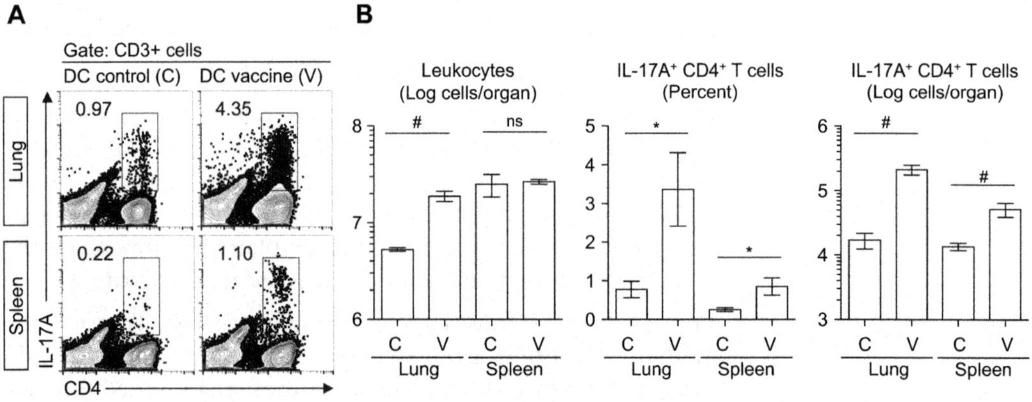

Fig. 2 Th17 cells increase in the immunized mice at day 7 after immunization. (**a**) Representative profile obtained by flow cytometry. The lungs and spleen were isolated from three mice that received unpulsed DCs or antigen-loaded DCs. Leukocytes were stimulated with PMA/ionomycin for 3 h and the cells were then stained with the following antibodies: anti-CD4 mAb (clone GK1.5), anti-CD3 mAb (clone 145-2C11), and anti-IL-17A mAb (clone TC11-18H10.1). Extracellular and intracellular staining was performed according to the general instructions. The gates for flow cytometry were set for $CD3^+$ cells, and $CD4^+$ T cells expressing intracellular IL-17A were evaluated using FlowJo software (TreeStar Inc.). (**b**) Statistical analysis. Cell numbers and the population rate were measured. Representative data are shown from two separate experiments, which are expressed as the mean ± SD, *$p < 0.05$ by unpaired t-test, #$p < 0.05$ by unpaired t-test with Welch's correction, C: DC control, V: DC vaccine, ns: no significant difference

6. Prepare a sterile 50 mL conical tube and a 70 μm cell strainer, and set the strainer on the conical tube. Suspend the marrow clumps in the third dish and pass the suspension through the cell strainer. The marrow clumps will be trapped on the cell strainer and a single cell suspension will be collected in the conical tube.
7. Mash the marrow clumps on the cell strainer using the piston of a 2.5 mL syringe. Rinse the second and third dishes with 10 mL of the complete medium and pass the lavage fluid through the cell strainer. Cells retained on the mesh will be washed out in this step.
8. Centrifuge (300 × *g*, 5 min, 4 °C) the cell suspension. Resuspend the collected cells in 3 mL of RBC lysis buffer and incubate for 5 min at room temperature to burst the erythrocytes. Add 27 mL of the complete medium to stop hemolysis.
9. Centrifuge (300 × *g*, 5 min, 4 °C) the suspension. Resuspend the collected cells in 10 mL of complete medium. Pass the suspension through a 70 μm cell strainer set on a 50 mL conical tube to remove any debris. Rinse the conical tube with 10 mL of complete medium and then pass the lavage fluid through the cell strainer. Finally, 20 mL of cell suspension will be obtained.
10. Centrifuge (300 × *g*, 5 min, 4 °C) the cell suspension. Resuspend in 10 mL of complete medium. Count the viable cells using trypan blue dye. Approximately 1.2×10^8 BM cells can be obtained from three mice (*see* **Note 4**).

3.2 Differentiation of BMDCs

1. Adjust the density of BM cells to 3×10^6 cells/mL with complete medium and then add GM-CSF at 10 ng/mL. Transfer 10 mL of the suspension (3×10^7 cells) to a sterile 10 cm diameter dish. Thirty dishes can be prepared from the BM suspension derived from three mice.
2. Incubate the dishes at 37 °C under 5% CO_2. On day 3, remove 6 mL of the culture medium from a dish and add 7 mL of the complete medium containing 10 ng/mL GM-CSF to the dish.
3. On day 5, add 5 mL of the complete medium containing 10 ng/mL GM-CSF (*see* **Note 5**).
4. On day 6, collect nonadherent cells from each dish by flushing the medium against the dish with a pipette. Rinse each dish with 5 mL of the complete medium without GM-CSF and pool the rinse fluid together with the initially collected suspension.
5. Cells harvested by centrifugation (300 × *g*, 5 min, 4 °C) can be used as BMDCs. Resuspend the collected cells in 10 mL of complete medium without GM-CSF. Count the viable cells using trypan blue dye. Approximately 3×10^8 BMDCs can be obtained from three mice (*see* **Note 6**).

3.3 Immunization with Antigen-Pulsed BMDCs

1. Prepare BMDCs and heat-killed *C. gattii* as the following concentrations: 1×10^6 cells/mL BMDCs and 5×10^6 cells/mL heat-killed *C. gattii* (Δ*cap60* acapsular cells as a vaccination antigen). Pour 10 mL of the suspension into a sterile 10 cm diameter dish (untreated for cell culture) and prepare 12 dishes (*see* **Note 7**).
2. Incubate BMDCs with heat-killed *C. gattii* in complete medium with 10 ng/mL GM-CSF for 24 h at 37 °C and under 5% CO_2.
3. After incubation, BMDCs engulfing several Δ*cap60* acapsular cells can be observed by microscopy. Collect nonadherent cells from each dish by flushing the medium against the dish with a pipette. Rinse each dish with 10 mL of DPBS and pool the lavage fluid with the initially collected suspension.
4. Centrifuge ($300 \times g$, 5 min, 4 °C) the cell suspension, and wash the harvested cells twice with sterile DPBS to remove any residual GM-CSF.
5. Count the viable BMDCs using trypan blue dye. Approximately 3×10^7 cells can be harvested from 12 dishes to inject 60 mice. Adjust the density of the antigen-pulsed BMDCs to 2.5×10^6 cells/mL with sterile DPBS. Keep the tube containing the suspension in crushed ice (*see* **Notes 8** and **9**).
6. Intravenously inject 200 μL of the suspension (5×10^5 cells) as DC vaccine using a 27 G needle and 1 mL syringe. DC vaccines are administered twice every 2 weeks.

3.4 Preparation of Lung Leukocytes

1. Euthanize the mice by carbon dioxide inhalation. Isolate their left and right lung lobes with forceps and scissors. Transfer the lungs into a 15 mL conical tube containing 10 mL DPBS. Gently roll the lungs in the conical tube containing DPBS to wash the lung-attached blood. Keep the conical tubes in crushed ice (*see* **Note 10**).
2. Sterilize by soak the forceps and ophthalmic scissors with two sharp tips in 70% ethanol, and then soak them in the 2R medium to remove any excess ethanol.
3. Transfer the lungs into an ice-cold 1.5 mL microtube using forceps and mince the lungs quickly in the microtube using the scissors. The lungs can easily be minced in the narrow space in the microtube.
4. Wash the scissors in the dish with 5 mL of 2R medium and transfer the minced lungs using 5 mL of the lavage fluid into a 15 mL conical tube. Add each enzyme solution to the 5 mL solution containing minced lung at the following concentration: 2 mg/mL collagenase-D, 1 mg/mL hyaluronidase, and 10 μg/mL DNase I.

5. Rotate the conical tube containing the minced lung and enzyme solution using a tube rotator at 37 °C for 60 min to dissociate the tissue (*see* **Note 11**).
6. Add 250 μL of 100 mM EDTA solution to the solution to stop the digestion reaction.
7. Set a 70 μm cell strainer on the dish and add 250 μL of 100 mM EDTA solution. Transfer the digestion solution onto the mesh, before rinsing the conical tube and its cap with 4 mL of 2R medium to collect any remaining pieces of the lungs. Transfer the lavage fluid onto the mesh (*see* **Note 12**).
8. Mash the pieces of lungs on the mesh using the piston of a 2.5 mL syringe. Collect the homogenates in a 14 mL round-bottom tube. Rinse the mesh with 3 mL of 2R medium and pool the rinse fluid together with the initially collected homogenates. Finally, 12 mL of cell suspension can be obtained (*see* **Note 13**).
9. Centrifuge (300 × *g*, 5 min, 4 °C) the cell suspension. Resuspend the cells in 2 mL of 30% Percoll solution. Prepare two sets each comprising a 20 mL syringe with an indwelling needle, and collect 44% Percoll solution in one and 70% Percoll solution in the other. Insert the indwelling needle into the bottom of the 30% Percoll solution and carefully pour 4 mL of 44% Percoll solution under the 30% Percoll layer. The Percoll solution can be poured repeatedly for up to four samples after cleaning the needle using cotton wool with alcohol. Similarly, pour 3 mL of 70% Percoll solution under the 44% Percoll layer. Finally, three layers of Percoll are obtained in 9 mL of solution (*see* **Note 14**).
10. Centrifuge (1000 × *g*, 20 min, 25 °C) the Percoll solution without acceleration and deceleration. Ensure that the tube is handled carefully so the layers are not disturbed.
11. Aspirate the 30% layer including the epithelial cells and dead cells using an aspirator pipette with a vacuum pump, and transfer the suspension at the 44–70% interface into the 15 mL conical tube using a 3 mL transfer pipette, which includes the lung leukocytes. Erythrocytes are precipitated at the bottom of the tube.
12. Add 10 mL of the ice-cold washing buffer to the conical tube and gently mix the suspension by inverting. Centrifuge (700 × *g*, 5 min, 4 °C) the suspension and resuspend the cells in 10 mL of complete medium.
13. Centrifuge (300 × *g*, 5 min, 4 °C) the suspension and carefully collect the supernatant to remove the residual EDTA. Resuspend the cells in complete medium.

14. Count the viable cells using trypan blue dye. Approximately 2×10^6 lung leukocytes can be obtained from a naive mouse. A greater number of lung leukocytes can be obtained from the early phase mice that receive the control DCs or antigen-pulsed DCs (Fig. 2).

3.5 Induction of Cytokine-Producing T Cells by Polyclonal Stimulation

1. Mix equal volumes of 2× cell suspension and 2× PMA/ionomycin medium in a dish or 96-well round-bottom plate (*see* **Note 15**).
2. Incubate the cell suspension at 37 °C under 5% CO_2 for 1.5 h.
3. Add 1:10 volume of 10× brefeldinA/monensin medium to stop cytokine release.
4. Incubate the cell suspension at 37 °C under 5% CO_2 for 1.5 h (*see* **Note 16**).
5. Centrifuge (300 × *g*, 5 min, 4 °C) the suspension. Resuspend the harvested cells in cell staining buffer (*see* **Note 17**).
6. If necessary, transfer the cell suspension to a 96-well V-bottom plate for cell staining. Ideally, one staining sample contains 1×10^6 cells (*see* **Note 18**).

4 Notes

1. Select the mouse's sex according to the experimental design. If the DCs will be transferred to female mice, then female mice should preferably be used to prepare the BMDCs.
2. It is recommended to use untreated Petri dishes, which are generally used to prepare agar plates for microbial cultivation, for cell culture. If cell culture-grade dishes are used, BMDCs will adhere strongly to the dishes and the yield of BMDCs will be decreased.
3. After the epiphyses are cut off, the bone shaft appears to be a tube filled with red marrow. After flushing out the marrow suspension, it should not be aspirated again with the needle and syringe because repeated flushing through the thin needle might damage the cells. The first dish should receive the uncut bone, the second dish is a reservoir for the fresh medium and cut bone, and the third dish receives the marrow suspension flushed with fresh medium from the second dish.
4. BM cells contain progenitor cells for BMDCs and a number of unstimulated granulocytes.
5. Add 10 mL of the complete medium at this point if BMDCs are harvested on day 7. One dish will contain 20 mL of medium.
6. In general, the adherent cells are macrophages. The harvested nonadherent cells comprise $CD11c^+$ and $CD11c^-$ cells.

Depending on the experimental design, $CD11c^+$ DCs should be enriched using a cell sorting system such as a MACS® Cell Separator (Miltenyi Biotec) or MojoSort Magnetic Cell Separation system (BioLegend).

7. To prepare the antigen unpulsed DCs as the control for immunization, BMDCs are cultivated in the complete medium containing 10 ng/mL GM-CSF without any antigens. In general, use the heat-killed capsule-deficient mutant (Δ*cap60*) as the vaccine antigen because protein antigens that can induce protective T cells have not yet been identified. BMDCs are unable to take up capsulated *C. gattii* cells, so capsular strains cannot be used as vaccine antigens. Heat-killed Δ*cap60* cells are prepared as described previously [18, 24]. It is not always necessary to add toll-like receptor ligands or vaccine adjuvant such as lipopolysaccharide to boost the DC vaccine.
8. Unloaded *C. gattii* cells are also precipitated with the BMDCs after centrifugation. BMDCs and *C. gattii* cells differ in terms of their cell size, so the BMDCs can be counted separately.
9. Antigen-pulsed BMDCs tend to adhere to the bottom of the dish, which tends to greatly reduce the cell yield. Our study did not determine whether the adherent cells can be used for vaccination.
10. If necessary, the lungs may be perfused with DPBS to remove any circulating blood cells, but it is difficult to remove them completely. If the localization of leukocytes in the lungs must be strictly discriminated, an intravascular staining and intratracheal staining approach may be performed as described in previous studies [25, 26].
11. Enzymatic digestion may affect the expression levels of surface antigens on the lung leukocytes, so do not allow the enzymatic reaction to continue for more than the specified time.
12. Lung cells tend to adhere to other cells or the bottom of dish when the lung tissues are mashed. The concentration of EDTA should be maintained at 2 mM in each step.
13. The indwelling needle does not reach the bottom of the 15 mL conical tube, so short tubes are preferable.
14. Some time might be required for the upper layering approach using Percoll solution. Alternatively, the collected cells can be resuspended in 6 mL of 37% Percoll/EDTA solution and the suspension is then centrifuged (1000 × *g*, 20 min, 25 °C) with acceleration and deceleration. Leukocytes and erythrocytes will be precipitated at the bottom of the conical tube. After removing the supernatant, the erythrocytes can be burst using RBC lysis buffer, as described above. In the single-layer approach, some of the aggregated dead cells are unavoidably incorporated in the target fraction.

15. Cells might be aggregated and adhere to the bottom of the container after chemical stimulation. Thus, it might be better to use larger culture containers for harvesting the stimulated cells. All leukocytes can be stimulated by chemical stimulators such as PMA and ionomycin. It is not always necessary to adjust the cell density with this approach. Cytokine-producing T cells can also be induced in medium containing 100 ng/mL of anti-CD3 monoclonal antibody (mAb, clone 145-2C11) and anti-CD28 mAb (clone 37.51). Alternatively, antigen-specific T cells can be activated by overnight coculture with Δ*cap60*-pulsed BMDCs. In a 96-well round-bottom plate, 5×10^5 antigen-loaded BMDCs and 1×10^6 lung leukocytes are cocultivated in 200 μL of medium.
16. Brefeldin A and monensin may affect the viability of cells, and long-term cultivation will downregulate the production of cytokines and the expression of cell-surface proteins. Thus, do not exceed the specified incubation period.
17. The cytokine levels in the culture supernatant could be determined using an enzyme-linked immunosorbent assay.
18. Refer to the manufacturer's protocol for details of how to stain cytokine-producing T cells and how to perform flow cytometry.

Acknowledgments

This chapter describes research supported by KAKENHI (15K21644, 16H05349, and 15K15383) from the Ministry of Education, Culture, Sports, Science and Technology of Japan, by the Research program on Emerging and Re-emerging Infectious Diseases from the Japan Agency for Medical Research and Development, AMED, and by LEGEND Research Grant Program 2015 from Tomy Digital Biology Co. Ltd.

References

1. Galanis E, MacDougall L, Kidd S et al (2010) Epidemiology of *Cryptococcus gattii*, British Columbia, Canada, 1999–2007. Emerg Infect Dis 16:251–257
2. Smith RM, Mba-Jonas A, Tourdjman M et al (2014) Treatment and outcomes among patients with *Cryptococcus gattii* infections in the United States Pacific Northwest. PLoS One 9:e88875
3. Lizarazo J, Escandón P, Agudelo CI et al (2014) Retrospective study of the epidemiology and clinical manifestations of *Cryptococcus gattii* infections in Colombia from 1997–2011. PLoS Negl Trop Dis 8:e3272
4. BCCDC (2011) Environmental pathogens, *Cryptococcus gattii*. British Columbia annual summary of reportable diseases 2011. pp 112–113
5. CDC (2010) Emergence of *Cryptococcus gattii*, Pacific Northwest, 2004–2010. Morb Mortal Wkly Rep 59:865–868
6. Okubo Y, Wakayama M, Ohno H et al (2013) Histopathological study of murine pulmonary cryptococcosis induced by *Cryptococcus gattii*

and *Cryptococcus neoformans*. Jpn J Infect Dis 66:216–221

7. Ngamskulrungroj P, Chang Y, Sionov E, Kwon-Chung KJ (2012) The primary target organ of *Cryptococcus gattii* is different from that of *Cryptococcus neoformans* in a murine model. MBio 3:e00103–e00112
8. Cheng P-Y, Sham A, Kronstad JW (2009) *Cryptococcus gattii* isolates from the British Columbia cryptococcosis outbreak induce less protective inflammation in a murine model of infection than *Cryptococcus neoformans*. Infect Immun 77:4284–4294
9. Brouwer AE, Siddiqui AA, Kester MI et al (2007) Immune dysfunction in HIV-seronegative, *Cryptococcus gattii* meningitis. J Infect 54:e165–e168
10. Einsiedel L, Gordon DL, Dyer JR (2004) Paradoxical inflammatory reaction during treatment of *Cryptococcus neoformans* var. *gattii* meningitis in an HIV-seronegative woman. Clin Infect Dis 39:e78–e82
11. Urai M, Kaneko Y, Ueno K et al (2015) Evasion of innate immune responses by the highly virulent *Cryptococcus gattii* by altering capsule glucuronoxylomannan structure. Front Cell Infect Microbiol 5:101
12. Leongson K, Cousineau-Côté V, Goupil M et al (2013) Altered immune response differentially enhances susceptibility to *Cryptococcus neoformans* and *Cryptococcus gattii* infection in mice expressing the HIV-1 transgene. Infect Immun 81:1100–1113
13. Gibson JF, Johnston SA (2014) Immunity to *Cryptococcus neoformans* and *C. gattii* during cryptococcosis. Fungal Genet Biol 78:76–86
14. Saijo T, Chen J, Chen SC-A et al (2014) Anti-granulocyte-macrophage colony-stimulating factor autoantibodies are a risk factor for central nervous system infection by *Cryptococcus gattii* in otherwise immunocompetent patients. MBio 5:e00912–e00914
15. Mershon KL, Vasuthasawat A, Lawson GW et al (2009) Role of complement in protection against *Cryptococcus gattii* infection. Infect Immun 77:1061–1070
16. Hole CR, Wormley FL (2012) Vaccine and immunotherapeutic approaches for the prevention of cryptococcosis: lessons learned from animal models. Front Microbiol 3:291
17. Chaturvedi AK, Hameed RS, Wozniak KL et al (2014) Vaccine-mediated immune responses to experimental pulmonary *Cryptococcus gattii* infection in mice. PLoS One 9:e104316
18. Ueno K, Kinjo Y, Okubo Y et al (2015) Dendritic cell-based immunization ameliorates pulmonary infection with highly virulent *Cryptococcus gattii*. Infect Immun 83:1577–1586
19. Murdock BJ, Huffnagle GB, Olszewski MA, Osterholzer JJ (2014) Interleukin-17A enhances host defense against cryptococcal lung infection through effects mediated by leukocyte recruitment, activation, and gamma interferon production. Infect Immun 82:937–948
20. Hill JO (1992) $CD4^+$ T cells cause multinucleated giant cells to form around *Cryptococcus neoformans* and confine the yeast within the primary site of infection in the respiratory tract. J Exp Med 175:1685–1695
21. Okubo Y, Tochigi N, Wakayama M et al (2013) How histopathology can contribute to an understanding of defense mechanisms against cryptococci. Mediat Inflamm 2013:465319–465311
22. Decken K, Köhler G, Palmer-Lehmann K et al (1998) Interleukin-12 is essential for a protective Th1 response in mice infected with *Cryptococcus neoformans*. Infect Immun 66:4994–5000
23. Kawakami K, Qureshi MH, Zhang T et al (1999) Interferon-gamma (IFN-gamma)-dependent protection and synthesis of chemoattractants for mononuclear leucocytes caused by IL-12 in the lungs of mice infected with *Cryptococcus neoformans*. Clin Exp Immunol 117:113–122
24. Ueno K, Urai M, Ohkouchi K et al (2016) Dendritic cell-based vaccine against fungal infection. Methods Mol Biol 1403:537–549
25. Anderson KG, Mayer-Barber K, Sung H et al (2014) Intravascular staining for discrimination of vascular and tissue leukocytes. Nat Protoc 9:209–222
26. Zhao J, Zhao J, Mangalam AK et al (2016) Airway memory CD4(+) T cells mediate protective immunity against emerging respiratory coronaviruses. Immunity 44:1379–1391

Part V

Translation to Clinical Use

Chapter 23

Testing Antifungal Vaccines in an Animal Model of Invasive Candidiasis and in Human Mucosal Candidiasis

Esther Segal

Abstract

The following article will concentrate on the NDV-3 anti-*Candida* and *Staphylococcus* vaccine. The vaccine is composed of the N-terminal portion of the *Candida albicans* agglutinin-like sequence 3 protein (Als3p) and aluminum hydroxide as adjuvant. The vaccine conferred protection to mice against experimental vaginal, oral, and intravenous challenge with *C. albicans*. Due to the sequence and structural homology of the Als3p with *Staphylococcus aureus* surface proteins, the vaccine also protected against experimental skin and IV infection with *S. aureus*. The vaccine has reached the stage of human trials: phase 1 clinical studies have shown that the vaccine is safe and immunogenic. The latest brief conference abstract reports of vaccination in women suffering from recurrent vaginal candidiasis, indicating that the recurrence rates were lower in the women receiving the vaccine.

Key words Vaccine, *Candida albicans*, *Staphylococcus aureus*, NDV-3 vaccine, Als3p

1 Introduction

The overall impact of infectious diseases on human health and wellbeing is known since antiquity [1]. Although the burden of these diseases has greatly decreased due to the development of specific vaccines to prevent infections, awareness and availability of improved personal and general hygiene, and use of antimicrobial drugs to combat active infections, they still are a significant component of current medicine [1, 2]. Infectious diseases are considered a major cause of death even in developed countries [2, 3]. Although fungal infections—the mycoses, were among the earliest infectious diseases with known etiology to be recognized in men and animals [4], effective prevention of the latter by the use of antifungal vaccines is still lacking. Development of vaccines against mycoses is less advanced than those against bacteria and viruses, probably due to the eukaryotic nature and the biological complexity of the fungi and the target population to be vaccinated, often immunocompromised.

Markus Kalkum and Margarita Semis (eds.), *Vaccines for Invasive Fungal Infections: Methods and Protocols*, Methods in Molecular Biology, vol. 1625, DOI 10.1007/978-1-4939-7104-6_23, © Springer Science+Business Media LLC 2017

Candidiasis, caused by the yeasts of the genus *Candida*, is among the most common human fungal infections [5, 6]. Candidiasis can be manifested as a superficial cutaneous-mucosal infection, with very high prevalence, affecting skin, nails, oral and vaginal mucosa [6, 7]. It can also be manifested as a deep-seated, invasive infection, mostly in immunocompromised or otherwise debilitated individuals [6]. *Candida species* are the third or fourth most common blood-stream microbial isolates in hospitalized patients [8, 9]. Invasive candidiasis is associated with high mortality, even under treatment with the current available antifungal drugs [10]. Thus, invasive candidiasis still poses a medical problem, for which prevention by vaccination could be considered a worthwhile endeavor.

Despite the difficulties mentioned above to develop antifungal vaccines, numerous attempts to develop anti-*Candida* vaccines have been undertaken, as reviewed previously [11]. These studies revealed that immunizations with live organisms afford protection to the immunized animals. However, considering the risks associated with the use of live non-attenuated vaccines, it is unlikely that these preparations can be of practical value. As for the non-viable immunogens, some of these afforded partial protection as well, particularly those composed of subcellular components, which led to the best results. The protective ability of these subcellular components was assessed in different experimental animal models by challenge of the vaccinated animals with the live fungi.

Of the studies with subcellular components, the investigations of Segal and colleagues [12–20] employing a ribosomal fraction of *C. albicans* were among the most extensive and continuous. These investigators isolated by differential centrifugation a ribosomal fraction from a *C. albicans* cell extract [12]. The ribosomes were used as an immunogen, which was supplemented with Freund's incomplete adjuvant (IFA) and administered by sub-cutaneous (SC) injection. The vaccinations were carried out in three murine models: naive ICR mice [12, 13], mice immunocompromised by pretreatment with cyclophosphamide [14], and the F1 of black C57 × BALB/c mice bearing a lymphatic tumor (EL4) [15]. The efficacy of the ribosomal vaccine in protecting the mice against invasive candidiasis induced by a challenge with live particles of a virulent *C. albicans* strain was assessed during 30 days post-challenge. Vaccination of non-compromised mice rendered them significantly immune to the lethal challenge with *C. albicans* [12, 13]. The compromised animals were also partially protected [14], and even among the tumor-bearing mice, immunization induced some protection, as expressed by the lower *Candida*-kidney colonization [15], this being the only valid criterion for evaluating efficacy of vaccination in this model, since the tumor itself was lethal. Immunization with *C. albicans* ribosomes also afforded protection against the antigenically related pathogenic *Candida* species, such as *C. tropicalis* [16]. The induced protection was accompanied by appearance of specific humoral and cell-mediated immune (CMI) responses [17–19]. Thus, the *Candida* ribosomal preparation described by Segal and coworkers apparently revealed the merits of an effective vaccine to protect animals against experimental invasive candidiasis. A later study of this group [20] investigated the use of liposomes as adjuvants, by incorporating the ribosomes into liposomes. The data showed that the efficacy of the liposomes containing ribosomes was similar to that of ribosomes with IFA. Hence, the feasibility of using ribosomes incorporated into liposomes as adjuvants, which are suitable for use in humans, was indicated. Unfortunately, circumstances prevented further experiments leading to evaluation in human trials.

The following article will concentrate on a more recent, different vaccine: the NDV-3 anti-*Candida* and *Staphylococcus* vaccine developed by the group of investigators headed by Edwards and colleagues [21–30]. The vaccine is based on the studies of Ibrahim et al. [22, 23] and Spellberg et al. [24] with the *C. albicans* adhesin Als1p (agglutinin-like sequence protein) which demonstrated improved survival against an intravenous challenge with *C. albicans* in immunocompetent and immunocompromised mice.

The NDV-3 anti-*Candida* and *Staphylococcus* vaccine described herewith is composed of the N-terminal portion of the *Candida albicans* agglutinin-like sequence 3 protein (Als3p) and aluminum hydroxide as adjuvant. The vaccine conferred protection to mice against experimental vaginal, oral and intravenous (IV) challenge with *C. albicans* [25–27]. Due to the sequence and structural homology of the Als3p with *Staphylococcus aureus* surface proteins, the vaccine also protected against experimental skin and IV infection with *S. aureus* [27, 28].

This vaccine has reached the stage of human trials [29, 30]. Phase 1 clinical studies have shown that the vaccine is safe and immunogenic [29]. The latest brief report [30] documents a study of vaccination in women suffering from recurrent vulvo-vaginal candidiasis (RVVC), indicating that the recurrence rates were lower in the women receiving the vaccine.

1.1 General Concepts

1. Vaccines are means of prevention of infectious diseases. The basis for development of vaccines is an immunizing antigen, which can be either a whole attenuated or killed microorganism, a subcellular fraction, or component of the etiological agent of the infection. Such antigens are generally associated with the pathogenesis process of the particular infection, such as molecules that act as adhesins. This is the case in the vaccine described herewith: Als1p functions as an adhesin and invasin of *Candida albicans* and is part of the pathogenesis of candidiasis [21].

2. The development of vaccines involves an experimental preclinical stage that assesses in an experimental animal model the elicited immunity following vaccination with the immunizing antigen. This should also be associated with the assessment of the protective efficacy of the vaccine toward the respective infection.
3. Protective efficacy is evaluated through exposure of laboratory animals to the live virulent-specific infectious agent—a process termed challenge. Protective efficacy may be expressed as survival following challenge, as prolongation of time to death or as amelioration of morbidity, which can be measured by different parameters, such as microbial colonization of tissues or organs.
4. Those vaccines, which pass successfully these experimental steps, are on the verge of clinical trials. Human trials are limited as to evaluation of efficacy of vaccine, as obviously, no challenge with live microbial agents can be undertaken.

   Thus, the following sections of this chapter dedicated to the NDV-3 vaccine, both in the experimental phase and partial human trials, are presented considering these general concepts. The sections include the materials, methodology, and outline of the experimental and human trials.

2 Materials

2.1 Murine Models (Refs. 22–28)

1. Female BALB/c immunocompetent mice (inbred mice).

   Juvenile mice: 8–10 weeks old and retired breeders: >6 month (end-result not different).
2. Female BALB/c immunocompromised mice by intraperitoneal (IP) injection of 200 mg/kg of cyclophosphamide.
3. Female CD1 mice (outbred mice) (*see* **Note 1**).

2.2 Vaccine

1. Immunizing antigen: Recombinant N-terminal domain of Als1p (r-Als1p-N) (amino acids 17–432 of Als1p) produced in *Saccharomyces cerevisiae* purified by gel filtration and N-nitrilotriacetic acid matrix affinity purification.
2. Complete Freund's adjuvant (CFA) in the BALB/c and CD1 model.
3. Incomplete Freund's adjuvant (IFA) in the BALB/c model and CD1 (booster injection).
4. Alum (2% alhydrogel) adjuvant in the CD1 model (*see* **Note 2**).

2.3 Organism Used for Challenge

1. *Candida albicans* SC5314 in BALB/c and CD1 models.
2. In BALB/c also other *C. albicans* strains and *C. glabrata*, *C. krusei*, *C. parapsilosis*, and *C. tropicalis* strains.

2.4 Clinical Trials

2.4.1 Immunizing Antigen

The active component of the NDV-3 vaccine was a recombinant version of the N-terminal region of *C. albicans* Als3p formatted with aluminum hydroxide as adjuvant (1 mg Al/mL in PBS, pH 7).

2.4.2 Analysis of Immune Responses

1. Flat-bot.5tom microtiter plates.
2. Horse radish peroxidase (HRP)-conjugated mouse anti-human IgG (Pierce).
3. HRP-conjugated mouse anti-human IgA1 (Pierce).
4. Microplate spectrophotometer.
5. 96-well plates for ELISpot.
6. Appropriate ELISpot antibody pairs.
7. ImmunoSpot® S5 Core Analyzer.

3 Methods

3.1 Vaccination Protocol

3.1.1 The BALB/c Mice Model

1. Inject immunocompetent or immunocompromised mice IP with r-Als1p-N (20 μg) mixed with CFA. Boost on day 21 by injecting r-Als1p-N (20 μg) mixed with IFA.
2. For another group of immunocompetent or immunocompromised mice inject subcutaneously (S.C) r-Als1p-N (20 μg) mixed with CFA. Administer a booster injection on day 21 with r-Als1p-N (20 μg) mixed with IFA.

3.1.2 The CD1 Mice Model

1. Immunize the CD1 mice S.C using the same adjuvants and time schedule as in the BALB/c model.
2. In addition, vaccinate one group with r-Als1p-N and allum as adjuvant, using the same time schedule as vaccination with the r-Als1p-N +CFA and IFA.

3.2 Immuno-suppression

BALB/c mice were rendered neutropenic by intraperitoneal administration of 200 mg/kg of cyclophosphamide on day −2 (relevant to vaccination).

3.3 Challenge

Challenge mice with live 2.5×10^5 to 5×10^5 blastospores of the challenge organisms by intravenous (IV) inoculation into the tail vein 14 days following the boost (*see* **Note 3**).

3.4 Follow-Up and Evaluation Criteria

3.4.1 Evaluation of Immunogenicity

Two weeks after the boost inoculation the immunogenicity of the vaccine was evaluated by

1. Antibody titers to rAls1p were determined by an enzyme-linked immunosorbent assay (ELISA) in 96-well plates coated with r-Als1p-N (5 μg/mL), using goat anti-mouse secondary antibody conjugated with horseradish peroxidase.

2. Cell-mediated immunity was assessed by:

   (a) Detection of delayed type hypersensitivity (DTH) by evaluating the intensity of the foot-pad swelling reaction of the immunized mice as response to injection with rAls1p-N.

   (b) *C. albicans*-induced cytokine profile*s* of splenocytes from immunized mice.

3.4.2 Evaluation of Efficacy

Criteria included:

1. Survival rate during a 30-day follow-up.
2. Candida kidney burden—kidneys were harvested prior to onset of death in the control group. Quantitative colonization was established by enumeration of colony-forming units (CFU) in the tissue homogenates of the kidneys (*see* **Note 4**).

3.5 Clinical Trials (Refs. 29, 30)

3.5.1 Phase 1: Healthy Individuals—Evaluation of Safety and Immunogenicity of the Vaccine

1. *Outline*: Two double blind studies including 150 adult volunteers, men and women; aged 18–50, were conducted.

   (a) *Single dose vaccination.* Single dose of 0.5 mL vaccine containing 30 or 300 μg of immunizing antigen (r-Als1p-N), and 0.5 mL of sterile saline (placebo group) was administered intra-muscular (IM) in the upper right or left deltoid muscle. The subjects were divided into two groups: vaccinated with 30 or 300 mg of vaccine; each group included a placebo subgroup (administered with saline).

   Evaluation was carried out on days 3, 7, 14, 28, 90, and 180 post-vaccination.

   Subjects recorded temperature, injection site reaction, and other adverse effects and were evaluated by study personnel at the specified dates (*see* above).

   Blood samples were collected on the specified dates for the analysis of the immune responses (*see* below), including day 0 (vaccination day).

   (b) *Two dose vaccination.* On day 180 post-vaccination with a single dose, subjects who gave consent to receive a second dose were administered with 30 mg or 300 μg as above.

   Evaluation was carried out on days 7, 14, and 90 post-vaccination.

2. *Analysis of immune responses*: Plasma and peripheral blood mononuclear cells (PBMC) were separated.

   (a) *Anti-Als3p total IgG and IgA1 titers.* Plasma samples were analyzed for the presence of anti-Als3p total IgG and IgA1 titers, using an enzyme-linked immunosorbent assay (ELISA). The ELISA assays were carried out in flat-bottom microtiter plates coated 24 h prior to the assay with Als3p (5 ug/mL). The plasma samples were with fourfold serial dilutions. The total IgG of anti-Als3p was detected using the HRP-conjugated mouse anti-human IgG, and the total IgA—with mouse anti-human IgA1 HRP conjugate. Absorbance readings were done at 450 and 570 nm.

(b) *Measurement of PBMC of Als3p-specific IFN-gamma and IL-17A Secretion*. PBMC separated on the specific collection dates indicated above were processed and stored in cryovials in liquid nitrogen until testing. The PBMC samples were evaluated by enzyme-linked immunosorbent spot (ELISpot) test to determine the production of IFN-gamma or IL-17A using an ImmunoSpot® S5 Core Analyzer.

3.5.2 Phase 2: Vaccination of Women with Recurrent Vulvo-Vaginal Candidiasis (RVVC)

This is an exploratory double blind, placebo controlled Phase 1b/2a human proof-of-concept clinical study.

1. *Outline*: The study included women who had at least three episodes of VVC in the past 12 months, a *C. albicans* culture-confirmed episode of VVC at the time of screening and confirmation that the episode was resolved by fluconazole by the day of vaccination.
2. *Vaccination*: All patients who met the inclusion criteria received one dose of either NDV-3A or placebo on study day 0.
3. *Evaluation of vaccination*: Patient follow-up consisted of scheduled and patient-initiated unscheduled visits for 1 year post-vaccination.

   The study protocol included evaluation of safety, immunogenicity, and efficacy after 6 months post-vaccination including a planned physician visit.

3.6 Results

3.6.1 Murine Models

1. Protection to a lethal challenge of Candida elicited by the vaccine
   (a) Intraperitoneal vaccination of BALB/c mice with 20 μg of rAls1p and CFA/IFA improved survival of mice challenged with a lethal inoculum of *C. albicans* (2×10^5 blastospores).
   (b) Subcutaneous vaccination of BALB/c and CD1 mice with 20 μg of rAls1p and CFA/IFA or allum improved survival of mice challenged with a lethal inoculum of *C. albicans.*
   (c) Subcutaneous vaccination of BALB/c mice with 20 μg of rAls1p and CFA/IFA improved survival of mice challenged with lethal inocula of various strains *C. albicans, C. glabrata, C. krusei, C. parapsilosis, C. tropicalis.*
   (d) Subcutaneous vaccination of BALB/c mice with 20 μg of rAls1p and CFA/IFA was active in immunocompetent and

immunocompromised mice (neutropenic and corticosteroid treated) challenged with lethal inoculum of *C. albicans* by: improving survival, prolonging time to death and reducing fungal burden in the kidneys.

2. Immunity elicited by the vaccine

Vaccination of BALB/c mice with 20 μg of rAls1p stimulated cell-mediated immunity, rather than humoral immunity, specifically:

(a) Increased stimulation of Th1 splenocytes.
(b) Increased in-vivo delayed hypersensitivity.
(c) The vaccine requires T cells and not B cells to induce protection.
(d) Antibodies did not correlate with protection.

3.6.2 Clinical Trials

1. Phase 1: Healthy individuals—Evaluation of Safety and Immunogenicity of the Vaccine

(a) Safety:
- Safe and generally well tolerated after 1 or 2 vaccination doses.
- Complaints included: injection site pain, disappearing within 2–3 days.
- Adverse effects (systemic and at injection site) in a small proportion of vaccinated subjects.
- In vaccinated subjects receiving 2 vaccine doses the most common adverse effects were fatigue and headache.

(b) Immune responses:
- Seroconversion was noted in all vaccinated subjects.
- The IgG and IgA levels were higher in subjects vaccinated with 300ug of vaccine.
- Anti Als3p total IgG and IgA1 reached peak levels by day 14 post-vaccination in subjects administered with 1 or 2 doses of vaccine.
- In the subjects receiving 2 doses, the second dose caused a significant boost of IgG and IgA titers.
- The vaccine elicited PBMC production of IFN-gamma and IL 17A.
- Subjects vaccinated with 300 ug of vaccine responded more rapidly regarding PBMC production of IFN-gamma.

2. Phase 2: Vaccination of women with recurrent vulvo-vaginal candidiasis (RVVC)

The published interim results can be summarized as follows: the safety and immunogenicity of the vaccine is similar in women with RVVC as was previously seen in healthy women: no serious adverse events associated with the vaccine.

Recurrence rates of VVC defined as patient-reported symptom severity scores of >2 on a scale of 0–9 were significantly lower in the patients receiving the vaccine vs. placebo group.

The results with NDV-3A vaccine indicate statistically significant and clinically relevant benefits to patients with RVVC.

3.7 Summary and Conclusions

1. Very few, if any, of fungal vaccines have reached human trials. Hence, the fact that the NDV-3 vaccine reached this stage is an achievement in itself.
2. The human trials aiming to reduce morbidity of patients suffering from recurrent vaginal candidiasis appear promising.
3. However, thus far, no human trials to protect patients against invasive candidiasis have been carried out.
4. Thus, the major goal—development of an anti-*Candida* vaccine for the prevention of invasive candidiasis, which endangers life of patients at risk, has not been achieved.
5. It should be added that human trials of vaccines for the assessment of protection against invasive infections, particularly in immunocompromised patients, are hampered by numerous difficulties, including among others problems of financial funding.
6. It is of interest that the NDV-3 vaccine has a protective capacity both against the fungal pathogen, *Candida albicans*, as well as against the bacterial pathogen *Staphylococcus aereus*. This feature adds further value to the vaccine, making it a valuable tool in the fight against life-threatening infections in patients at risk, should it be successful in human trials.

4 Notes

1. Experimental infections are mostly done in inbred mice, which permit easier evaluation of the data due to the uniformity of the studied population. On the other hand, outbred animals are of importance, since they parallel human populations, which are not homogenous.
2. Most vaccines use adjuvants to increase the efficacy of the vaccine. Experimental vaccines use frequently Freund's complete or incomplete adjuvant (CFA or IFA, respectively). Both CFA and IFA cannot be used in humans due to toxicity. In human vaccines Alum is used as adjuvant.

3. It is of great importance to pay attention to the challenge dose. Too low dose might result in an infection only in part of the control group and therefore would not be reliable as a comparison for the evaluation of efficacy of the vaccine. A too high challenge dose, which would lead to a fast killing in the control group, is also not recommended. Hence, the infecting dose has to be established in preliminary experiments.
4. Systemic experimental candidiasis induced by IV inoculation of *Candida* is characterized by colonization of most visceral organs of the experimental animal. Most prominent colonization is noted in the kidneys, which can be related to the severity of the infection. Thus, most models use *Candida* kidney burden as a measurement of *Candida* colonization and index of infection.

References

1. Dye C (2014) After 2015: infectious diseases in a new era of health and development. Phil Trans R Soc B 369:20130426
2. Murraya KA, Prestonc N, Allend T et al (2015) Global biogeography of human infectious diseases. Proc Natl Acad Sci U S A 112: 12746–12751
3. Europe PMC Funders Group; Author Manuscript (2015) Global, regional, and national age-sex specific all-cause and cause-specific mortality for 240 causes of death, 1990-2013: a systematic analysis for the global burden of disease study. Lancet 385:117–171
4. Drouhet E (1998) Historical introduction: evolution of knowledge of the fungi and mycoses from Hipocrates to the twenty- first century. In: Ajello L, Hay R (eds) Topley & Wilson's microbiology and microbial infections, Medical mycology, vol 4, 9th edn. Arnold, London, pp 3–42
5. Edwards J (2015) Candida species. In: Mandell, Douglas and Bennett's principles and practice of infectious diseases, 8th edn. Saunders, Philadelphia, pp 2879–2894
6. Segal E, Elad D (2005) Candidiasis. In: Merz WG, Hay RJ (eds) Topley &Wilson's Microbiology & Microbial Infections, Medical mycology, vol 5, 10th edn. ASM, Washington, DC, pp 579–623
7. Richardson MD, Warnock DW (2012) Superficial candidosis. In: Fungal infection diagnosis and management, 4th edn. Blackwell Publishing Ltd, Chichester, pp 121–137
8. Wisplinghoff H, Bischoff T, Tallent SM et al (2004) Nosocomial bloodstream infections in US hospitals: analysis of 24,179 cases from a prospective nationwide surveillance study. Clin Infect Dis 39:309–317
9. Wisplinghoff H, Seifert H, Wenzel RP et al (2003) Current trends in the epidemiology of nosocomial bloodstream infections in patients with hematological malignancies and solid neoplasms in hospitals in the United States. Clin Infect Dis 36:1103–1110
10. Bailly S, Leroy O, Montravers P et al (2015) Antifungal de-escalation was not associated with adverse outcome in critically ill patients treated for invasive candidiasis: post hoc analyses of the AmarCAND2 study data. Intensive Care Med 41:1931–1940
11. Segal E, Elad D (2006) Fungal vaccines and immunotherapy. J Med Mycol 16:134–151
12. Levy R, Segal E, Eylan E (1981) Protective immunity against murine candidiasis elicited by Candida albicans ribosomal fractions. Infect Immun 31:874–878
13. Levy R, Segal E (1986) Induction of candidacidal activity in mice by immunization with Candida albicans ribosomes. FEMS Microbiol Lett 36:213–217
14. Segal E, Sandovsky-Losica H (1981) Experimental vaccination with Candida albicans ribosomes in cyclophosphamide treated animals. Sabouraudia 19:267–274
15. Segal E, Spongin A, Levy R et al (1987) Induction of protection against candidiasis in tumor bearing mice by vaccination with Candida albicans ribosomes. J Med Vet Mycol 25:355–363
16. Segal E, Nussbaum S, Barr-Nea L (1985) Protection against systemic infections with various Candida species elicited by vaccination

with Candida albicans ribosomes. J Med Vet Mycol 235:275–285

17. Levy R, Segal E, Eylan E (1984) Detection of antibodies against Candida albicans ribosomes by the enzyme linked immunosorbent assay. Mycopathologia 87:167–170
18. Levy R, Segal E, Eylan E et al (1983) Cell-mediated immunity following experimental vaccinations with Candida albicans ribosomes. Mycopathologia 83:161–168
19. Segal E, Sandovsky-Losica H, Nussbaum S (1985) Immune responses elicited by Candida albicans ribosomes in cyclophosphamide treated animals. Mycopathologia 89:113–118
20. Eckstein M, Barenholz Y, Bar LK, Segal E (1997) Liposomes containing Candida albicans ribosomes as a prophylactic vaccine against disseminated candidiasis in mice. Vaccine 15:220–224
21. Edwards JE (2012) Fungal cell wall vaccines: an update. J Med Microbiol 61:895–903
22. Ibrahim AS, Spellberg BJ, Avanesian V et al (2005) Vaccination with recombinant N-terminal domain of Als1p improves survival during murine disseminated candidiasis by enhancing cell-mediated, not humoral, immunity. Infect Immun 73:999–1005
23. Ibrahim AS, Spellberg BJ, Avanesian V et al (2006) The anti-Candida vaccine based on the recombinant N-terminal domain of Als1p is broadly active against disseminated candidiasis. Infect Immun 74:3039–3041
24. Spellberg BJ, Ibrahim AS, Avenissian V et al (2005) The anti-Candida albicans vaccine composed of the recombinant N terminus of Als1p reduces fungal burden and improves survival in both immunocompetent and immunocompromised mice. Infect Immun 73:6191–6193
25. Ibrahim AS, Gebremariam LG, Lee H et al (2013) NDV-3 protects mice from vulvovaginal candidiasis through T- and B-cell immune response. Vaccine 31:5549–5556
26. Luo G, Ibrahim AS, French SW et al (2011) Active and passive immunization with rHyr1p-N protects mice against hematogenously disseminated candidiasis. PLoS One 6:e25909. doi:10.1371/journal.pone.0025909
27. Lin L, Ibrahim AS, Xu X et al (2009) Th1-Th17 cells mediate protective adaptive immunity against Staphylococcus aureus and Candida albicans infection in mice. PLoS Pathog 5(12):e1000703. doi:10.1371/journal.ppat.1000703
28. Spellberg B, Ibrahim AS, Yeaman MR et al (2008) The antifungal vaccine derived from the recombinant N terminus of Als3p protects mice against the bacterium Staphylococcus aureus. Infect Immun 76:4574–4580
29. Schmidt CS, White CJ, Ibrahim AS et al (2012) NDV-3, a recombinant alum-adjuvanted vaccine for Candida and Staphylococcus aureus, is safe and immunogenic in healthy adults. Vaccine 30:7594–7600
30. Edwards JE, Schwarz MW, Schmidt, CS et al (2016) NDV-3A vaccine reduces recurrences of vaginitis in patients with recurrent vulvovaginal candidiasis. ASM Conference on "Candida and Candidiasis"

INDEX

Markus Kalkum and Margarita Semis (eds.), *Vaccines for Invasive Fungal Infections: Methods and Protocols*, Methods in Molecular Biology, vol. 1625, DOI 10.1007/978-1-4939-7104-6, © Springer Science+Business Media LLC 2017

E

F

G

H

I

K

L

M

Printed by Printforce, the Netherlands